T0263803

Hypertensive Heart Disease

Editors

RAGAVENDRA R. BALIGA
GEORGE L. BAKRIS

HEART FAILURE CLINICS

www.heartfailure.theclinics.com

Consulting Editor
EDUARDO BOSSONE

Founding Editor
JAGAT NARULA

October 2019 • Volume 15 • Number 4

ELSEVIER

1600 John F. Kennedy Boulevard • Suite 1800 • Philadelphia, Pennsylvania, 19103-2899

http://www.theclinics.com

HEART FAILURE CLINICS Volume 15, Number 4
October 2019 ISSN 1551-7136, ISBN-13: 978-0-323-68123-0

Editor: Stacy Eastman
Developmental Editor: Laura Fisher

© 2019 Elsevier Inc. All rights reserved.

This periodical and the individual contributions contained in it are protected under copyright by Elsevier, and the following terms and conditions apply to their use:

Photocopying
Single photocopies of single articles may be made for personal use as allowed by national copyright laws. Permission of the Publisher and payment of a fee is required for all other photocopying, including multiple or systematic copying, copying for advertising or promotional purposes, resale, and all forms of document delivery. Special rates are available for educational institutions that wish to make photocopies for non-profit educational classroom use. For information on how to seek permission visit www.elsevier.com/permissions or call: (+44) 1865 843830 (UK)/(+1) 215 239 3804 (USA).

Derivative Works
Subscribers may reproduce tables of contents or prepare lists of articles including abstracts for internal circulation within their institutions. Permission of the Publisher is required for resale or distribution outside the institution. Permission of the Publisher is required for all other derivative works, including compilations and translations (please consult www.elsevier.com/permissions).

Electronic Storage or Usage
Permission of the Publisher is required to store or use electronically any material contained in this periodical, including any article or part of an article (please consult www.elsevier.com/permissions). Except as outlined above, no part of this publication may be reproduced, stored in a retrieval system or transmitted in any form or by any means, electronic, mechanical, photocopying, recording or otherwise, without prior written permission of the Publisher.

Notice
No responsibility is assumed by the Publisher for any injury and/or damage to persons or property as a matter of products liability, negligence or otherwise, or from any use or operation of any methods, products, instructions or ideas contained in the material herein. Because of rapid advances in the medical sciences, in particular, independent verification of diagnoses and drug dosages should be made.

Although all advertising material is expected to conform to ethical (medical) standards, inclusion in this publication does not constitute a guarantee or endorsement of the quality or value of such product or of the claims made of it by its manufacturer.

Heart Failure Clinics (ISSN 1551-7136) is published quarterly by Elsevier Inc., 360 Park Avenue South, New York, NY 10010-1710. Months of publication are January, April, July, and October. Business and editorial offices: 1600 John F. Kennedy Boulevard, Suite 1800, Philadelphia, PA 19103-2899. Periodicals postage paid at New York, NY, and additional mailing offices. Subscription prices are USD 261.00 per year for US individuals, USD 501.00 per year for US institutions, USD 100.00 per year for US students and residents, USD 300.00 per year for Canadian individuals, USD 580.00 per year for Canadian institutions, USD 315.00 per year for international individuals, USD 580.00 per year for international institutions, and USD 100.00 per year for Canadian and foreign students/residents. To receive student and resident rate, orders must be accompanied by name of affiliated institution, date of term, and the *signature* of program/residency coordinator on institution letterhead. Orders will be billed at individual rate until proof of status is received. Foreign air speed delivery is included in all *Clinics* subscription prices. All prices are subject to change without notice. **POSTMASTER:** Send address changes to *Heart Failure Clinics*, Elsevier Health Sciences Division, Subscription Customer Service, 3251 Riverport Lane, Maryland Heights, MO 63043. **Customer Service: 1-800-654-2452 (US and Canada). From outside of the US and Canada, call 314-447-8871. Fax: 314-447-8029. For print support, E-mail: JournalsCustomerService-usa@elsevier.com. For online support, E-mail: JournalsOnlineSupport-usa@elsevier.com.**

Reprints. For copies of 100 or more of articles in this publication, please contact the Commercial Reprints Department, Elsevier Inc., 360 Park Avenue South, New York, NY 10010-1710. Tel.: 212-633-3874; Fax: 212-633-3820; E-mail: reprints@elsevier.com.

Heart Failure Clinics is covered in *MEDLINE/PubMed (Index Medicus)*.

Contributors

CONSULTING EDITOR

EDUARDO BOSSONE, MD, PhD, FCCP, FESC, FACC
Division of Cardiology, A. Cardarelli Hospital, Naples, Italy

EDITORS

RAGAVENDRA R. BALIGA, MD, MBA, FACC, FRCP, FACP
Division of Cardiovascular Medicine, Professor, Department of Internal Medicine, The Ohio State University College of Medicine, Director, Cardio-Oncology Center of Excellence, The Ohio State University Wexner Medical Center, Columbus, Ohio, USA

GEORGE L. BAKRIS, MD, MA, FAHA, FASH
Professor of Medicine and Director, American Heart Association Comprehensive Hypertension Center, Department of Medicine, University of Chicago Medicine, Chicago, Illinois, USA

AUTHORS

MUHAMMAD R. AFZAL, MD, FACC
Division of Cardiovascular Medicine, The Ohio State University Wexner Medical Center, Columbus, Ohio, USA

GEORGE L. BAKRIS, MD, MA, FAHA, FASH
Professor of Medicine and Director, American Heart Association Comprehensive Hypertension Center, Department of Medicine, University of Chicago Medicine, Chicago, Illinois, USA

RAGAVENDRA R. BALIGA, MD, MBA, FACC, FRCP, FACP
Division of Cardiovascular Medicine, Professor, Department of Internal Medicine, The Ohio State University College of Medicine, Director, Cardio-Oncology Center of Excellence, The Ohio State University Wexner Medical Center, Columbus, Ohio, USA

JENNIFER BALLARD-HERNANDEZ, DNP, FAHA, AACC, FAANP
Department of Medicine, Cardiology Division, U.S. Department of Veterans Affairs, VA Long Beach Healthcare System, Long Beach, California, USA

ANTONIO BELLASI, MD, PhD
Department of Nephrology and Dialysis, ASST Lariana, S. Anna Hospital, Como, Italy

HANNAH F. BENSIMHON, MD
Clinical Fellow, Division of Cardiology, Department of Medicine, The University of North Carolina at Chapel Hill, Chapel Hill, North Carolina, USA

JAVED BUTLER, MD, MPH, MBA
Patrick H. Lehan Chair in Cardiovascular Research, Professor and Chairman, Department of Medicine, University of Mississippi Medical Center, Jackson, Mississippi, USA

MATTHEW A. CAVENDER, MD, MPH
Assistant Professor, Division of Cardiology, Department of Medicine, The University of North Carolina at Chapel Hill, Chapel Hill, North Carolina, USA

LUCA DI LULLO, MD, PhD
Department of Nephrology and Dialysis, L. Parodi – Delfino Hospital, Colleferro, Roma, Italy

CLIVE GOULBOURNE, MD
Cardiology Fellow, Division of Cardiology,
Department of Medicine, Stony Brook
University Medical Center, Stony Brook,
New York, USA

GMERICE HAMMOND, MD, MPH
Cardiologist, Research Fellow Cardiovascular
Division, Washington University School of
Medicine, St Louis, Missouri, USA

LAUREN J. HASSEN, MD, MPH
Chief Medical Resident, Department of
Internal Medicine, The Ohio State University
Wexner Medical Center, Columbus, Ohio,
USA

KONSTANTINOS IMPRIALOS, MD
VAMC and Georgetown University,
Washington, DC, USA

DIPTI ITCHHAPORIA, MD, FACC, FESC
Department of Medicine, Cardiology
Division, Hoag Memorial Hospital, University of
California, Irvine, Irvine, California,
USA

STEVEN J. KALBFLEISCH, MD, FHRS
Professor of Medicine, Division of
Cardiovascular Medicine, The Ohio State
University Wexner Medical Center, Columbus,
Ohio, USA

**ANDREAS P. KALOGEROPOULOS, MD,
MPH, PhD**
Associate Professor of Medicine, Division of
Cardiology, Department of Medicine, Stony
Brook University Medical Center, Stony Brook,
New York, USA

BRENT C. LAMPERT, DO, FACC
Associate Professor of Clinical Medicine,
Medical Director, Heart Transplantation and
Mechanical Circulatory Support, The Ohio
State University Wexner Medical Center,
Columbus, Ohio, USA

DANIEL J. LENIHAN, MD, FACC, FESC
Cardiovascular Division, Professor of
Medicine, John T. Milliken Department of
Internal Medicine, Director, Cardio-Oncology
Center of Excellence, Washington University
School of Medicine, St Louis, Missouri,
USA

JIM X. LIU, MD, FACC
Assistant Professor, Division of
Cardiovascular Medicine, Department of
Internal Medicine, The Ohio State University
Wexner Medical Center, Columbus, Ohio,
USA

SCOTT MAFFETT, MD
Associate Professor of Cardiovascular
Medicine, Interim Director of the Division of
Cardiovascular Medicine, Director of
Cardiovascular Fellowship Program, The Ohio
State University Wexner Medical Center,
Columbus, Ohio, USA

OMAR MOHAMED, MD
Division of Cardiovascular Medicine, The Ohio
State University Wexner Medical Center,
Columbus, Ohio, USA

AAYAH MOHAMED-OSMAN, MD
Division of Cardiovascular Medicine, The Ohio
State University Wexner Medical Center,
Columbus, Ohio, USA

VASILIOS PAPADEMETRIOU, MD
VAMC and Georgetown University,
Washington, DC, USA

VIREN PATEL, MD, FACC
Assistant Professor, Division of
Cardiovascular Medicine, Department of
Internal Medicine, The Ohio State University
Wexner Medical Center, Columbus, Ohio,
USA

TAMAR S. POLONSKY, MD, MSCI
Department of Medicine, Section of
Cardiology, The University of Chicago
Medicine, Chicago, Illinois, USA

MICHAEL W. RICH, MD
Professor of Medicine, Cardiovascular
Division, Washington University School
of Medicine, St Louis, Missouri,
USA

CLAUDIO RONCO, MD, PhD
International Renal Research Institute,
S. Bortolo Hospital, Vicenza, Italy

L. JOSEPH SALIBA, MD
Clinical Instructor Housestaff, Department of
Internal Medicine, The Ohio State University
Wexner Medical Center, Columbus, Ohio,
USA

SALVATORE SAVONA, MD
Division of Cardiovascular Medicine, The Ohio
State University Wexner Medical Center,
Columbus, Ohio, USA

JEREMY SLIVNICK, MD
Cardiovascular Fellow, The Ohio State
University Wexner Medical Center, Columbus,
Ohio, USA

**MATTHEW J. SORRENTINO, MD, FACC,
FAHA**
Vice Chair for Clinical Operations, Professor,
Department of Medicine, Section of
Cardiology, The University of Chicago
Medicine, Chicago, Illinois, USA

KONSTANTINOS STAVROPOULOS, MD
VAMC and Georgetown University,
Washington, DC, USA

SAURAV UPPAL, MD
Cardiovascular Medicine Fellow, Division of
Cardiovascular Medicine, Department of
Internal Medicine, The Ohio State University
Wexner Medical Center, Columbus, Ohio, USA

Contents

Epidemiology and Natural History

Elevated blood pressure (BP) has a strong and continuous association with Stage B and C heart failure (HF) and carries the highest attributable risk for HF. Intensive treatment of hypertension is crucial, as progression from hypertension (Stage A HF) to left ventricular hypertrophy (LVH) or other structural damage (Stage B HF) is common despite therapy. Echo cardiography is the modality of choice to detect Stage B HF. Ideally, Stage B HF should be prevented. However, regression of established LVH and other structural damage is feasible and improves prognosis. Despite differences among antihypertensive agents, control of BP remains the most important goal.

Hypertensive heart disease includes the development of diastolic dysfunction, left ventricular hypertrophy, and heart failure with preserved and reduced ejection fraction. The development of heart failure can occur because of complications of ischemic heart disease or from progression of diastolic dysfunction to heart failure with preserved ejection fraction degenerating to a dilated heart with systolic dysfunction or heart failure with reduced ejection fraction. Hypertension clinical trials have shown that the treatment of hypertension can prevent the development of heart failure. In addition, lifestyle modification with exercise and weight loss can improve diastolic function and reduce the risk for heart failure.

Pathophysiology and Natural History

The kidney is a regulatory organ and accommodates changes in cardiac function. There is cross-talk between the kidney and the heart. In heart failure, the kidney acts as a bystander but also contributes to several maladaptive processes. The pathophysiology of worsening kidney function and its association with prognosis are discussed, as are other aspects of how worsening kidney function contributes to increased cardiovascular risk. Data suggest that morbidity and mortality reduction in people with heart failure and kidney disease requires use of a renin angiotensin system blocker, beta blocker, and mineralocorticoid receptor antagonist, as well as an SGLT 2 inhibitor.

Patients with acute or chronic decompensated heart failure (ADHF) present with various degrees of heart and kidney dysfunction characterizing cardiorenal syndrome (CRS). CRS can be generally defined as a pathophysiologic disorder of the heart and kidneys whereby acute or chronic dysfunction of 1 organ may induce acute or chronic dysfunction of the other. ADHF is a challenge in the management of heart failure. This review provides an overview the pathophysiology of type 1 CRS together with new approaches to treatment in patients with heart failure with worsening renal function or acute kidney disease.

Special Populations

The incidence and prevalence of both hypertension (HTN) and heart failure (HF) increase progressively with age. As a result, hypertensive HF (HHF) is highly prevalent among older adults and is one of the most common phenotypes of HF in the very old. In this article, the authors provide an overview of the epidemiology, pathophysiology, clinical features, diagnosis, management, prognosis, and prevention of HHF in the elderly population. Reducing the prevalence of HTN and ameliorating the progression from HTN to HF hold the greatest promise for limiting the impact of HHF on the health and well-being of older adults.

As cancer therapies improve, the population of survivors of cancer has increased, and the long-term effects of cancer treatments have become more apparent. Cardiotoxicity is a well-established adverse effect of many antineoplastic agents. Hypertension is common in survivors of cancer, can be caused or worsened by certain agents, and has been shown to increase the risk of other cardiovascular diseases including heart failure. Pretreatment risk assessment and careful monitoring of blood pressure during therapy is essential. Aggressive management of preexisting or incident hypertension in survivors of cancer is paramount to decrease the risk of heart failure and other cardiovascular diseases in these patients.

Heart failure (HF) is a significant cause of cardiovascular morbidity and mortality for women in the United States. There are clear sex-specific differences between men and women in etiology, disease progression, and outcomes. HF with preserved ejection fraction is the most common type of HF in women, with hypertensive heart disease playing a pivotal role in its etiology. The Practice Guidelines do not endorse sex-specific recommendations for standard medical therapy of HF management. Women are underrepresented in HF clinical trials, leading to a lacking evidence base supporting sex-specific therapy. Further studies are needed to evaluate targeted HF therapies in women.

Metabolic syndrome is an increasingly prevalent constellation of disease processes among the global population. Hypertension and obesity are among the contributing etiologies, and obesity increases the likelihood of hypertensive heart disease by creating a proinflammatory state, as well as increasing sympathetic tone and formation of reactive oxygen species. Hypertensive heart disease is characterized by myocardial fibrosis, which portends higher risk of developing reduced ejection fraction, diastolic dysfunction, ischemia, and arrhythmias, making early diagnosis and treatment essential to the prevention of cardiac events.

Prognostic Markers and Management

The prevalence of diabetes mellitus and heart failure is increasing. The novel sodium-glucose cotransporter-2 (SGLT2) inhibitors offer multidimensional ameliorating effects on cardiovascular and heart failure risk factors. Several studies have assessed the impact on cardiovascular events, with data suggesting beneficial effects on cardiovascular events in high-risk patients with diabetes in patients with heart failure. The reverse J-curve pattern between blood pressure levels and mortality has emerged as an important topic in the field of heart failure. There is no significant evidence to propose any potential effect of SGLT2 inhibitors on the J-shape-suggested mortality in patients with heart failure.

Hypertensive heart disease represents a spectrum of illnesses from uncontrolled hypertension to heart failure. The authors discuss the natural history and pathogenesis of heart failure owing to hypertensive heart disease, reviewing the important role of left ventricular hypertrophy as the inciting process leading to diastolic dysfunction and heart failure with preserved ejection fraction. They describe the various mechanisms by which a subset of patients ultimately develops systolic heart failure. They discuss management strategies for hypertensive heart disease at all stages of the disease process. Treatment in the initial stages before onset of heart failure may result in regression of disease.

Hypertension is the most common cardiovascular risk factor and underlies heart failure, coronary artery disease, stroke, and chronic kidney disease. Hypertensive heart disease can manifest as cardiac arrhythmias. Supraventricular and ventricular arrhythmias may occur in the hypertensive patients. Atrial fibrillation and hypertension contribute to an increased risk of stroke. Some antihypertensive drugs predispose to electrolyte abnormalities, which may result in atrial and ventricular arrhythmias. A multipronged strategy involving appropriate screening, aggressive lifestyle modifications, and optimal pharmacotherapy can result in improved blood pressure control and prevent the onset or delay progression of heart failure, coronary artery disease, and cardiac arrhythmias.

Hannah F. Bensimhon and Matthew A. Cavender

Diabetes is strongly associated with development of cardiovascular disease and poor cardiovascular outcomes. Management of hypertension reduces cardiovascular outcomes among patients with diabetes. Many studies have examined the benefits of various classes of antihypertensives among patients with diabetes. Based on these, the American Diabetes Association has advised that all patients (particularly those with microalbuminuria) be treated first with an angiotensin-converting enzyme inhibitor or an aldosterone receptor blocker followed by a calcium channel blocker or diuretic. Recently, sodium glucose transporter 2 inhibitors have been identified for their benefit in blood pressure control and cardiovascular risk reduction in patients with diabetes.

Jim X. Liu, Saurav Uppal, and Viren Patel

Heart failure presents a particularly difficult public health challenge. Of the heart failure presentations, acute hypertensive heart failure represents a distinct clinical phenotype and is characterized by sudden-onset systemic hypertension and pulmonary edema. The pathophysiology of acute hypertensive heart failure is primarily driven by an abnormal ventricular-vascular relationship, and the medical management is aimed at improving this relationship.

HEART FAILURE CLINICS

SERIES OF RELATED INTEREST

Cardiology Clinics
http://www.cardiology.theclinics.com/

THE CLINICS ARE AVAILABLE ONLINE!
Access your subscription at:
www.theclinics.com

Preface

Hypertensive Heart Failure: Sprinting to the Finish Line to Prevent End-Organ Damage

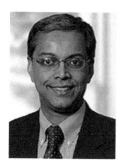

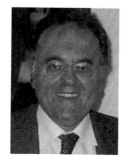

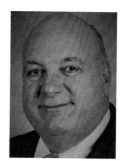

Ragavendra R. Baliga, MD, MBA, FACC, FRCP, FACP

Eduardo Bossone, MD, PhD, FCCP, FESC, FACC

George L. Bakris, MD, MA, FAHA, FASH

Editors

Hypertension affects a billion individuals globally,[1] and with the aging population (79% of men and 85% of women >75 years old have high blood pressure [BP]), this number continues to grow,[2,3] and the consequences of hypertension are expected to increase. High BP is second only to cigarette smoking as a preventable cause of death in the United States,[4] and uncontrolled hypertension results in heart failure, coronary artery disease, kidney disease, stroke, and aortic dissection.[5] Progress over the last few decades has led to better understanding and a new knowledge of this growing worldwide epidemic of high BP. In 2017, based on epidemiologic studies, including the findings of the SPRINT trial, the American College of Cardiology/American Heart Association (ACC/AHA)/Multisociety Guidelines[3,6,7] categorized BP into 3 major categories: elevated (120-129/<80 mm Hg), stage 1 (systolic blood pressure [SBP] 130-139 or diastolic blood pressure [DBP] 80-89 mm Hg), and stage 2 (SBP $\geq$140 mm Hg or DBP $\geq$90 mm Hg), based on strong evidence that generally there is a linear relationship between lower SBP and DBP and cardiovascular risk. These new thresholds will increase the number of individuals who will now be categorized with this diagnosis, with regard to age of the patient or comorbidity. These guide-

lines also raised the bar for therapeutic targets for BP and recommended tailoring therapy to a combination of both BP and accompanying 10-year estimated risk of atherosclerotic cardiovascular disease.[8] Pharmacologic intervention is recommended (a) when BP is $\geq$130/80 mm Hg in those at high risk for cardiovascular disease or (b) when BP is $\geq$140/90 mm Hg in those without risk or low risk for cardiovascular disease. These guidelines continue the Seventh Report of the Joint National Committee recommendations for the use of 2 first-line agents of different classes in patients with stage 2 hypertension and an average BP of >20/10 mm Hg above their BP target. The 2018 ACC/AHA and European Society of Cardiology/European Society of Hypertension (ESC/ESH) guidelines interpreted similar data with a fundamental difference of 2 different BP goals: <130/80 mm Hg for ACC/AHA and <140/90 mm Hg for ESC/ESH (**Fig. 1**).[6] The caution in the ESC/ESH guidelines stems from possible harm due to antihypertensive therapy. In the ACCORD trial, there was an increase in serious adverse events attributable to antihypertensive medications (3.3% vs 1.27%; $P<.001$).[9] Even though there was no overall increase in adverse events in the SPRINT trial, there were increases in low BP (2.4% vs 1.4%; $P<.001$) and syncope

Heart Failure Clin 15 (2019) xiii–xv
https://doi.org/10.1016/j.hfc.2019.07.001
1551-7136/19/© 2019 Published by Elsevier Inc.

Guideline Differences	American College of Cardiology/American Heart Association (ACC/AHA)			European Society of Cardiology/European Society of Hypertension (ESC/ESH)		
Level of blood pressure (BP) defining hypertension	Systolic (mm Hg)	and/ or	Diastolic (mm Hg)	Systolic (mm Hg)	and/ or	Diastolic (mm Hg)
Office/Clinic BP	≥130		≥80	≥140		≥90
Daytime mean	≥130		≥80	≥135		≥85
Nighttime mean	≥110		≥65	≥120		≥70
24–h mean	≥125		≥75	≥130		≥80
Home BP mean	≥130		≥80	≥135		≥85
BP targets for treatment	<130/80 mm Hg			Systolic targets <140 mm Hg and close to 130 mm Hg		
Initial Combination Therapy	Initial single-pill combination therapy in patients > 20/10 mm Hg above BP goal			Initial single-pill combination therapy in patients ≥140/90 mm Hg		
Hypertensive requiring intervention	>130/80 mm Hg			≥140/90 mm Hg		

Guideline Similarities	ACC/AHA	ESC/ESH
Importance of home BP monitoring	• Take BP at home, twice in the morning and twice in the evening, in the week before clinic • Bring the BP machine in annually for validation	
Therapy	• Restrict beta blockers to patients with comorbidities or other indications • Initial single pill combination as initial therapy	
Follow-up	• Detect poor adherence and focus on improvement • BP telemonitoring and digital health solutions recommended	

Fig. 1. Comparison of American and European Society definitions and management of hypertension. (*Reprinted from* Journal of the American College of Cardiology, Volume 73, Issue 23, George Bakris, Waleed Ali, Gianfranco Parati, ACC/AHA versus ESC/ESH on hypertension guidelines: JACC guideline comparison, Pages 3018-3026, Copyright 2019, with permission from Elsevier.)

(2.3% vs 1.7%; $P = .05$).[10] Other differences include the approach to assess risk and goals in older people at 130/70 to 139/79 mm Hg for ESC/ESH but <130/80 mm Hg for ACC/AHA. Guideline implementation should include patient participation and cooperation. This is a large part of the ESC/ESH guideline and mentioned but not emphasized in the ACC/AHA guideline. The more aggressive BP targets in the ACC/AHA guideline are, in part, due to realism regarding applying lifestyle changes.

Management of BP is a marathon and a sprint— it is a marathon when it comes to managing the BP in an individual patient but, when managing the BP in the whole population, the need to reduce risk of CVD is urgent[11] and, therefore, a sprint. Keeping this in mind, we have assembled an outstanding group of contributors to discuss key issues that are of interest to the practicing physician who manages BP every day in their patients with heart failure. We hope the articles in this issue will better prepare the physician managing BP to reach the finish line of reducing the burden of end-organ damage due to hypertension worldwide.

Ragavendra R. Baliga, MD, MBA, FACC, FRCP, FACP
Cardio-Oncology Center of Excellence
Division of Cardiovascular Medicine
Department of Internal Medicine
The Ohio State University
Wexner Medical Center
200 Davis Heart and Lung Research Institute
473 West 12th Avenue
Columbus, OH 43210-1267, USA

Eduardo Bossone, MD, PhD, FCCP, FESC, FACC
Division of Cardiology
Cardarelli Hospital
Via A. Cardarelli, 9
Naples 80131, Italy

George L. Bakris, MD, MA, FAHA, FASH
Department of Medicine
American Heart Association
Comprehensive Hypertension Center
University of Chicago Medicine
5841 S. Maryland Avenue, MC1027
Chicago, IL 60637, USA

E-mail addresses:
ragavendra.baliga@osumc.edu (R.R. Baliga)
ebossone@hotmail.com (E. Bossone)
gbakris@uchicago.edu (G.L. Bakris)

REFERENCES

1. Bakris GL, Baliga RR. Hypertension. New York: Oxford University Press; 2012.
2. Forouzanfar MH, Liu P, Roth GA, et al. Global burden of hypertension and systolic blood pressure of at least 110 to 115 mm Hg, 1990-2015. JAMA 2017; 317(2):165–82.
3. Whelton PK, Carey RM, Aronow WS, et al. 2017 ACC/AHA/AAPA/ABC/ACPM/AGS/APhA/ASH/ASPC/NMA/PCNA Guideline for the prevention, detection, evaluation, and management of high blood pressure in adults: a report of the American College of Cardiology/American Heart Association Task Force on Clinical Practice Guidelines. J Am Coll Cardiol 2018;71(19):e127–248.
4. Danaei G, Ding EL, Mozaffarian D, et al. The preventable causes of death in the United States: comparative risk assessment of dietary, lifestyle, and metabolic risk factors. PLoS Med 2009;6(4): e1000058.
5. Bossone E, Gorla R, LaBounty TM, et al. Presenting systolic blood pressure and outcomes in patients with acute aortic dissection. J Am Coll Cardiol 2018;71(13):1432–40.
6. Bakris G, Ali W, Parati G. ACC/AHA versus ESC/ESH on hypertension guidelines: JACC guideline comparison. J Am Coll Cardiol 2019;73(23): 3018–26.
7. Ali W, Bakris G. The management of hypertension in 2018: what should the targets be? Curr Hypertens Rep 2019;21(6):41.
8. Baliga RR, Cannon CP. Dyslipidemia. New York: Oxford University Press; 2012.
9. Group AS, Cushman WC, Evans GW, et al. Effects of intensive blood-pressure control in type 2 diabetes mellitus. N Engl J Med 2010;362(17): 1575–85.
10. Group SR, Wright JT Jr, Williamson JD, et al. A randomized trial of intensive versus standard blood-pressure control. N Engl J Med 2015; 373(22):2103–16.
11. Baliga RR, Smith SC Jr, Narula J. Protecting a billion hearts. Glob Heart 2014;9(4):361–2.

Epidemiology and Natural History

Diagnosis and Prevention of Hypertensive Heart Failure

Andreas P. Kalogeropoulos, MD, MPH, PhD[a],*, Clive Goulbourne, MD[a],
Javed Butler, MD, MPH, MBA[b]

KEYWORDS

- Hypertension • Blood pressure • Heart failure • Left ventricular hypertrophy
- Left ventricular systolic dysfunction • Echocardiography • Epidemiology • Guidelines

KEY POINTS

- Blood pressure has a strong and continuous association with heart failure (HF) risk down to the less than 120/80 mm Hg target and carries the highest attributable risk.
- Progression from hypertension (stage A HF) to left ventricular hypertrophy or other structural damage (stage B HF) compounds HF risk for clinical (stage C) HF.
- Echocardiography, potentially aided by biomarkers as a screening tool for patient selection, can detect patients with hypertension and stage B HF who need aggressive therapy.
- Prevention of hypertension, control of high blood pressure to contemporary targets, and aggressive treatment of structural heart damage significantly reduces HF risk.
- Although efficiency differs between antihypertensive classes, with evidence favoring angiotensin-modulating agents and diuretics, priority should be given to intensive BP control.

INTRODUCTION

Prolonged exposure of the heart to elevated blood pressure (BP) causes a variety of changes in the myocardial structure, coronary vasculature, and conduction system of the heart, collectively known as hypertensive heart disease. The resulting left ventricular (LV) dysfunction, ischemia, and arrhythmias, in conjunction with adverse changes in renal function, predispose patients with elevated BP to development of heart failure (HF). Because of high prevalence in the population, hypertension carries the highest attributable (and therefore potentially preventable) risk for HF at the population level, together with coronary artery disease (CAD).[1] For these reasons, the American College of Cardiology (ACC) and the American Heart Association (AHA) consider hypertension a

Disclosure: A.P. Kalogeropoulos has received research support from the National Heart, Lung, and Blood Institute, the American Heart Association, the American Society of Echocardiography, the Centers of Disease Control and Prevention, and Critical Diagnostics. C. Goulbourne has no relevant disclosures. J. Butler has received research support from the National Institutes of Health, the Patient-Centered Outcomes Research Institute, and the European Union. He serves on the speaker bureau for Novartis, Janssen, and NovoNordisk. He serves as a consultant and/or on steering committee, clinical events committee, or data safety monitoring boards for Abbott, Adrenomed, Amgen, Array, Astra Zeneca, Bayer, BerlinCures, Boehringer Ingelheim, Bristol Myers Squib, Cardiocell, CVRx, G3 Pharmaceutical, Innolife, Janssen, Lantheus, LinaNova, Luitpold, Medtronic, Merck, Relypsa, Roche, Sanofi, StealthPeptide, SC Pharma, V-Wave Limited, Vifor, and ZS Pharma.

[a] Division of Cardiology, Department of Medicine, Stony Brook University, Stony Brook University Medical Center, Health Sciences Center, 101 Nicolls Road, T-16, Rm 080, Stony Brook, NY 11794-8167, USA; [b] Department of Medicine, University of Mississippi Medical Center, 2500 North State Street, Jackson, MS 39216-4505, USA
* Corresponding author.
E-mail address: andreas.kalogeropoulos@stonybrook.edu
; @Andreas_SBU (A.P.K.)

Heart Failure Clin 15 (2019) 435–445
https://doi.org/10.1016/j.hfc.2019.05.001
1551-7136/19/© 2019 Elsevier Inc. All rights reserved.

precursor to HF and designate patients with elevated BP as having stage A HF, that is, being at risk for HF even in the absence of detectable structural damage to the heart.[2] The underlying goal of this classification ("stages") of HF is to stress the importance of prevention, because development of stage B HF (structural damage without symptoms) has a high propensity of evolving into clinical (stages C and D) HF, **Fig. 1**.

In this review, we use the framework proposed by ACC and AHA for the prevention of HF to summarize (1) the current trends in the prevalence of hypertension (and the impact of the recently revised definitions) and left ventricular hypertrophy (LVH); (2) the evidence that links elevated BP and BP-induced structural heart damage to HF risk; and (3) detection and diagnosis of preclinical and

clinical hypertensive HF; and (4) current preventive strategies.

STAGE A: HYPERTENSION WITHOUT STRUCTURAL HEART DAMAGE
Definitions

The main body of contemporary scientific evidence on hypertension has been derived by clinical trials and health care databases that used the Seventh Report of the Joint National Committee (JNC-7) definitions,[3] which defined elevated systolic BP (SBP) as ≥140 mm Hg (≥130 mm Hg for those with diabetes or renal dysfunction) or diastolic BP ≥90 mm Hg (≥80 mm Hg), **Table 1**. The recently revised US definitions set forth by ACC and AHA designate BP levels above ≥130/

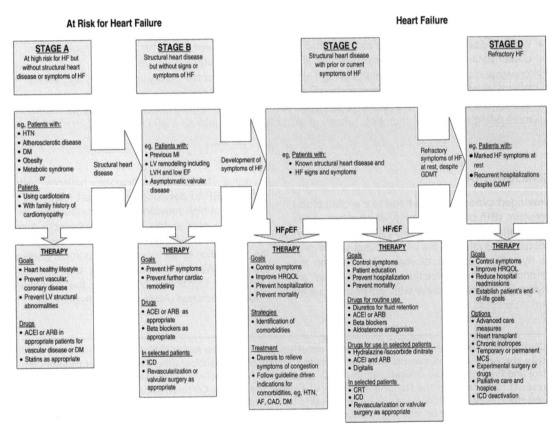

Fig. 1. Stages in the development of HF and recommended therapy by stage. ACEI, angiotensin-converting enzyme inhibitor; AF, atrial fibrillation; ARB, angiotensin receptor blocker; CAD, coronary artery disease; CRT, cardiac resynchronization therapy; DM, diabetes mellitus; EF, ejection fraction; GDMT, guideline-directed medical therapy; HF, heart failure; HFpEF, heart failure with preserved ejection fraction; HFrEF, heart failure with reduced ejection fraction; HRQOL, health-related quality of life; HTN, hypertension; ICD, implantable cardioverter-defibrillator; LV, left ventricular; LVH, left ventricular hypertrophy; MCS, mechanical circulatory support; MI, myocardial infarction. (*Adapted from* Hunt SA, Abraham WT, Chin MH, et al. 2009 focused update incorporated into the ACC/AHA 2005 guidelines for the diagnosis and management of heart failure in adults: a report of the American College of Cardiology Foundation/American Heart Association Task Force on Practice Guidelines. J Am Coll Cardiol. 2009;53:e9; with permission.)

Table 1
Current American College of Cardiology/ American Heart Association (ACC/AHA) versus the Seventh Report of the Joint National Committee (JNC VII) classification of hypertension and blood pressure thresholds

BP Category	SBP (mm Hg)		DBP (mm Hg)
ACC/AHA Guidelines (2018)			
Normal	<120	And	<80
Elevated	120–129	And	<80
Hypertension[a]			
Stage 1	130–139	Or	80–89
Stage 2	≥140	Or	≥90
JNC VII Guidelines (2003)			
Normal	<120	And	<80
Prehypertension	120–139	Or	80–89
Hypertension[a]			
Stage 1	140–159	Or	90–99
Stage 2	≥160	Or	≥100

Abbreviations: DBP, diastolic blood pressure; SBP, Systolic blood pressure.

[a] Diagnosis of hypertension is based on ≥2 readings obtained on ≥2 occasions.

Data from Whelton PK, Carey RM, Aronow WS, et al. 2017 ACC/AHA/AAPA/ABC/ACPM/AGS/APhA/ASH/ASPC/ NMA/PCNA guideline for the prevention, detection, evaluation, and management of high blood pressure in adults: executive summary: a report of the American College of Cardiology/American Heart Association Task Force on Clinical Practice Guidelines. J Am Coll Cardiol. 2018;71(19):2199-2269; and Chobanian AV, Bakris GL, Black HR, et al. The Seventh Report of the Joint National Committee on Prevention, Detection, Evaluation, and Treatment of High Blood Pressure: the JNC 7 report. JAMA. 2003;289(19):2560-2572.

80 mm Hg as elevated (stage 1 hypertension) and recommend pharmacotherapy for those with elevated cardiovascular risk.[4] This approach, which is based on clinical studies showing that risk does not plateau below the 140/90 mm Hg threshold (bur rather below 120/80 mm Hg)[5] and clinical trials demonstrating benefit with lower BP targets,[6] substantially changes the epidemiology of hypertension,[7] **Fig. 2**.

Epidemiology

In a global collaboration incorporating data from 19.1 million adults (18 years or older),[8] the age-standardized prevalence of elevated BP using the JNC-7 definition was 20.1% in women and 24.1% in men in 2015. Although the prevalence of elevated BP decreased in high-income and some middle-income countries, the number of adults with elevated BP increased from 594 million in 1975 to 1.13 billion in 2015, largely attributed to low- and middle-income countries.[8] Despite a decrease in age-specific prevalence, population growth and aging are driving the global increase in the number of adults with elevated BP.

Hypertension and Risk for Heart Failure

Hypertension and CAD consistently carry the highest population attributable risk for HF. In the Olmsted County data, hypertension was the most common risk factor for HF (66% of patients).[9] Although the relative risk for HF was particularly high for CAD and diabetes, the population attributable risk was highest for CAD and hypertension, each accounting for approximately 20% of HF cases in the population, with CAD accounting for the greatest proportion of cases in men (23%) and hypertension for the greatest proportion of cases in men (28%).[9]

Although elevated BP contributes to development of HF regardless of LV systolic function, hypertension is consistently more prevalent in HF presenting with midrange (defined as 40%–41% to 50%) and preserved ejection fraction compared with those with reduced ejection fraction. In a European registry of ambulatory patients with HF,[10] treated hypertension was present in 55.6%, 60.1%, and 67.0% of patients with reduced, midrange, and preserved ejection fraction, respectively. Similar findings have been reported by other well-characterized cohorts.[11]

Despite the need to categorize BP for public health and health policy purposes, the association between BP and HF risk is continuous. Among 4400 older adults (age, 73 ± 5 years; 82% white, 18% black; 53% women) enrolled in 2 large population-based studies in the United States,[12] there was a continuous positive association between SBP and HF risk for levels of SBP as low as less than 115 mm Hg (**Fig. 3**); over half of HF events occurred in enrollees with SBP less than 140 mm Hg.

Diagnosis

Diagnosis of stage A hypertensive HF amounts to diagnosis of hypertension. Although the detection and diagnosis of hypertension is outside the scope of the current review, it is worth mentioning that the latest American and European guidelines offer detailed guidance on use of alternative diagnostic methods besides traditional office-based BP measurements and highlight the need for confirmation before classifying elevated BP.[4,13]

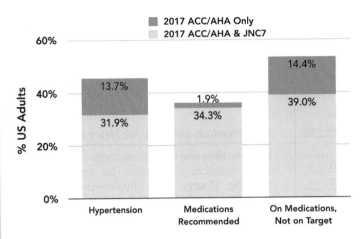

Fig. 2. Impact of the 2017 American College of Cardiology/American Heart Association (ACC/AHA) versus Seventh Report of the Joint National Committee (JNC-7) guidelines on the prevalence of hypertension, recommendation for pharmacologic antihypertensive treatment, and blood pressure above goal among US adults. (*Adapted from* Muntner P, Carey RM, Gidding S, et al. Potential US population impact of the 2017 ACC/AHA High Blood Pressure guideline. Circulation 2018;137:117; with permission.)

STAGE B: HYPERTENSION WITH SUBCLINICAL HEART DAMAGE
Definitions

The most common cardiac abnormality associated with elevated BP is LVH. Although functional LV abnormalities, including diastolic dysfunction, subclinical systolic dysfunction, and ischemia (which can lead to diastolic and systolic dysfunction), can be induced and/or aggravated by hypertension, LVH is considered the hallmark of hypertension-induced structural heart damage. This is because hypertension is by far the most common and clinically important acquired risk factor for LVH and, conversely, other abnormalities are multifactorial. However, the presence of any structural abnormality in the presence of elevated BP, including LV systolic dysfunction (impaired LV ejection fraction) or silent myocardial ischemia/infarct puts the patient at higher risk for HF and should be considered as stage B HF as well (see **Fig. 1**).

The most common method for detection of LVH is echocardiography. Although electrocardiographically detected LVH is strongly associated with subsequent HF risk, the sensitivity of electrocardiogram (ECG) for screening purposes is inadequate and specificity is not optimal either. Therefore, estimates of LVH as an indicator of stage B hypertensive HF should ideally rely on echocardiography. According to the latest joint American/European echocardiographic guidelines,[14] a body surface area-indexed LV mass greater than 115 g/m^2 in men or greater than 95 g/m^2 in women indicates LVH. Because initial LV remodeling associated with elevated BP usually manifests as increased wall thickness and subsequently concentric LVH, further classification of LVH into concentric or eccentric using the relative wall thickness (**Fig. 4**) is helpful.[15]

Epidemiology

In a systematic review of studies published in 2000 to 2010, which encompassed 37,700 untreated and treated patients with hypertension (80.3% white, 52.4% men, 9.6% with diabetes, 2.6% with cardiovascular disease), LVH prevalence was 36% using conservative criteria to 41% with more liberal criteria in the entire population and was not different between women and men, but was higher among treated patients.[16] Concentric LVH was present in approximately 20% of patients regardless of gender, indicating that LVH is a still highly prevalent despite substantial progress in the detection and treatment of hypertension.

The association between BP and LVH is continuous. In a meta-analysis of 73,556 subjects from 20 studies, LV mass index and relative wall thickness were greater in the 17,314 participants with prehypertension (JNC-7 definition) compared with the 44,170 normotensive participants.[17] The same meta-analysis reported higher E/e' ratio and left atrium diameter in participants with prehypertension than in normotensive subjects.[17] In a longitudinal analysis of 880 untreated participants without LVH at baseline, the 10-year incidence of LVH increased progressively from normotensive to prehypertension and hypertension (9.0%, 23.2%, and 36.5%, respectively).[18] These data taken together suggest that alterations in cardiac structure and function already begin with suboptimal BP even without overt hypertension.

Besides LVH, subclinical CAD including silent myocardial infarction (which constitutes structural cardiac damage and hence stage B HF[19]) is more common among patients with hypertension, especially smokers and those with additional metabolic risk factors.[20] Although hypertension is associated with increased risk for silent myocardial infarction to a lesser degree compared with diabetes or

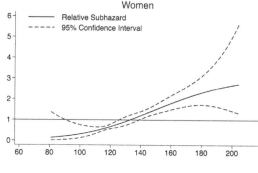

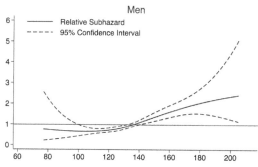

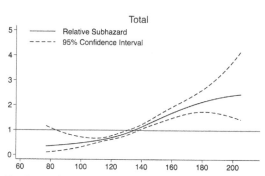

Fig. 3. Nonlinear association of systolic blood pressure and heart failure risk. (*From* Butler J, Kalogeropoulos AP, Georgiopoulou VV, et al. Systolic blood pressure and incident heart failure in the elderly. The Cardiovascular Health Study and the Health, Ageing and Body Composition Study. Heart 2011;97:1309; with permission.)

known cardiovascular disease, the risk increases with age.[21] Prevalence estimates of silent myocardial infarcts in patients with hypertension are hard to obtain, because ECG detection is rather insensitive (1–2 per 1000 patient-years in clinical trials[21]) and mass functional imaging is impractical for population-based studies or large clinical trials.

Structural Findings and Risk for Stage C Heart Failure

The presence of LVH significantly compounds risk for HF among patients with hypertension. In the

Multi-Ethnic Study of Atherosclerosis study, among 4745 enrollees (age, 61 ± 10 years, 53.5% women, 61.7% non-whites), ECG-detected LVH (6.1% of participants) and MRI-detected LVH (10.5% of participants) were associated with approximately 2.5- and 4-fold higher risk for HF, respectively. The pattern of LVH plays also into risk for HF, with eccentric LVH carrying higher risk for HF versus concentric LVH in the Framingham Heart Study.[22] Also, participants with eccentric LVH had a higher propensity for HF with reduced ejection fraction, whereas those with concentric hypertrophy were more prone to HF with preserved ejection fraction.[22]

Although asymptomatic LV systolic dysfunction, another stage B HF manifestation, is far less common than LVH among patients with hypertension, it is associated with significantly increased risk for HF. Among 2384 initially untreated subjects with hypertension, an echocardiographic ejection fraction less than 50% was found in 3.6% of subjects[23]; in these patients the risk for new onset HF requiring hospitalization was 10-fold higher during follow-up (mean, 6 years; range, 0–17).

Interestingly, in a real-world registry from Europe, hypertension was identified as the underlying cause in 30% of patients with HF and midrange ejection fraction (compared with 16% in those with reduced and 49% in those with preserved ejection fraction).[11] These data suggest that hypertension can cause progression of stage B disease from LVH to systolic dysfunction in a substantial proportion of patients before becoming clinically manifest as HF.

Diagnosis of Stage B Disease (Asymptomatic Structural Heart Damage)

In patients with primary hypertension, an ECG is recommended as part of the initial evaluation, whereas echocardiography is optional and reserved for younger patients (≤18 years of age) or those who have evidence of secondary hypertension, chronic uncontrolled hypertension, or symptoms of HF.[4] The recently released appropriate use criteria for multimodality imaging in nonvalvular heart disease classify echocardiography as an appropriate modality (score 8 out of 9) for initial evaluation of suspected hypertensive heart disease and potentially appropriate (score 5 out of 9) for asymptomatic patients.[24] However, most patients with hypertension remain asymptomatic for a long time even in the presence of LVH or other structural damage. Therefore, echocardiography at initial evaluation of hypertension might be a reasonable option for most patients. The recent update in American guidelines for HF offers further

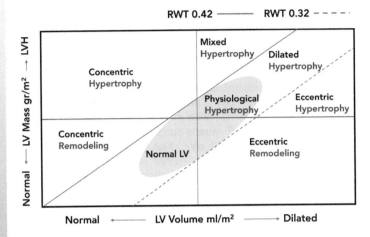

Fig. 4. Left ventricular (LV) geometric patterns classified according to LV mass, LV volume, and relative wall thickness (RWT). (*From* Marwick TH, Gillebert TC, Aurigemma G, et al. Recommendations on the use of echocardiography in adult hypertension: A report from the European Association of Cardiovascular Imaging (EACVI) and the American Society of Echocardiography (ASE). J Am Soc Echocardiogr. 2015;28:736; with permission.)

guidance on this topic,[25] introducing biomarker-based screening for patient selection based on the results of a large-scale study.[26] In that unblinded single-center study,[26] patients with hypertension, diabetes, or vascular disease, but without established LV systolic dysfunction or symptomatic HF, randomly received screening with B-type natriuretic peptide (BNP) or usual care, and those with BNP ≥50 pg/mL underwent echocardiography and were referred to a cardiovascular specialist; all patients received coaching on adherence to medications and healthy lifestyle. BNP-based screening reduced the composite endpoint of asymptomatic LV dysfunction (systolic or diastolic) with or without newly diagnosed HF.[26]

Electrocardiography

Although LVH can be detected by ECG, the sensitivity and specificity is suboptimal unless body mass index and age are taken into account. In the Framingham Heart Study,[27] the adjusted voltage sum of R in aVL and S in V3, alone and in combination with QRS duration, had a specificity of 32% and 39%, respectively, in men, and 46% and 51%, respectively, in women at 95% sensitivity. An ECG can also detect other high-risk elements, including rhythm disturbances and previous silent myocardial infarction; however, ECG has overall low sensitivity for the detection of nonischemic stage B HF, especially in older adults.[28]

Echocardiography

Although LV mass can be approximately calculated with several echocardiographic methods, including M-mode, 2D, and 3D echocardiography, the basic principle is the same; LV mass is calculated by subtracting the volume of the LV cavity from the volume encompassed by the epicardium,

multiplied by the estimated specific density of myocardium.[14]

The 2D echocardiographic methods can accommodate for the shape of LV, and therefore are advantageous compared with M-mode for patients with known cardiac disease and altered LV geometry. On the other hand, the M-mode method is simple and subject to less measurement variability, and therefore it is best suited for screening populations in whom altered LV geometry is uncommon.[14] The best documented methods based on 2D LV measurements are the area-length method and the truncated ellipsoid method.[14] However, M-mode and 2D methods suffer from assumptions about the shape of the LV; hence the mass of asymmetric LV cannot be accurately estimated. Use of 3D echocardiography significantly improves the accuracy and reproducibility of LV volume and mass measurements, but requires additional resources and therefore is not yet suitable for population-based applications.[14]

Echocardiography is also useful to assess LV systolic dysfunction (usually defined as ejection fraction <50% for practical purposes), which clearly puts the patient at elevated risk of HF, and LV diastolic function. Diastolic dysfunction should be assessed with multiple echocardiographic parameters to improve diagnostic classification, including left atrial volume, which is prognostic for the development of HF and atrial fibrillation.[29] Other, early signs of LV dysfunction, including impaired LV mechanics, have been associated with hypertension, but are unsuitable for wide clinical practice application.

Cardiac magnetic resonance

Although cardiac magnetic resonance (CMR) is the most reproducible noninvasive modality for detection of LVH and LV systolic dysfunction and serial measurements of LV dimensions, it is not suitable for population-based applications to prevent hypertensive HF, because of limited availability and considerable cost, especially in middle- and low-income settings. Also, CMR is problematic in patients with claustrophobia, atrial fibrillation, and some implantable devices. However, CMR is an excellent option to assess LV structure for clinical study purposes.

STAGE C: CLINICAL HYPERTENSIVE HEART FAILURE

The diagnosis of clinical (stage C) HF secondary to long-standing hypertension does not differ from HF due to other causes. Also, because hypertension is present in most patients who develop HF,[9] especially those with HF and preserved ejection fraction,[30] it is often difficult to attribute new HF cases solely to hypertension. Because hypertension and LVH are highly prevalent among older adults, and dyspnea can be multifactorial in these patients, biomarkers are useful in the diagnosis of HF, especially when systolic function is preserved. For this reason, the updated American HF guidelines recommend natriuretic peptide testing (class I) for patients presenting with dyspnea to support a diagnosis or exclusion of HF.[25] The European guidelines provide a more detailed diagnostic algorithm,[31] where BNP less than 35 pg/mL or N-terminal pro-BNP less than 125 pg/mL render the diagnosis of HF unlikely; if both symptoms and natriuretic peptides concur, echocardiography is recommended.

The onset of symptoms among patients with stage B disease is often insidious, and heightened clinical awareness is required to detect the transition to stage C, because symptomatic status is not always straightforward to assess. In this aspect, functional testing may provide additional information. In a study of 510 asymptomatic patients (age, 58 ± 12 years) with type 2 diabetes mellitus, hypertension, or obesity, asymptomatic left ventricular impairment (LVH, elevated LV filling pressures, or abnormal myocardial deformation) was independently associated with impaired exercise capacity.[32]

PREVENTION OF HYPERTENSIVE HEART FAILURE

Controlling BP dramatically reduces the risk of structural heart damage, for example, LVH and clinical HF among patients with hypertension (stage A HF), and prevents progression to clinical HF among patients with existing structural damage as a result of long-standing hypertension (stage B HF). In the pivotal SPRINT trial, tighter control of BP led to reduced rates of cardiovascular events across the board, but the most profound effect was on HF incidence.[6] However, detection and control of high BP in the population requires public awareness, access to care, and substantial health care resources as a result of high prevalence. The recently revised US guidelines for the diagnosis and treatment of hypertension continue to shift actionable BP levels from what is common in the population to what is optimal for cardiovascular disease prevention.[4] Although this approach has merit from a public health standpoint, it compounds the health care system issues described above and creates new challenges. The problem is even more complex with regard to stage B HF. Detection of structural heart damage secondary to hypertension, most commonly manifesting as LVH, requires some form of cardiac imaging (usually echocardiography), because ECG-based detection is insensitive. Although patients with LVH or other structural damage benefit the most from interventions, population screening is not feasible. In this aspect, biomarker-guided selection of high-risk patients with hypertension is a reasonable strategy and supported by evidence.[26]

Preventing Hypertension (Stage A Disease)

Although more than 300 genetic loci have been associated with hypertension, genetic variants collectively explain less than 3.5 of total BP variance.[33] Therefore, the risk for hypertension is largely determined by modifiable environmental and lifestyle factors,[33] most importantly excess weight, unhealthy diet, excessive dietary sodium, and inadequate potassium intake, insufficient physical activity, and consumption of alcohol (**Table 2**). Prevention strategies applied early in childhood and early adult life carry the greatest long-term potential for benefit.

Preventing Structural Heart Alterations (Stage B Disease)

The cornerstone of preventing hypertension-induced cardiac damage and clinical HF is treating BP to appropriate targets (see **Table 1**). Cardiovascular risk is higher in patients with LVH compared with those with persistently normal LV mass, even after LVH regression.[34] Therefore, preventing LVH is an important therapeutic goal. Adherence to lifestyle changes (see **Table 2**) is crucial before and after medication initiation.

The need for intensive BP control to prevent structural heart damage is supported by many observational and interventional studies. In a meta-analysis of 20 studies, the prevalence of

Table 2
Lifestyle modifications to prevent and control hypertension

Lifestyle Factor	Recommendation
Diet	Follow a DASH-type dietary pattern: • Rich in fruits, vegetables, whole grains, nuts, legumes, lean protein, low-fat dairy products • Low in refined sugar, saturated fat, and cholesterol
Sodium intake	Reduce sodium intake below 2300 mg daily (6 g of salt); ≥70% of sodium intake comes from processed foods, including breads, salted meats, canned goods, cereals, pastries, and food preparation (fast-food and sit-down restaurants)
Potassium intake	Increase potassium intake to 4700 mg daily; a DASH-type diet is preferred over dietary supplements to achieve this goal
Physical activity	Engage in regular aerobic physical activity, of at least moderate intensity, most days of the week; aim for at least 150 min/wk total
Weight	Aim at a body mass index <25 kg/m²
Alcohol intake	For those who drink alcohol, consume: • ≤2 alcoholic drinks daily (men) • ≤1 alcoholic drink daily (women)

Data from Carey RM, Muntner P, Bosworth HB, et al. Prevention and control of hypertension: JACC health promotion series. J Am Coll Cardiol. 2018;72(11):1278-1293; and the American Heart Association.

structural and functional cardiac changes among patients with JNC-7 "prehypertension" (120–139/80–89 mm Hg) was higher compared with normotensive patients.[17] In a recent longitudinal study, the 10-year incidence of LVH was higher among those with baseline prehypertension versus normotensive particpants.[18] In SPRINT, intensive BP lowering (target SBP <120 mm Hg) led to 46% lower risk of ECG-detected LVH within 4 years of follow-up compared with standard BP lowering (target SBP <140 mm Hg), providing more definitive support for intensive BP control.[35]

Preventing Clinical Heart Failure (Stage C Disease)

Treatment of hypertension to intensive BP targets with appropriate agents along with lifestyle modifications dramatically reduces risk for HF, especially among high-risk patients. In addition, intensive therapy can reverse existing structural heart damage and reduce risk for progression to clinical HF among patients with existing LVH, LV systolic dysfunction, or silent ischemia.

Treating hypertension to prevent heart failure risk

Little doubt exists as to the value of treating hypertension to "traditional" BP targets (<140/90 mm Hg) to prevent cardiovascular disease and HF. In a network meta-analysis of studies in patients with hypertension and high cardiovascular risk with over 220,000 patients, all antihypertensive medication classes except beta-blockers reduced HF risk compared with placebo, with diuretics (odds ratio [OR] = 0.59; 95% CI, 0.47–0.73), angiotensin-converting enzyme inhibitors (OR = 0.71; 95% CI, 0.59–0.85), and angiotensin receptor blockers (OR = 0.76; 95% CI, 0.62–0.90) being the most efficient.[36] In the same meta-analysis, diuretic-based therapies were the more efficient approach for the prevention of HF.[36] The impressive results of SPRINT,[6] which demonstrated a 38% risk reduction for HF after a median of 3.8 years of intensive (target BP <120/80 mm Hg) versus standard (target BP <140/90 mm Hg) strategy among patents at increased cardiovascular risk but without diabetes, have provided strong evidence in favor of intensive targets for patients at high risk. In SPRINT, intensive treatment started with a combination of thiazide-type diuretic, angiotensin-modulating agent, or calcium channel blocker, with beta-blockers initially reserved for compelling indications. Patients were followed up monthly with appropriate medication titration or addition of unused classes to reach the less than 120/80 mm Hg target. Spironolactone and alpha-blockers were allowed in resistant cases.[6]

Treating left ventricular hypertrophy

All classes of antihypertensive medications have been shown to reduce LVH compared with placebo,[37] albeit to a different degree. In a meta-analysis of 75 trials involving 6000 patients, regression of LV mass was significantly less with beta-blockers than with angiotensin receptor blockers, but none of the other comparisons between medication classes (which included angiotensin receptor blockers, calcium channel blockers, and diuretics) revealed significant differences.[38] Beta-blockers showed less regression than other classes combined, and regression was more pronounced with angiotensin receptor blockers versus the others.[38] However, it should be noted that patients with LVH often have stage 2 hypertension (BP $\geq$140/90 mm Hg) and need more than 1 agent to reach optimal BP (<120/80 mm Hg),[4] and therefore combination therapy is common. As thiazide diuretics potentiate the effects of angiotensin-modulating agents, a combination of these agents is probably the most reasonable option for patients with known LVH.[39]

Intensive BP control is probably the most important goal. In SPRINT,[35] among participants with baseline ECG-detected LVH (605 patients, 7.4% of the cohort), those assigned to the intensive BP target (<120/80 mm Hg) were 66% more likely to regress or improve their LVH versus those assigned to the standard BP target (<140/90 mm Hg) after a median of 3.8 years.

Left ventricular systolic dysfunction

Although not specific to systolic dysfunction induced by long-standing hypertension, studies have shown that beta-blocker and angiotensin-modulating therapy can reverse LV remodeling and improve LV geometry and function.[40,41]

SUMMARY

Intensive treatment of hypertension to appropriate BP targets together with lifestyle changes is crucial in the prevention of and therapy for hypertensive HF. Regression of LVH or other structural heart alterations secondary to hypertension is feasible and associated with improved prognosis. The results of the SPRINT trial suggest that an intensive target (<120/80 mm Hg) is appropriate for the prevention of HF and for the prevention and reversal of subclinical cardiac damage. Because the yield of preventive interventions is optimal before the development of symptoms, a biomarker-guided strategy to direct echocardiographic screening at high-risk patients might be worth considering for most patients with newly discovered hypertension. There are differences in the properties and the effectiveness of antihypertensive agents in preventing and reversing structural cardiac alterations, with angiotensin-modulating agents having the strongest evidence for benefit. However, as many patients will require combination therapy to achieve BP targets, the most important goal in the prevention of hypertensive HF remains appropriate control of BP.

REFERENCES

1. Kalogeropoulos A, Georgiopoulou V, Kritchevsky SB, et al. Epidemiology of incident heart failure in a contemporary elderly cohort: the health, aging, and body composition study. Arch Intern Med 2009; 169(7):708–15.

2. Yancy CW, Jessup M, Bozkurt B, et al. 2013 ACCF/AHA guideline for the management of heart failure: a report of the American College of Cardiology Foundation/American Heart Association Task Force on Practice Guidelines. J Am Coll Cardiol 2013; 62(16):e147–239.

3. Chobanian AV, Bakris GL, Black HR, et al. The seventh report of the joint national committee on prevention, detection, evaluation, and treatment of high blood pressure: the JNC 7 report. JAMA 2003; 289(19):2560–72.

4. Whelton PK, Carey RM, Aronow WS, et al. 2017 ACC/AHA/AAPA/ABC/ACPM/AGS/APhA/ASH/ASPC/NMA/PCNA guideline for the prevention, detection, evaluation, and management of high blood pressure in adults: executive summary: a report of the American College of Cardiology/American Heart Association Task Force on clinical practice guidelines. J Am Coll Cardiol 2018;71(19):2199–269.

5. Rapsomaniki E, Timmis A, George J, et al. Blood pressure and incidence of twelve cardiovascular diseases: lifetime risks, healthy life-years lost, and age-specific associations in 1.25 million people. Lancet 2014;383(9932):1899–911.

6. Group SR, Wright JT Jr, Williamson JD, et al. A randomized trial of intensive versus standard blood-pressure control. N Engl J Med 2015; 373(22):2103–16.

7. Muntner P, Carey RM, Gidding S, et al. Potential US population impact of the 2017 ACC/AHA high blood pressure guideline. Circulation 2018;137(2): 109–18.

8. NCD Risk Factor Collaboration (NCD-RisC). Worldwide trends in blood pressure from 1975 to 2015: a pooled analysis of 1479 population-based measurement studies with 19.1 million participants. Lancet 2017;389(10064):37–55.

9. Dunlay SM, Weston SA, Jacobsen SJ, et al. Risk factors for heart failure: a population-based case-control study. Am J Med 2009;122(11):1023–8.

10. Chioncel O, Lainscak M, Seferovic PM, et al. Epidemiology and one-year outcomes in patients with chronic heart failure and preserved, mid-range and reduced ejection fraction: an analysis of the ESC Heart failure long-term registry. Eur J Heart Fail 2017;19(12):1574–85.

11. Guisado-Espartero M, Salamanca-Bautista P, Aramburu-Bodas Ó, et al. Heart failure with mid-range ejection fraction in patients admitted to internal medicine departments: findings from the RICA Registry. Int J Cardiol 2018;255:255124–8.

12. Butler J, Kalogeropoulos AP, Georgiopoulou VV, et al. Systolic blood pressure and incident heart failure in the elderly. The Cardiovascular Health Study

and the Health, Ageing and Body Composition Study. Heart 2011;97(16):1304–11.

13. Williams B, Mancia G, Spiering W, et al. 2018 ESC/ESH Guidelines for the management of arterial hypertension. Eur Heart J 2018;39(33):3021–104.

14. Lang RM, Badano LP, Mor-Avi V, et al. Recommendations for cardiac chamber quantification by echocardiography in adults: an update from the American Society of Echocardiography and the European Association of Cardiovascular Imaging. J Am Soc Echocardiogr 2015;28(1):1–39 e14.

15. Marwick TH, Gillebert TC, Aurigemma G, et al. Recommendations on the use of echocardiography in adult hypertension: a report from the European Association of Cardiovascular Imaging (EACVI) and the American Society of Echocardiography (ASE). J Am Soc Echocardiogr 2015;28(7):727–54.

16. Cuspidi C, Sala C, Negri F, et al. Prevalence of left-ventricular hypertrophy in hypertension: an updated review of echocardiographic studies. J Hum Hypertens 2012;26(6):343–9.

17. Cuspidi C, Sala C, Tadic M, et al. Pre-hypertension and subclinical cardiac damage: a meta-analysis of echocardiographic studies. Int J Cardiol 2018; 270:270302–8.

18. Cuspidi C, Facchetti R, Bombelli M, et al. High normal blood pressure and left ventricular hypertrophy echocardiographic findings from the PAMELA population. Hypertension 2019;73(3):612–9.

19. Soliman EZ. Silent myocardial infarction and risk of heart failure: current evidence and gaps in knowledge. Trends Cardiovasc Med 2019;29(4):239–44.

20. Rendina D, Ippolito R, De Filippo G, et al. Risk factors for silent myocardial ischemia in patients with well-controlled essential hypertension. Intern Emerg Med 2017;12(2):171–9.

21. Valensi P, Lorgis L, Cottin Y. Prevalence, incidence, predictive factors and prognosis of silent myocardial infarction: a review of the literature. Arch Cardiovasc Dis 2011;104(3):178–88.

22. Velagaleti RS, Gona P, Pencina MJ, et al. Left ventricular hypertrophy patterns and incidence of heart failure with preserved versus reduced ejection fraction. Am J Cardiol 2014;113(1):117–22.

23. Verdecchia P, Angeli F, Gattobigio R, et al. Asymptomatic left ventricular systolic dysfunction in essential hypertension: prevalence, determinants, and prognostic value. Hypertension 2005;45(3):412–8.

24. Writing Group M, Doherty JU, Kort S, et al. ACC/AATS/AHA/ASE/ASNC/HRS/SCAI/SCCT/SCMR/STS 2019 appropriate use criteria for multimodality imaging in the assessment of cardiac structure and function in nonvalvular heart disease: a report of the American College of Cardiology Appropriate Use Criteria Task Force, American Association for Thoracic Surgery, American Heart Association, American Society of Echocardiography, American Society of Nuclear Cardiology, Heart Rhythm Society, Society for Cardiovascular Angiography and Interventions, Society of Cardiovascular Computed Tomography, Society for Cardiovascular Magnetic Resonance, and the Society of Thoracic Surgeons. J Am Coll Cardiol 2019;73(4):488–516.

25. Yancy CW, Jessup M, Bozkurt B, et al. 2017 ACC/AHA/HFSA focused update of the 2013 ACCF/AHA guideline for the management of heart failure: a report of the American College of Cardiology/American Heart Association Task Force on Clinical Practice Guidelines and the Heart Failure Society of America. J Card Fail 2017;23(8):628–51.

26. Ledwidge M, Gallagher J, Conlon C, et al. Natriuretic peptide-based screening and collaborative care for heart failure: the STOP-HF randomized trial. JAMA 2013;310(1):66–74.

27. Norman JE Jr, Levy D. Improved electrocardiographic detection of echocardiographic left ventricular hypertrophy: results of a correlated data base approach. J Am Coll Cardiol 1995;26(4):1022–9.

28. Yang H, Marwick TH, Wang Y, et al. Association between electrocardiographic and echocardiographic markers of stage B heart failure and cardiovascular outcome. ESC Heart Fail 2017;4(4):417–31.

29. Nagueh SF, Smiseth OA, Appleton CP, et al. Recommendations for the evaluation of left ventricular diastolic function by echocardiography: an update from the American Society of Echocardiography and the European Association of Cardiovascular Imaging. J Am Soc Echocardiogr 2016;29(4):277–314.

30. Georgiopoulou VV, Velayati A, Burkman G, et al. Comorbidities, sociodemographic factors, and hospitalizations in outpatients with heart failure and preserved ejection fraction. Am J Cardiol 2018; 121(10):1207–13.

31. Ponikowski P, Voors AA, Anker SD, et al. 2016 ESC guidelines for the diagnosis and treatment of acute and chronic heart failure: the task force for the diagnosis and treatment of acute and chronic heart failure of the European Society of Cardiology (ESC) developed with the special contribution of the Heart Failure Association (HFA) of the ESC. Eur Heart J 2016;37(27):2129–200.

32. Kosmala W, Jellis CL, Marwick TH. Exercise limitation associated with asymptomatic left ventricular impairment: analogy with stage B heart failure. J Am Coll Cardiol 2015;65(3):257–66.

33. Carey RM, Muntner P, Bosworth HB, et al. Prevention and control of hypertension: JACC health promotion series. J Am Coll Cardiol 2018;72(11):1278–93.

34. Angeli F, Reboldi G, Poltronieri C, et al. The prognostic legacy of left ventricular hypertrophy: cumulative evidence after the MAVI study. J Hypertens 2015;33(11):2322–30.

35. Soliman EZ, Ambrosius WT, Cushman WC, et al. Effect of intensive blood pressure lowering on left

ventricular hypertrophy in patients with hypertension: SPRINT (Systolic Blood Pressure Intervention Trial). Circulation 2017;136(5):440–50.

36. Sciarretta S, Palano F, Tocci G, et al. Antihypertensive treatment and development of heart failure in hypertension: a Bayesian network meta-analysis of studies in patients with hypertension and high cardiovascular risk. Arch Intern Med 2011;171(5):384–94.

37. Schmieder RE, Martus P, Klingbeil A. Reversal of left ventricular hypertrophy in essential hypertension. A meta-analysis of randomized double-blind studies. JAMA 1996;275(19):1507–13.

38. Fagard RH, Celis H, Thijs L, et al. Regression of left ventricular mass by antihypertensive treatment: a meta-analysis of randomized comparative studies. Hypertension 2009;54(5):1084–91.

39. Mimran A, Weir MR. Angiotensin-receptor blockers and diuretics–advantages of combination. Blood Press 2005;14(1):6–11.

40. Konstam MA. Angiotensin converting enzyme inhibition in asymptomatic left ventricular systolic dysfunction and early heart failure. Eur Heart J 1995;16(Suppl):N59–64.

41. Colucci WS, Kolias TJ, Adams KF, et al. Metoprolol reverses left ventricular remodeling in patients with asymptomatic systolic dysfunction: the REversal of VEntricular Remodeling with Toprol-XL (REVERT) trial. Circulation 2007;116(1):49–56.

The Evolution from Hypertension to Heart Failure

Matthew J. Sorrentino, MD

KEYWORDS

- Diastolic dysfunction • Left ventricular hypertrophy (LVH)
- Heart failure with preserved ejection fraction (HFpEF)
- Heart failure with reduced ejection fraction (HFrEF)

KEY POINTS

- Hypertensive heart disease includes diastolic dysfunction, left ventricular hypertrophy, and heart failure with preserved and reduced ejection fraction.
- Diastolic dysfunction is the first manifestation of hypertensive heart disease.
- Diastolic dysfunction can progress to the development of heart failure with preserved ejection fraction (HFpEF).
- An instigating factor, such as an ischemic event, can cause HFpEF to progress to heart failure with a reduced ejection fraction (HFrEF).
- The treatment of hypertension can reduce left ventricular mass, improve diastolic function, and reduce the incidence of heart failure.

Hypertension is the most common risk factor for the development of heart failure. The Framingham Heart Study observed that hypertension preceded the onset of heart failure in 91% of individuals during a 20-year follow-up.[1] More than 70 million US adults have hypertension using 140/90 or greater as the definition. An additional 30 million are defined as having hypertension using the American College of Cardiology/American Heart Association definition of hypertension as 130/80 or greater.[2] By 2030, it is estimated that more than 41% of Americans will have hypertension. More than 6.5 million adults currently have heart failure in the United States and this is estimated to increase by 46% from 2012 to 2030.[3] The increase in prevalence of longstanding hypertension is one of the key underlying risk factors driving the growing incidence of heart failure in this country.

Hypertensive heart disease is a term used to describe patients with clinical manifestations of heart disease caused by the impact of hypertension on the heart. Hypertensive heart disease includes the development of diastolic dysfunction, left ventricular hypertrophy (LVH), and heart failure with preserved and reduced ejection fraction (HFpEF, HFrEF) (**Table 1**).[4] The development of heart failure can occur because of complications of ischemic heart disease (eg, following a myocardial infarction) or from progression of diastolic dysfunction to HFpEF degenerating to a dilated heart with systolic dysfunction or HFrEF.

DIASTOLIC DYSFUNCTION

Left ventricular diastolic dysfunction is typically the first manifestation of hypertensive heart disease. Diastolic dysfunction refers to abnormalities in diastolic filling, distensibility, or relaxation of the left ventricle (LV). Many patients may show abnormalities in diastolic parameters but remain

The author has nothing to disclose.
Department of Medicine, Section of Cardiology, University of Chicago Medicine, 5841 South Maryland Avenue, MC 6080, Room B607, Chicago, IL 60637, USA
E-mail address: msorrent@medicine.bsd.uchicago.edu

Heart Failure Clin 15 (2019) 447–453
https://doi.org/10.1016/j.hfc.2019.06.005
1551-7136/19/© 2019 Elsevier Inc. All rights reserved.

Table 1
Staging of severity of hypertensive heart disease

Degree I	Diastolic dysfunction
Degree II	Left ventricular hypertrophy
Degree III	Heart failure with preserved ejection fraction
Degree IV	Heart failure with reduced ejection fraction

Adapted from Messerli FH, Rimoldi SF, Bangalore S. The Transition From Hypertension to Heart Failure: Contemporary Update. JACC Heart Fail 2017;5(8):546; with permission.

asymptomatic. These patients are classified as having diastolic dysfunction. Once symptoms of breathlessness and exercise intolerance develop along with signs of fluid retention, patients are classified as having HFpEF as long as systolic function remains normal.[5]

Diastole begins with relaxation of the LV. Isovolumic relaxation is an energy-dependent process that begins at aortic valve closure and ends with mitral valve opening. When the mitral valve opens, a volume and pressure gradient between the left atrium and LV results in early rapid filling of the LV. Volume and pressure between the left atrium and LV equilibrate (diastasis) until left atrial contraction results in further LV filling at the end of diastole. In a normal heart at a normal heart rate, left atrial contraction is not essential for adequate LV filling because the LV will have nearly reached its maximum end-diastolic volume before atrial contraction begins.

Box 1 lists some of the common abnormalities in structure and function of the heart with diastolic dysfunction. LV relaxation is slowed or delayed leading to impaired rate and extent of filling of the LV. The LV becomes stiff with decreased distensibility. With reduced early diastolic filling, the LV diastolic volume and cardiac output

Box 1
Common abnormalities of diastolic dysfunction

Delayed LV relaxation

Impairment in LV filling

Increased late diastolic filling dependent on left atrial contraction

Increased left atrial, pulmonary venous, and LV diastolic pressure

Chamber remodeling: increased LV wall thickness, normal or reduced end-diastolic volume, left atrial enlargement

becomes more dependent on late diastolic filling supplied by left atrial contraction (referred to as the atrial kick). The left atrial contribution to filling increases and in more advanced states may account for more than 30% of the cardiac output. Left atrial pressure increases causing the left atrium to dilate. Dilation of the left atrium is an early sign of increased LV filling pressures and diastolic dysfunction. With time, pulmonary venous pressures increase and can cause pulmonary congestion and signs and symptoms of heart failure.

There are several factors that can predispose to diastolic dysfunction noted in **Box 2**. Common factors include myocardial ischemia, infiltrative heart diseases with myocardial fibrosis, pericardial constriction, and left ventricular pressure overload with the development of LVH caused by such conditions as aortic stenosis or increased afterload caused by systemic hypertension.[6] Chronic longstanding hypertension is the most common cause of diastolic dysfunction and is a disease of chronic increased afterload leading to the development of LVH. Hypertension is also a major atherosclerosis risk factor and may contribute to myocardial ischemia and fibrosis.

The prevalence of diastolic dysfunction is estimated to be as high as 27% in the general population.[7] A higher risk of developing diastolic dysfunction has been associated with older age, obesity, hypertension, diabetes, and renal insufficiency. The presence of diastolic dysfunction predicts the development of heart failure. A Mayo clinic population-based cohort study showed a marked progression of diastolic dysfunction with age with persistent or worsening diastolic dysfunction an independent risk factor for subsequent heart failure.[8]

LEFT VENTRICULAR HYPERTROPHY

LVH is a common finding in patients with increased blood pressure and may be present before the diagnosis of hypertension. LVH is diagnosed by voltage criteria on an electrocardiogram or by measurement of LV wall thickness and calculation of LV mass by echocardiography or MRI.

Box 2
Factors that predispose diastolic dysfunction

Myocardial ischemia

Infiltrative heart disease (myocardial fibrosis)

Pericardial constriction

LV pressure overload (aortic stenosis, increased afterload caused by hypertension)

Echocardiography and MRI are more sensitive in diagnosing LVH than using electrocardiogram criteria, which can only identify more advanced LVH. LVH is defined as an increase in LV mass usually caused by increased wall thickness secondary to a chronic increase in afterload. Initially, hypertension causes a concentric thickening of the LV walls with a normal or mildly diminished LV cavity. With progression of hypertensive heart disease, the LV can begin to dilate causing eccentric hypertrophy.[9]

It has long been observed that the presence of LVH is associated with an increase in cardiovascular mortality.[10] The Multi-Ethnic Study of Atherosclerosis (MESA) study used MRI to evaluate LV mass and geometry and found that LVH is associated with a significantly elevated risk for heart failure.[11] LVH commonly precedes the development of heart failure. More than two-thirds of patients with heart failure meet echocardiographic criteria for LVH.

The development of pathologic LVH is associated with an increase in interstitial fibrosis, which can cause increasing stiffness of the LV, diastolic dysfunction, and increased LV filling pressures.[12] LVH can develop early in response to hypertension. There is a higher incidence of LVH in patients who do not have a nocturnal fall in blood pressure (nondippers).[13] Activation of certain hormonal systems, such as the adrenergic nervous system and the renin angiotensin system (RAS), may promote LVH.[14] Angiotensin II is a known factor promoting myocyte hypertrophy. In addition, genetic factors are likely involved in the development of LVH especially in black patients.[15]

HEART FAILURE WITH PRESERVED EJECTION FRACTION

Patients presenting with the signs and symptoms of heart failure but with preserved systolic cardiac function are classified as having HFpEF. Typical patients with HFpEF have an ejection fraction that is 50% or higher, a normal LV end-diastolic volume, diastolic dysfunction, and LVH. Common associated findings include left atrial enlargement, increased pulmonary pressures, right ventricular dilation, and tricuspid regurgitation. Patients with compensated heart failure will continue to show findings of diastolic dysfunction despite treatment.

The progression of diastolic dysfunction can lead to the development of HFpEF. An episode of heart failure may be triggered by an increase in intravascular volume or pressure. Studies using continuous measurements of intracardiac pressures show that a significant increase in diastolic pressure precedes an acute decompensation in

heart failure and that these changes occur greater than 2 weeks before hospitalization for heart failure.[16] Potential triggers that can cause acute decompensation of HFpEF are listed in **Box 3** and include uncontrolled hypertension, salt and fluid overload, onset of atrial fibrillation, myocardial ischemia, progressive kidney disease, anemia, chronic obstructive pulmonary disease, and infections.[17]

The prevalence of HFpEF increases with age. Additional risk factors for HFpEF include hypertension, obesity, and myocardial ischemia. A chronic increase in afterload causing diastolic dysfunction and LVH seems to be the most common mechanism leading to HFpEF. The addition of obesity and insulin resistance to chronic hypertension seems to augment the cardiac changes increasing the incidence of heart failure. Approximately two-thirds of patients with HFpEF also have coronary artery disease, which may further contribute to myocardial fibrosis and adverse outcomes.[18] LVH is about three times more prevalent in black patients compared with whites and is an independent risk factor associated with cardiovascular risk.

HFpEF accounts for more than 50% of heart failure presentations. Unlike HFrEF, however, treatment trials have not found a universal treatment that significantly improves outcomes. This may be caused by the heterogeneic nature of HFpEF. HFpEF presents as a diverse syndrome associated with a variety of comorbidities. A matrix configuration of predisposition phenotypes with clinical presentations has recently been proposed to classify patients with HFpEF to guide research and care (**Table 2**).[19] In this configuration, overweight/obesity and insulin resistance are the most common predisposition phenotype for HFpEF. Arterial hypertension, renal insufficiency, and coronary artery disease are additional predisposing phenotypes. Most patients with HFpEF

Box 3
Triggers of acute decompensated heart failure in patients with HFpEF

Uncontrolled hypertension

Increased sodium intake and volume expansion

New-onset atrial fibrillation

Myocardial ischemia

Progressive kidney disease

Anemia

Chronic obstructive pulmonary disease

Infection

Table 2
HFpEF predisposition phenotypes and clinical presentation phenotypes

HFpEF Predisposition Phenotypes	HFpEF Clinical Presentation Phenotypes
Obesity/insulin resistance	Lung congestion
+ Hypertension	+ Chronotropic incompetence
+ Renal dysfunction	+ Pulmonary hypertension
+ Coronary artery disease	+ Skeletal muscle weakness + Atrial fibrillation

Adapted from Shah SJ, Kitzman DW, Borlaug BA, et al. Phenotype-Specific Treatment of Heart Failure With Preserved Ejection Fraction: A Multiorgan Roadmap. Circulation 2016;134(1):76; with permission.

present with breathlessness and signs of lung congestion. Additional clinical presentations that may require specific treatments include chronotropic incompetence, pulmonary hypertension, skeletal muscle weakness, and atrial fibrillation.

HEART FAILURE WITH REDUCED EJECTION FRACTION

Hypertension and coronary artery disease are the most common causes of heart failure. The incidence of heart failure increases with age. Racial differences in risk factors for heart failure have been identified with black patients having a greater proportion of heart failure risk caused by hypertension. The Framingham study showed that the lifetime risk of developing heart failure is twice as high in individuals having a blood pressure of 160/100 or greater compared with a normal blood pressure.[20] The Prevention of Renal and Vascular End-Stage Disease (PREVEND) study evaluated predictors of the two types of heart failure.[21] Patients with HFpEF tended to be older, female, and have obesity and hypertension. Male sex, smoking, and a prior myocardial infarction were preferentially associated with HFrEF. This suggests that HFpEF and HFrEF may be distinct syndromes.

HFpEF can progress to HFrEF but this is not common unless an instigating factor intervenes, such as an ischemic event. The Cardiovascular Health Study reported the natural history of individuals with LVH and found that over a 7-year period only 7% transitioned to eccentric hypertrophy.[22] The development of eccentric hypertrophy was associated with a previous myocardial infarction or significant above-median LV mass. A small study of predominantly black patients with LVH and a normal ejection fraction found that 18% eventually presented with a reduced ejection fraction with a coronary event as the common precipitating cause.[23] Coronary artery disease, however, is common in patients with HFpEF and is the predominant risk factor for disease progression and increased mortality.[18]

DIAGNOSIS/EVALUATION OF HEART FAILURE

The diagnosis of heart failure is considered in patients presenting with the classic clinical manifestations of heart failure including dyspnea, fatigue, and fluid retention. Patients with preserved and reduced ejection fraction can present with similar symptoms and the physical examination may not be able to determine which syndrome is present. Therefore, all patients presenting with heart failure need to have an evaluation of the LV ejection fraction to diagnose which type of heart failure is present. Echocardiography is useful in determining if HFpEF is the cause of symptoms. Common echocardiographic findings of HFpEF include LVH, left atrial enlargement, elevated pulmonary artery pressures, and Doppler evidence for diastolic dysfunction. B-type natriuretic peptide (BNP) measurements can help confirm the diagnosis of heart failure but need to be cautiously evaluated in patients with renal dysfunction where BNP levels may be elevated and in obesity where BNP levels are lower.

TREATMENT

Heart failure is categorized into four stages (**Table 3**). Patients with risk factors for heart failure are classified as stage A. Treatment of stage A patients target risk factors to prevent progression to structural heart disease and symptomatic heart failure. Patients with structural heart disease but no heart failure signs or symptoms are classified as stage B heart failure. Patients with diastolic

Table 3
Stages of heart failure

Stage A	Risk factors for heart failure without structural heart disease or symptoms
Stage B	Structural heart disease without signs or symptoms of heart failure
Stage C	Symptomatic heart failure
Stage D	Refractory heart failure

dysfunction, therefore, are considered to have stage B heart failure. Treatment should focus on prevention of progression of diastolic dysfunction to symptomatic heart failure (stage C). The term heart failure with mid-range ejection fraction has been used for patients with ejection fractions measured between 40% and 50%. These patients more closely represent patients with HFrEF and have a higher prevalence of coronary artery disease than patients with HFpEF.[24]

Hypertension clinical trials have shown that the treatment of hypertension can prevent the development of heart failure. The Systolic Hypertension in the Elderly (SHEP) trial showed that treatment of isolated systolic hypertension with chlorthalidone achieved a significant reduction in the development of heart failure compared with placebo.[25] Similar findings were noted with a calcium channel blocker in the Systolic Hypertension in Europe (Syst-Eur) trial[26] and with indapamide in the Hypertension in the Very Elderly Trial (HYVET).[27] Chlorthalidone was shown to be superior to doxazosin and amlodipine in preventing heart failure in the Antihypertensive and Lipid-Lowering Treatment to Prevent Heart Attack Trial (ALLHAT).[28,29] A reduction in blood pressure to a target of 120 mm Hg systolic compared with 140 mm Hg systolic in the Systolic Blood Pressure Intervention (SPRINT) trial achieved a significant 38% reduction in heart failure.[30] Finally, targeting risk factors for heart failure in patients without definite hypertension may prevent heart failure as shown in the Heart Outcomes Prevention Evaluation (HOPE) trial where treatment with an angiotensin-converting enzyme inhibitor in a high-risk cohort reduced the risk of developing heart failure.[31]

The mechanisms by which a reduction in blood pressure prevents heart failure are likely multifactorial. There is evidence that optimal blood pressure control may prevent or cause regression of diastolic dysfunction.[32] Reduction in blood pressure with a lifestyle modification program and antihypertensive agents can cause a regression of LVH and a reduction in cardiac mass. Regression of LVH is associated with an improvement in diastolic and systolic LV function, a reduction in premature ventricular contractions and arrhythmias, and a reduced incidence of atrial fibrillation. The Losartan Intervention for Endpoint Reduction in Hypertension (LIFE) study evaluated the effect of antihypertensive treatment on patients with significant LVH.[33] Both systolic and diastolic parameters were improved in patients that exhibited LVH regression.[34,35] Regression of LVH is associated with a reduction in cardiovascular risk.

Regression of LVH is seen within months of effective antihypertensive therapy and may continue over several years. RAS blockers, calcium channel blockers, and diuretics seem to be the most effective agents in producing LVH regression. β-Blockers are less effective and are associated with a less reduction in outcomes compared with a RAS blocker as noted in the LIFE trial. It seems to be more important, however, to achieve optimal blood pressure control to realize significant LV mass reduction than choosing a particular treatment regimen.[36]

Clinical trials of patients with HFpEF have not shown the advantage of one specific therapy over another, unlike trials of patients with HFrEF where treatment with such agents as RAS blockers and β-blockers give a survival advantage. Therefore, treatment that targets symptoms and risk factors is recommended for patients with HFpEF. Most patients with HFpEF present with symptoms of dyspnea and signs of fluid retention. Diuretics improve symptoms in part by lowering LV filling pressures. Chlorthalidone is a long-acting thiazide-like diuretic and is an excellent agent for lowering blood pressure and mobilization of fluid. Loop diuretics may be needed for patients with more significant volume overload. Spironolactone may have a role in treatment for its mild diuretic effects and possible effects on myocardial fibrosis. The Treatment of Preserved Cardiac Function Heart Failure with an Aldosterone Antagonist (TOP-CAT) trial with spironolactone failed to reduce the primary end point in the overall population but showed benefit in patients with an elevated BNP level.[37] Finally, there is some evidence suggesting treatment with a combination of an angiotensin-receptor blocker valsartan with the neprilysin inhibitor sacubitril may decrease BNP levels and certain diastolic parameters in patients with HFpEF.[38] Treatment of HFrEF has been well established by clinical trials and is not reviewed here. Until clinical trials are completed, patients with heart failure with mid-range ejection fraction should be treated the same as patients with HFrEF.

Lifestyle modification is a crucial and important aspect of care of patients with diastolic dysfunction, LVH, and HFpEF. Physical inactivity and obesity are associated with the risk of HFpEF. Improvement in physical activity may lead to a lower risk of developing heart failure. The Cooper Center Longitudinal Study suggested that a 1-MET improvement in physical fitness was associated with a 17% lower incidence of heart failure.[39] Weight loss has also been associated with improvements in diastolic function and a lower risk of heart failure.[40] A program of caloric and sodium restriction with increased physical activity has great potential for improving symptoms and outcomes in patients with HFpEF.

SUMMARY

The incidence of hypertension and hypertensive heart disease is increasing. New definitions of hypertension have the potential of identifying individuals at risk for developing heart failure at an earlier time so that preventive measures can be adopted. The development of diastolic dysfunction and LVH are risk factors for progression to heart failure. HFpEF accounts for more than 50% of heart failure cases and is strongly associated with hypertension, obesity, and insulin resistance. Unfortunately, outcomes of patients with HFpEF are no different from patients with a reduced ejection fraction. There is emerging evidence that a lifestyle modification program with more aggressive blood pressure targets can help prevent the progression to heart failure and improve outcomes.

REFERENCES

1. Levy D, Larson MG, Vasan RS, et al. The progression from hypertension to congestive heart failure. JAMA 1996;275(20):1557–62.

2. Muntner P, Carey RM, Gidding S, et al. Potential US population impact of the 2017 ACC/AHA high blood pressure guideline. Circulation 2018;137(2):109–18.

3. Benjamin EJ, Virani SS, Callaway CW, et al. Heart disease and stroke statistics-2018 update: a report from the American Heart Association. Circulation 2018;137(12):e67–492.

4. Messerli FH, Rimoldi SF, Bangalore S. The transition from hypertension to heart failure: contemporary update. JACC Heart Fail 2017;5(8):543–51.

5. Aurigemma GP, Gaasch WH. Clinical practice. Diastolic heart failure. N Engl J Med 2004;351(11):1097–105.

6. Bonow RO, Udelson JE. Left ventricular diastolic dysfunction as a cause of congestive heart failure. Mechanisms and management. Ann Intern Med 1992;117(6):502–10.

7. Kuznetsova T, Herbots L, Lopez B, et al. Prevalence of left ventricular diastolic dysfunction in a general population. Circ Heart Fail 2009;2(2):105–12.

8. Kane GC, Karon BL, Mahoney DW, et al. Progression of left ventricular diastolic dysfunction and risk of heart failure. JAMA 2011;306(8):856–63.

9. Devereux RB, Roman MJ, Ganau A, et al. Cardiac and arterial hypertrophy and atherosclerosis in hypertension. Hypertension 1994;23(6 Pt 1):802–9.

10. Vakili BA, Okin PM, Devereux RB. Prognostic implications of left ventricular hypertrophy. Am Heart J 2001;141(3):334–41.

11. Bluemke DA, Kronmal RA, Lima JA, et al. The relationship of left ventricular mass and geometry to incident cardiovascular events: the MESA (Multi-Ethnic Study of Atherosclerosis) study. J Am Coll Cardiol 2008;52(25):2148–55.

12. van Hoeven KH, Factor SM. A comparison of the pathological spectrum of hypertensive, diabetic, and hypertensive-diabetic heart disease. Circulation 1990;82(3):848–55.

13. Fagard RH, Celis H, Thijs L, et al. Daytime and nighttime blood pressure as predictors of death and cause-specific cardiovascular events in hypertension. Hypertension 2008;51(1):55–61.

14. Harrap SB, Dominiczak AF, Fraser R, et al. Plasma angiotensin II, predisposition to hypertension, and left ventricular size in healthy young adults. Circulation 1996;93(6):1148–54.

15. Drazner MH, Dries DL, Peshock RM, et al. Left ventricular hypertrophy is more prevalent in blacks than whites in the general population: the Dallas Heart Study. Hypertension 2005;46(1):124–9.

16. Zile MR, Bennett TD, St John SM, et al. Transition from chronic compensated to acute decompensated heart failure: pathophysiological insights obtained from continuous monitoring of intracardiac pressures. Circulation 2008;118(14):1433–41.

17. Yancy CW, Lopatin M, Stevenson LW, et al. Clinical presentation, management, and in-hospital outcomes of patients admitted with acute decompensated heart failure with preserved systolic function: a report from the Acute Decompensated Heart Failure National Registry (ADHERE) Database. J Am Coll Cardiol 2006;47(1):76–84.

18. Hwang SJ, Melenovsky V, Borlaug BA. Implications of coronary artery disease in heart failure with preserved ejection fraction. J Am Coll Cardiol 2014; 63(25 Pt A):2817–27.

19. Shah SJ, Kitzman DW, Borlaug BA, et al. Phenotype-specific treatment of heart failure with preserved ejection fraction: a multiorgan roadmap. Circulation 2016;134(1):73–90.

20. Lloyd-Jones DM, Larson MG, Leip EP, et al. Lifetime risk for developing congestive heart failure: the Framingham Heart Study. Circulation 2002;106(24):3068–72.

21. Brouwers FP, de Boer RA, van der Harst P, et al. Incidence and epidemiology of new onset heart failure with preserved vs. reduced ejection fraction in a community-based cohort: 11-year follow-up of PREVEND. Eur Heart J 2013;34(19):1424–31.

22. Desai RV, Ahmed MI, Mujib M, et al. Natural history of concentric left ventricular geometry in community-dwelling older adults without heart failure during seven years of follow-up. Am J Cardiol 2011;107(2):321–4.

23. Rame JE, Ramilo M, Spencer N, et al. Development of a depressed left ventricular ejection fraction in patients with left ventricular hypertrophy and a normal ejection fraction. Am J Cardiol 2004;93(2):234–7.

24. Nauta JF, Hummel YM, van Melle JP, et al. What have we learned about heart failure with mid-range ejection fraction one year after its introduction? Eur J Heart Fail 2017;19(12):1569–73.

25. Prevention of stroke by antihypertensive drug treatment in older persons with isolated systolic hypertension. Final results of the Systolic Hypertension in the Elderly Program (SHEP). SHEP Cooperative Research Group. JAMA 1991;265(24):3255–64.

26. Staessen JA, Fagard R, Thijs L, et al. Randomised double-blind comparison of placebo and active treatment for older patients with isolated systolic hypertension. The Systolic Hypertension in Europe (Syst-Eur) Trial Investigators. Lancet 1997; 350(9080):757–64.

27. Beckett NS, Peters R, Fletcher AE, et al. Treatment of hypertension in patients 80 years of age or older. N Engl J Med 2008;358(18):1887–98.

28. Major cardiovascular events in hypertensive patients randomized to doxazosin vs chlorthalidone: the antihypertensive and lipid-lowering treatment to prevent heart attack trial (ALLHAT). ALLHAT Collaborative Research Group. JAMA 2000;283(15): 1967–75.

29. Major outcomes in high-risk hypertensive patients randomized to angiotensin-converting enzyme inhibitor or calcium channel blocker vs diuretic: the Antihypertensive and Lipid-Lowering Treatment to Prevent Heart Attack Trial (ALLHAT). JAMA 2002; 288(23):2981–97.

30. Wright JT Jr, Williamson JD, Whelton PK, et al. A randomized trial of intensive versus standard blood-pressure control. N Engl J Med 2015; 373(22):2103–16.

31. Effects of ramipril on cardiovascular and microvascular outcomes in people with diabetes mellitus: results of the HOPE study and MICRO-HOPE substudy. Heart Outcomes Prevention Evaluation Study Investigators. Lancet 2000;355(9200):253–9.

32. Bergstrom A, Andersson B, Edner M, et al. Effect of carvedilol on diastolic function in patients with diastolic heart failure and preserved systolic function. Results of the Swedish Doppler-echocardiographic study (SWEDIC). Eur J Heart Fail 2004;6(4):453–61.

33. Dahlof B, Devereux RB, Kjeldsen SE, et al. Cardiovascular morbidity and mortality in the Losartan Intervention For Endpoint reduction in hypertension study (LIFE): a randomised trial against atenolol. Lancet 2002;359(9311):995–1003.

34. Wachtell K, Palmieri V, Olsen MH, et al. Change in systolic left ventricular performance after 3 years of antihypertensive treatment: the Losartan Intervention for Endpoint (LIFE) Study. Circulation 2002; 106(2):227–32.

35. Wachtell K, Bella JN, Rokkedal J, et al. Change in diastolic left ventricular filling after one year of antihypertensive treatment: the Losartan Intervention For Endpoint Reduction in Hypertension (LIFE) Study. Circulation 2002;105(9):1071–6.

36. Miller AB, Reichek N, St John SM, et al. Importance of blood pressure control in left ventricular mass regression. J Am Soc Hypertens 2010;4(6):302–10.

37. Pitt B, Pfeffer MA, Assmann SF, et al. Spironolactone for heart failure with preserved ejection fraction. N Engl J Med 2014;370(15):1383–92.

38. Solomon SD, Zile M, Pieske B, et al. The angiotensin receptor neprilysin inhibitor LCZ696 in heart failure with preserved ejection fraction: a phase 2 double-blind randomised controlled trial. Lancet 2012; 380(9851):1387–95.

39. Pandey A, Patel M, Gao A, et al. Changes in mid-life fitness predicts heart failure risk at a later age independent of interval development of cardiac and noncardiac risk factors: the Cooper Center Longitudinal Study. Am Heart J 2015;169(2):290–7.

40. Pandey A, Patel KV, Vaduganathan M, et al. Physical activity, fitness, and obesity in heart failure with preserved ejection fraction. JACC Heart Fail 2018; 6(12):975–82.

Pathophysiology and Natural History

Heart Failure and Changes in Kidney Function
Focus on Understanding, Not Reacting

Tamar S. Polonsky, MD, MSCI[a], George L. Bakris, MD, MA[b],*

KEYWORDS

- Kidney • Heart failure • Creatinine • Hypertension

KEY POINTS

- Reductions in blood pressure, especially if levels are above 140/90 will result in a reduction in kidney function as manifested by a rise in serum creatinine.
- Increases of up to 30% in serum creatinine in the absence of hyperkalemia should be tolerated with renin angiotensin system blockers as long as hyperkalemia is not present.
- People with HFrEF will be more vulnerable to increases in serum creatinine in response to renin angiotensin system blockers.

INTRODUCTION

The kidney is a regulatory organ and will try to maintain homeostasis under all conditions including extracellular volume, acid base, status and blood pressure.[1,2] There are extensive signaling pathways within the kidney that allow it to preserve kidney blood flow across a wide range of blood pressures, and in response to changes in sodium and chloride levels.[3] However, these tightly regulated processes are disrupted in the setting of heart failure, during which there is a reduction in cardiac output, elevation in central venous pressure, and neurohormonal activation. As a result, markers of kidney function (such as the serum creatinine and glomerular filtration rate) are vulnerable to hemodynamic changes or use of heart failure therapies, particularly diuretics, renin-angiotensin aldosterone system (RAAS) inhibitors, and neprilysin inhibitors.

It is well-described that adults with both heart failure and chronic kidney disease (CKD) have worse outcomes than adults with heart failure and normal kidney function.[4] In addition, some studies have suggested that worsening kidney function over time also portended a less favorable prognosis among adults with heart failure.[5,6] However, data from more recent epidemiologic studies and clinical trials demonstrate that it is crucial to consider the clinical context of any changes in kidney function.[7,8] For example, a modest increase of up to 30% in serum creatinine associated after initiation of an RAAS inhibitor is associated with a reduction in cardiovascular events.[9] This article describes the kidney's role in cardiovascular homeostasis. In particular, how the kidney contributes to progression of heart failure, and the clinical significance of changes in kidney function among patients with heart failure are highlighted.

Disclosure Statement: None (T.S. Polonsky). Member scientific advisory board or consultant for Merck, Janssen, Novo Nordisk, Astra Zeneca, Boehringer Ingelheim, Bayer, Relypsa, Reata. Steering Committee Member-Janssen, Bayer (principal investigator-kidney outcome trial) (G.L. Bakris).
[a] Department of Medicine, Section of Cardiology, University of Chicago Medicine, 5841 South Maryland Avenue, Chicago, IL 60637, USA; [b] Department of Medicine, Am. Heart Assoc. Comprehensive Hypertension Center, University of Chicago Medicine, 5841 South Maryland Avenue, MC1027, Chicago, IL 60637, USA
* Corresponding author.
E-mail address: gbakris@uchicago.edu

NORMAL KIDNEY PHYSIOLOGY

With autoregulation, the kidney is able to maintain a steady filtration fraction across a wide range of mean arterial pressures, ranging from 70 to 150 mm Hg.[1] In the macula densa, a collection of specialized epithelial cells in the distal convoluted tubule adjacent to the afferent arteriole of the nephron, the kidney is able to detect the sodium concentration of tubular fluid. The kidney monitors sodium and chloride levels in a process called tubuloglomerular feedback. When sodium or chloride levels increase, the kidney releases adenosine, to trigger vasoconstriction of the afferent arteriole and reduce glomerular filtration rate (GFR, **Fig. 1**).

There are also neurohumoral reflexes between the heart and kidney that help control volume status. For example, an increase in atrial pressure inhibits the release of arginine vasopressin, thus promoting a water diuresis.[3] A high atrial pressure also leads to an increase in the secretion of atrial natriuretic peptide, which leads to sodium loss and vasodilation.

PATHOPHYSIOLOGY OF KIDNEY AND HEART FAILURE

There are several pathways in the setting of heart failure that contribute to a decline in the GFR, reflected as an increase in the serum creatinine. First, heart failure and CKD share common risk factors – including obesity, diabetes, hypertension and tobacco use – which can independently lead to loss of glomeruli, making the kidney more vulnerable to the deleterious effects of heart failure. Once heart failure develops, central venous congestion itself is associated with a decrease in GFR by increases in venous pressure transmitted to the kidney and increased interstitial pressure. These changes can be further exacerbated if rapid diuresis leads to a drop in kidney blood flow.[10] An increase in norepinephrine levels, which is a hallmark of heart failure, causes vasoconstriction of the kidney arterioles, also leading to a decrease in kidney blood flow and GFR.[2] The vasoconstriction alters the driving pressures in the arterioles, causing a decrease in hydrostatic pressure and an increase in oncotic pressure, which further enhances sodium reabsorption.[11]

As sodium reabsorption increases, the chloride delivery to macula densa decreases. This results in prostaglandin release by the macula densa cells to trigger granular juxtaglomerular cells lining the afferent arterioles to release renin. Thus, levels of angiotensin II increase further and stimulate the release of catecholamines, even further stimulating sodium reabsorption. Additionally, in extreme cases, arginine vasopressin released by the posterior pituitary gland in the brain also increases (see **Fig. 1**). Additionally, chronically elevated atrial pressures blunt the normal reflexes to decrease vasopressin secretion.[3] Although treatment with diuretics is often a necessary component of heart failure therapy, it can further decrease chloride delivery to the macula densa, leading to the vicious cycle of neurohormonal activation.

WORSENING KIDNEY FUNCTION IN THE OUTPATIENT SETTING

Among people with longstanding poorly controlled hypertension, lowering of blood pressure can lead to a rise in the creatinine. This is independent of heart failure and best understood by a loss of autoregulation over long periods of time by high pressures, as well as underlying renal injury to the vasculature and parenchyma. Thus, reducing the pressure to appropriate levels will result in an inability of the kidney to fully adjust to change acutely. Based on the amount of underlying damage, in many cases there is a trend to return toward previous levels over a few months. Underlying heart failure further complicates the problem, and until cardiac function improves, kidney function may remain relatively depressed.

Many studies have shown that, after initiation of antihypertensive medication, increases in serum creatinine up to 30% are not associated with a long-term decline in kidney function, and acutely may result in further slowing of CKD progression.[9,12–15] A rise in serum creatinine is particularly common with the use of RAAS inhibitors given that they selectively dilate the efferent arteriole in the glomerulus, leading to a reduction in glomerular filtration.[15–17] Recently, in the Systolic Blood Pressure Intervention Trial (SPRINT), adults with elevated cardiovascular risk who were randomized to a blood pressure goal of 120 mm Hg were more likely to experience an increase in creatinine than those randomized to a blood pressure goal of 140 mm Hg (3.8% vs 2.3%, hazard ratio [HR] 1.64, 95% confidence interval [CI] 1.30–2.10, $P<.001$).[18] Complete or partial resolution of the rise was seen in 90.4% of the events in the intensive arm. Moreover, SPRINT participants with CKD showed no differences in biomarkers of kidney damage over follow-up between those randomized to intensive versus standard blood pressure lowering.[19] Additionally, among SPRINT participants randomized to the intensive blood pressure treatment arm who developed CKD during follow-up, they had greater

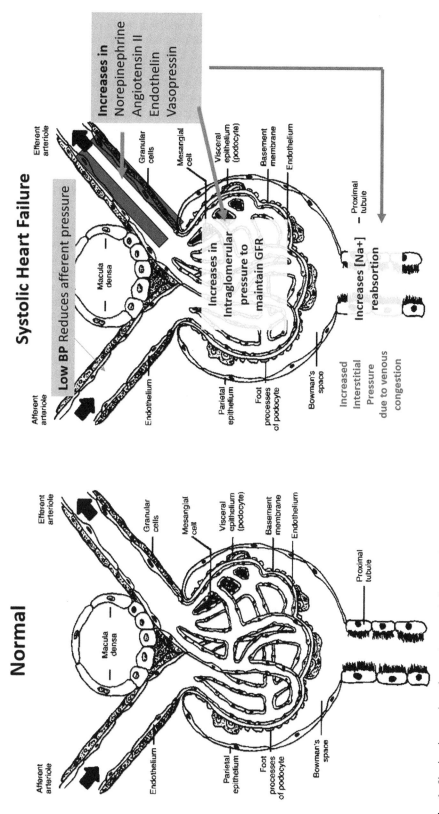

Fig. 1. Single glomerulus of a nephron and changes that ensue induced by hormonal changes and hemodynamics in heart failure.

decreases in biomarkers of kidney damage than controls, including albumin-creatinine ratio (ACR), interleukin-18, antichitinase-3-like protein 1 (YKL-40), and uromodulin.[20]

In a post hoc analysis of the Action to Control Cardiovascular Risk in Diabetes Blood Pressure (ACCORD-BP) trial, Collard and colleagues[21] evaluated those who experienced a greater than 30% rise in creatinine. In ACCORD BP, 4733 adults with diabetes were randomized to a goal systolic blood pressure (SBP) less than 140 mm Hg versus less than 120 mm Hg. In the post hoc analysis, the authors examined the association of a greater than 30% rise in creatinine with a composite outcome of major cardiovascular events, all-cause mortality, and kidney failure. Although the overall incidence of the composite outcome was similar between the 2 treatment groups, those randomized to the intensive blood pressure arm were more likely to die of cardiovascular death and all-cause mortality than those in the standard treatment group. In contrast, those randomized to intensive therapy were less likely to experience kidney failure than those randomized to standard therapy.

There are other clinical trials in advanced kidney disease that have demonstrated similar benefits of limited increases in serum creatinine in the presence of blood pressure control.[12–14] Taken together, these results suggest that limited increases in serum creatinine reflect changes in kidney blood flow and not injury.[9]

Studies of acute declines in kidney function among outpatients with heart failure also suggest a benign association if the reduction in kidney function develops in the setting of titration of medical therapy. For example, among participants in the Studies Of Left Ventricular Dysfunction (SOLVD) trial, a randomized controlled trial (RCT) of enalapril versus placebo in adults with heart failure with reduced ejection fraction, decline in kidney function was defined as a greater than 20% increase in serum creatinine 14 days after initiation of study medication.[22] In the overall population, early decline in kidney function was associated with increased mortality (adjusted HR 1.2, 95% CI 1.0–1.4, $P = .037$). When analysis was restricted to the placebo group, this association strengthened (adjusted HR = 1.4, 95% CI 1.1–1.8, $P = .004$). However, in the enalapril group, early declines in kidney function had no adverse prognostic significance (adjusted HR 1.0, 95% CI 0.8–1.3, $P = 1.0$, p interaction = 0.09). In patients who continued the study drug despite early decline in kidney function, a survival advantage remained with enalapril therapy (adjusted HR 0.66, 95% CI 0.5–0.9, $P = .018$). In a meta-analysis of participants in 5 RCTs of RAAS inhibitors in patients with HFrEF, Clark and colleagues[23] also found that early decline in kidney function should not necessarily deter providers from using RAAS inhibition. Compared with placebo, RAAS inhibitors reduced all-cause mortality overall (n = 20,573, relative risk ratio [RR] 0.91, 95% CI 0.86–0.95, $P = .0003$), including the group with no change in kidney function (n = 18,209, RR 0.91, 95% CI 0.83–0.99, $P = .04$), and in those with reduced kidney function group (n = 2364, RR 0.72, 95% CI 0.62–0.84, $P<.0001$).

WORSENING KIDNEY FUNCTION IN HEART FAILURE

Given the numerous pathophysiologic changes in the kidney that occur among patients with heart failure, these patients are at a particularly high risk of experiencing an elevation in serum creatinine with medication changes. Worsening kidney function (WKF) in the setting of heart failure is often defined as an increase in creatinine of at least 0.3 mg/dL or a 30% increase if serum creatinine is not 1 mg/dL. Risk factors for WKF among adults with heart failure include diabetes, pulmonary edema, and a baseline creatinine greater than 1.5 mg/dL.[24] Among patients admitted to the hospital for acute decompensated heart failure, WKF typically occurs in the first 3 to 4 days after admission, but can develop several days after discharge.[25]

Studies of adults with acute decompensated heart failure suggest that the prognosis associated with WKF largely depends on the clinical context. In a study combining individual participant data from 1233 adults in 6 cohorts, Salah compared how changes in kidney function related to the risk of all-cause mortality with changes in N-terminal pro-B-type natriuretic peptide (NT-proBNP).[26] They found that a reduction of NT-proBNP greater than 30% during hospitalization determined prognosis (all-cause mortality HR 1.81, 95% CI 1.32–2.50) regardless of changes in kidney function. Ibrahim and colleagues[7] confirmed the importance of decongestion in a randomized trial of standard care versus NT-pro-BNP guided diuresis for 151 adults admitted to the hospital with acute decompensated heart failure. Subjects with NT-proBNP less than 1000 pg/mL and WRF received higher doses of guideline-directed medical therapies, lower doses of loop diuretics, and had significantly lower CV event rates ($P<.001$).

Another study evaluating acute changes in serum creatinine with diuretic administration is the Diuretic Optimization Strategies Evaluation (DOSE) trial. This prospective multicenter trial investigated strategies of loop diuretic administration. They found that increases in serum creatinine were associated with a lower risk of death, emergency room visits within 60 days, or rehospitalization (HR 0.81 per 0.3 mg/dL increase, 95% CI 0.67–0.98, P = .026).[27] Moreover, compared to those with stable kidney function, there was a strong association between improved kidney function (n = 28) and the composite endpoint (HR 2.52, 95% CI 1.57–4.03, P<.001). Taken together, available data suggest that for acute and chronic management of HFrEF, it is important to prioritize decongestion and the use of evidence-based therapy, such as RAAS inhibitors even with modest degrees of WKF.

There are few studies comparing the risk of WKF in patients with HFpEF versus HFrEF. In a meta-analysis of 8 RCTs of RAAS inhibitors versus placebo (6 HFrEF, 1 HFpEF, 1 both), adults with HFrEF who were randomized to RAAS inhibitors and had WKF experienced higher rates of heart failure hospitalization, compared with patients who experienced no WKF (RR 1.19 [1.08–1.31], P<.001).[28] However, the risk associated with WKF in patients allocated to placebo was larger (RR 1.48 [1.35–1.62], P<.001) and significantly different from patients randomized to RAAS inhibitors with WKF (P for interaction = .005). Adults with HFpEF who were taking RAAS inhibitors also experienced a higher risk of hospitalization if they developed WKF compared to those without WKF (RR 1.78, 95% CI 1.43–2.21). However, unlike adults with HFrEF, WKF for those randomized to placebo did not result in increased hospitalization. Although is it possible that the pathophysiology of WKF differs between HFrEF and HFpEF, it is likely that the use of RAAS inhibitors simply unmasked greater disease severity.

CHANGES IN KIDNEY FUNCTION WITH NEPRILYSIN INHIBITORS

The clinical benefit of neprilysin inhibition among adults with HFrEF was established with the Prospective Comparison of ARNI with ACE inhibition to Determine Impact on Global Mortality and Morbidity in Heart Failure (PARADIGM-HF) trial.[29] In the study, 8399 patients with heart failure with reduced ejection fraction were randomized to treatment with sacubitril/valsartan or enalapril. The decrease in eGFR during follow-up was less with sacubitril/valsartan compared with enalapril, although the difference between the 2 groups was small (−1.61 mL/min/1.73 m2/y; [95% CI −1.77 to −1.44 mL/min/1.73 m2/y] vs −2.04 mL/min/1.73 m2/year [95% CI −2.21

to −1.88 mL/min/1.73 m2/year], P<.001).[30] There was also a greater increase in urinary albumin: creatinine excretion rate (UACR) with sacubitril/valsartan compared with enalapril (1.20 mg/mmol [95% CI 1.04–1.36 mg/mmol] vs 0.90 mg/mmol [95% CI 0.77–1.03 mg/mmol]; P<.001). The effect of sacubitril/valsartan on cardiovascular death or heart failure hospitalization was not modified by eGFR, UACR (p interaction = .70 and .34, respectively), or by change in UACR (p interaction = .38). The authors hypothesized that the increase in UACR was likely related to a direct effect from the accumulation of neprilysin inhibitors in the glomerulus, leading potentially to an increase in glomerular endothelial permeability and hydraulic conductivity, rather than an alteration in kidney arteriolar tone.

In contrast, use of sacubitril/valsartan was not associated with any improvement in kidney function among adults with CKD but without heart failure. In the United Kingdom Heart and Kidney Protection-III trial, 414 adults with a mean GFR of 34 mL/min/1.73 m2 were randomized to sacubitril/valsartan versus irbesartan.[31] After 12 months, there was no difference between groups in the estimated GFR or the UACR. However, those randomized to sacubitril/valsartan experienced greater improvement in their blood pressure control than those taking irbesartan, with an additional decrease in systolic and diastolic blood pressure by 5.4 (95% CI, 3.4–7.4) and 2.1 (95% CI, 1.0–3.3) mm Hg, respectively. The results suggest that there are different determinants of kidney disease progression among adults with CKD related to heart failure versus other etiologies.

SUMMARY

Understanding changes in kidney function in the context of heart failure is challenging and requires an understanding and knowledge of renal physiology, pharmacology of agents used, patients' hypertension history and level of control, and underlying diseases that can affect the kidney, the heart, or more commonly both such as diabetes. The kidney is a regulatory organ and as such can only adapt to changes within its functioning ability. The data presented here from trials focus on people with reasonable kidney function, as those with an estimated GFR of less than 30 were excluded from all trials. Moreover, this group is not well studied, and conclusions/assertions made in this article should not be extrapolated to those with stage 4 or 5 CKD or dialysis patients.

The heart and the kidney communicate through a neurohumoral network, and when cardiac function is altered, the kidney tries to adapt. When the kidney function is acutely depressed, as in a 50% or more reduction, the heart tries to compensate. In advanced heart or kidney disease, however, such compensations are not possible. Small changes in serum creatinine up to 30% above baseline, without hyperkalemia or acidosis ensuing, are safe and associated with lower mortality and better long-term kidney outcomes. It is not a sign of injury. Thus, patients should not be deprived of lifesaving medications in heart failure because of a rise in serum creatinine.

REFERENCES

1. Verbrugge FH, Dupont M, Steels P, et al. The kidney in congestive heart failure: 'are natriuresis, sodium, and diuretics really the good, the bad and the ugly? Eur J Heart Fail 2014;16(2):133–42.

2. Schefold JC, Filippatos G, Hasenfuss G, et al. Heart failure and kidney dysfunction: epidemiology, mechanisms and management. Nat Rev Nephrol 2016; 12(10):610–23.

3. Schrier RW. Role of diminished renal function in cardiovascular mortality: marker or pathogenetic factor? J Am Coll Cardiol 2006;47(1):1–8.

4. Hillege HL, Nitsch D, Pfeffer MA, et al. Renal function as a predictor of outcome in a broad spectrum of patients with heart failure. Circulation 2006; 113(5):671–8.

5. Ueda T, Kawakami R, Sugawara Y, et al. Worsening of renal function during 1 year after hospital discharge is a strong and independent predictor of all-cause mortality in acute decompensated heart failure. J Am Heart Assoc 2014;3(6):e001174.

6. Damman K, Valente MA, Voors AA, et al. Renal impairment, worsening renal function, and outcome in patients with heart failure: an updated meta-analysis. Eur Heart J 2014;35(7):455–69.

7. Ibrahim NE, Gaggin HK, Rabideau DJ, et al. Worsening renal function during management for chronic heart failure with reduced ejection fraction: results from the Pro-BNP Outpatient Tailored Chronic Heart Failure Therapy (PROTECT) Study. J Card Fail 2017; 23(2):121–30.

8. Testani JM, Brisco-Bacik MA. Worsening renal function and mortality in heart failure: causality or confounding? Circ Heart Fail 2017;10(2) [pii:e003835].

9. Bakris GL, Agarwal R. Creatinine bump following antihypertensive therapy. Hypertension 2018;72(6): 1274–6.

10. Metra M, Davison B, Bettari L, et al. Is worsening renal function an ominous prognostic sign in patients with acute heart failure? The role of congestion and its interaction with renal function. Circ Heart Fail 2012;5(1):54–62.

11. Schrier RW, De Wardener HE. Tubular reabsorption of sodium ion: influence of factors other than aldosterone and glomerular filtration rate. 1. N Engl J Med 1971;285(22):1231–43.

12. Agodoa LY, Appel L, Bakris GL, et al. Effect of ramipril vs amlodipine on renal outcomes in hypertensive nephrosclerosis: a randomized controlled trial. JAMA 2001;285(21):2719–28.

13. Wright JT Jr, Bakris G, Greene T, et al. Effect of blood pressure lowering and antihypertensive drug class on progression of hypertensive kidney disease: results from the AASK trial. JAMA 2002; 288(19):2421–31.

14. Bakris GL, Sarafidis PA, Weir MR, et al. Renal outcomes with different fixed-dose combination therapies in patients with hypertension at high risk for cardiovascular events (ACCOMPLISH): a prespecified secondary analysis of a randomised controlled trial. Lancet 2010;375(9721):1173–81.

15. Bakris GL, Weir MR. Angiotensin-converting enzyme inhibitor-associated elevations in serum creatinine: is this a cause for concern? Arch Intern Med 2000; 160(5):685–93.

16. Holtkamp FA, de Zeeuw D, Thomas MC, et al. An acute fall in estimated glomerular filtration rate during treatment with losartan predicts a slower decrease in long-term renal function. Kidney Int 2011;80(3):282–7.

17. Hirsch S, Hirsch J, Bhatt U, et al. Tolerating increases in the serum creatinine following aggressive treatment of chronic kidney disease, hypertension and proteinuria: pre-renal success. Am J Nephrol 2012;36(5):430–7.

18. Sprint Research Group, Wright JT Jr, Williamson JD, Whelton PK, et al. A randomized trial of intensive versus standard blood-pressure control. N Engl J Med 2015;373(22):2103–16.

19. Malhotra R, Craven T, Ambrosius WT, et al. Effects of intensive blood pressure lowering on kidney tubule injury in CKD: a longitudinal subgroup analysis in SPRINT. Am J Kidney Dis 2019;73(1):21–30.

20. Zhang WR, Craven TE, Malhotra R, et al. Kidney damage biomarkers and incident chronic kidney disease during blood pressure reduction: a case-control study. Ann Intern Med 2018;169(9):610–8.

21. Collard D, Brouwer TF, Peters RJG, et al. Creatinine rise during blood pressure therapy and the risk of adverse clinical outcomes in patients with type 2 diabetes mellitus. Hypertension 2018;72(6):1337–44.

22. Testani JM, Kimmel SE, Dries DL, et al. Prognostic importance of early worsening renal function after initiation of angiotensin-converting enzyme inhibitor therapy in patients with cardiac dysfunction. Circ Heart Fail 2011;4(6):685–91.

23. Clark H, Krum H, Hopper I. Worsening renal function during renin-angiotensin-aldosterone system inhibitor initiation and long-term outcomes in patients with left ventricular systolic dysfunction. Eur J Heart Fail 2014;16(1):41–8.

24. Klein L, Massie BM, Leimberger JD, et al. Admission or changes in renal function during hospitalization for worsening heart failure predict postdischarge survival: results from the Outcomes of a Prospective Trial of Intravenous Milrinone for Exacerbations of Chronic Heart Failure (OPTIME-CHF). Circ Heart Fail 2008;1(1):25–33.

25. Blair JE, Pang PS, Schrier RW, et al. Changes in renal function during hospitalization and soon after discharge in patients admitted for worsening heart failure in the placebo group of the EVEREST trial. Eur Heart J 2011;32(20):2563–72.

26. Salah K, Kok WE, Eurlings LW, et al. Competing risk of cardiac status and renal function during hospitalization for acute decompensated heart failure. JACC Heart Fail 2015;3(10):751–61.

27. Brisco MA, Zile MR, Hanberg JS, et al. Relevance of changes in serum creatinine during a heart failure trial of decongestive strategies: insights from the DOSE trial. J Card Fail 2016;22(10):753–60.

28. Beldhuis IE, Streng KW, Ter Maaten JM, et al. Renin-angiotensin system inhibition, worsening renal function, and outcome in heart failure patients with reduced and preserved ejection fraction: a meta-analysis of published study data. Circ Heart Fail 2017;10(2) [pii:e003588].

29. McMurray JJ, Packer M, Desai AS, et al. Angiotensin-neprilysin inhibition versus enalapril in heart failure. N Engl J Med 2014;371(11):993–1004.

30. Damman K, Gori M, Claggett B, et al. Renal effects and associated outcomes during angiotensin-neprilysin inhibition in heart failure. JACC Heart Fail 2018;6(6):489–98.

31. Haynes R, Judge PK, Staplin N, et al. Effects of sacubitril/valsartan versus irbesartan in patients with chronic kidney disease. Circulation 2018;138(15):1505–14.

Implication of Acute Kidney Injury in Heart Failure

Claudio Ronco, MD, PhD[a], Antonio Bellasi, MD, PhD[b],
Luca Di Lullo, MD, PhD[c],*

KEYWORDS

- Acute decompensated heart failure (ADHF) • Acute kidney injury (AKI) • Diuretics • Ultrafiltration
- Type 1 cardiorenal syndrome (CRS)

KEY POINTS

- The "cardiorenal axis" encompasses various interactions and feedback mechanisms that regulate the function of the heart and kidneys in health as well as pathologic conditions.
- In patients with chronic heart failure, renal hemodynamics is maintained through an increase in both glomerular afferent arteriole resistance and sodium reabsorption (at the site of the loop of Henle).
- Most heart-kidney cross-talk occurs in the setting of predisposing factors for chronic kidney disease and heart failure, such as obesity and metabolic syndrome, cachexia, diabetes mellitus and hypertension, proteinuria, uremia, and anemia.
- Response to acute and chronic pathologic noxae activate immune cells, resident fibroblasts, and myofibroblasts and induce procollagen and collagen deposition in the extracellular matrix leading to cardiac and renal fibrosis, further perpetuating the vicious cycle that binds heart and kidney in what is now recognized as cardiorenal syndrome.

INTRODUCTION

The "cardiorenal axis" encompasses various interactions and feedback mechanisms that regulate the function of heart and kidneys in health as well as pathologic conditions. In contrast to what was previously thought, kidney dysfunction in patients with heart failure (HF) may not be solely caused by low renal plasmatic flow in the context of low cardiac output.[1] Newer lines of evidence suggest that other pathophysiologic pathways are involved in kidney injury following HF.

In patients with chronic HF, renal hemodynamics is maintained through an increase in glomerular afferent arteriole resistance and sodium reabsorption (at the site of the loop of Henle).[1] These mechanisms are mediated by several neuro-hormonal factors, such as activation of the sympathetic nervous system (SNS) or the renin-angiotensin-aldosterone system (RAAS), which in turn lead to arginine, vasopressin, and endothelin release, resulting in systemic vasoconstriction, preservation of glomerular hydrostatic pressure and glomerular filtration rate (GFR), and salt and water retention.[1] Hence, both SNS and RAAS activation should be regarded as a compensatory response to preserve cardiac output, arterial blood pressure, and GFR.[1]

Most heart-kidney cross-talk occurs in the setting of predisposing factors for chronic kidney disease (CKD) and chronic HF, such as obesity and metabolic syndrome, cachexia, diabetes

Disclosure: The authors have nothing to disclose.
[a] International Renal Research Institute, S. Bortolo Hospital, Vicenza, Italy; [b] Department of Research, Innovation and Brand Reputation, ASST Papa Giovanni XXIII, Bergamo, Italy; [c] Department of Nephrology and Dialysis, L. Parodi – Delfino Hospital, Piazza Aldo Moro, 1, Colleferro, Roma 00034, Italy
* Corresponding author.
E-mail address: dilulloluca69@gmail.com

Heart Failure Clin 15 (2019) 463–476
https://doi.org/10.1016/j.hfc.2019.05.002
1551-7136/19/© 2019 Elsevier Inc. All rights reserved.

mellitus and hypertension, proteinuria, uremia, and anemia. Obesity and excess adiposity are linked to various chronic diseases, including type 2 diabetes mellitus, hypertension, obstructive sleep apnea, atrial fibrillation, HF, hyperuricemia, and CKD. It has been shown that adipocytes can undergo a tenfold increase in number and in size in obese individuals.[2] With such a dramatic increase in fat mass, cytokines and adipokines are produced in large quantities, and some of these such as interleukin 6 (IL-6) and tumor necrosis factor alpha (TNF-α) may mediate both renal and cardiac injury as well as promote high-sensitivity C-reactive protein (hs-CRP) and systemic inflammation.[3] Excess adiposity occurring in epicardial coronaries may be directly involved in cardiac function and structure abnormalities and play a role in the pathologic remodeling that occurs in patients with HF.[4] In contrast, some degree of heart and kidney dysfunction is observed in cachexia and sarcopenia. These conditions are likely related to inflammation.[5] However, the neurohormonal activation that characterizes CRS contributes to cachexia, ultimately affecting both cardiac and renal function.[3] Hypertension and type 2 diabetes mellitus are 2 of the most important risk factors for both HF and CKD in western countries. Lack of blood pressure control is directly related to accelerated loss of nephrons and reductions in the GFR as well as cardiac dysfunction.[4] Diabetes, through many mechanisms, contributes to glomerular dysfunction as well as arterial damage leading to CKD and cardiac damage.[4] Proteinuria as a result of endothelial, mesangial, and podocyte injury in the kidney is another potent predisposing factor for type 1 CRS. The large amount of albumin filtered in the urine increases the reabsorption workload of the proximal tubular cells of the functioning nephrons, leading to apoptosis, further nephron loss, and progression of kidney disease.[4] As well as its pathogenetic role in CKD, albuminuria is also predictive of the development of HF and is a risk marker for cardiovascular disease in both the general population and individuals with CKD.[4] Loss of skeletal and cardiac myocytes, impaired contraction, and cardiac dysfunction as well as adverse cardiac remodeling after myocardial infarction have been described in uremia caused by an abnormal intracellular calcium shift and excessive fibrosis. In this regard, restoration of renal function after kidney transplantation has been associated with improvement in left ventricular systolic function, reduction in left ventricular mass, and reduction in left ventricular size.[6] Other common risk factors link CKD and HF. For example, increased serum levels of uric acid are associated with uremia as well as accelerated

atherosclerosis and cardiovascular death.[5] Anemia is prevalent and portends morbidity and poor survival in patients with HF and CKD.[7] In CRS, anemia is probably related to hemodilution, impaired iron transport, inflammation/cytokine-induced erythropoietin deficiency and tissue resistance, malnutrition, cachexia, and vitamin deficiency. The presence of anemia is a consequence of CRS, and it can contribute to worsening of renal and cardiac function because the same neurohormonal and inflammatory pathways affecting endogenous erythropoietin production and resistance as well as iron utilization defect may ultimately impair heart and kidney function.[7]

Response to acute and chronic pathologic noxae activate immune cells, resident fibroblasts, and myofibroblasts and induce procollagen and collagen deposition in the extracellular matrix, leading to cardiac and renal fibrosis, further perpetuating the vicious cycle that binds heart and kidney in what is now recognized as cardiorenal syndrome (CRS).[8] In the following, all pathophysiologic "actors" of CRS are described together with data on the epidemiology and treatment of acute kidney injury (AKI) in the context of HF (type 1 CRS).

EPIDEMIOLOGY AND CLINICAL RELEVANCE OF CARDIORENAL SYNDROME

Accordingly to the RIFLE (risk, injury, failure, loss of kidney function, end-stage renal disease) criteria, between 20% and 40% of patients with acute decompensated heart failure (ADHF) eventually develop some degree of renal failure. One of the largest existing databases, the ADHERE (Acute Decompensated Heart Failure Registry) registry, has shown that one third of patients with HF present some degree of CKD and up to 20% of the enrolled subjects have serum creatinine (SCr) levels >2 mg/dL.[9]

Renal dysfunction in patients with ADHF usually develops in the context of other comorbid condition, such as hypertension, diabetes, dyslipidemia, and metabolic syndrome or obesity. However, regardless of the cause and case mix, renal function impairment in these fragile patients portends high risk of hospitalization as well as cardiovascular and all-cause mortality. The ADHERE also shows that patients with more advanced CKD present worse clinical outcomes as indicated by higher rates of admission to the intensive care unit (ICU), mechanical ventilation support, and higher mortality.[9]

According to the ESCAPE (Evaluation Study of Congestive Heart Failure and Pulmonary Artery Catheterization Effectiveness) trial, reduction in

GFR (<60 mL/min) was found in up to 30% patients with ADHF. Furthermore, baseline CKD and serum creatinine (SCr) level at discharge were both associated with higher rates of death and hospitalization.[10]

These findings were also reported in other series. In a retrospective study of more than 1000 hospitalized patients with HF, worsening renal function (WRF) occurred in 11% of patients during hospitalization and 16% of patients within the first 6 months after hospital discharge. Notably, WRF was strongly and significantly associated with the risk of rehospitalization and all-cause mortality.[11] In another retrospective observational study, the relationship between blood urea nitrogen (BUN), estimated glomerular filtration rate (eGFR; ie, a measure of renal function), and death at 2 months after hospital discharge for HF was evaluated. Lower eGFR and higher BUN levels (ie, worst renal function) at hospital admission were associated with poor outcomes at follow-up.[12] On the other hand, a smaller prospective study of 300 patients showed that modest increases of eGFR levels after hospital discharge for ADHF were associated with better long-term but worse short-term survival.[13] Although these findings may be confounded by selection or survival factors, available data support the notion that both serum BUN and the BUN/SCr ratio represent strong predictors of survival of patients with HF, both in the long term and the short term.[14]

If chronic renal and cardiac dysfunction are closely related and contribute to outcome, it is less clear how many patients with HF experience acute WRF or AKI because epidemiologic data suggest that variable incidence rate ranging between 17% and 30%. Similar to chronic kidney dysfunction, AKI in patients with HF is associated with a long-term risk of adverse events. In a seminal study, patients with HF admitted to the ICU who developed AKI presented an increased risk of all-cause death compared with peers with preserved renal function during hospitalization.[12] In another series of more than 600 patients with ADHF admitted to the ICU were stratified according to AKI onset and clinical course as stable early AKI, worsening early AKI, and late AKI (after discharge). Furthermore, based on RIFLE criteria, patients with AKI were also classified according to AKI severity: class R (risk), class I (injury), and class F (failure). After applying the Cox regression model, class I, class F, late AKI, and worsening early AKI were associated with in-hospital mortality. On the other hand, long-term survival rates (2 years median follow-up period) were lower in class I, class F, and worsening early AKI groups.[15]

Three large trials (ASCEND-HF [Acute Study of Clinical Effectiveness of Nesiritide in Decompensated Heart Failure], VERITAS, and EVEREST) have also investigated the relationship between HF and the rate of WRF. The ASCEND-HF trial tested nesiritide therapy in patients with acute HF, evaluating SCr levels both at admission and discharge, concluding that WRF was associated with higher rates of mortality and rehospitalization within 1 month from hospital discharge.[14] The VERITAS (Value of Endothelin Receptor Inhibition with Tezosentan in Acute Heart Failure Studies) evaluated the pharmacologic effects of endothelin receptor inhibition by tezosentan and concluded that increased levels of serum troponin, creatinine, and BUN were associated with a longer hospitalization period.[16] The EVEREST (Efficacy of Vasopressin Antagonism in Heart Failure Outcome Study with Tolvaptan) trial has evaluated the effects of tolvaptan on patients with ADHF. Tolvaptan increases fluid loss and allows conventional diuretic therapy doses to be reduced. In the study, the incidence of WRF was 13.8% in hospital and 11.9% after discharge. Of note, AKI episodes were similar in both in the tolvaptan and placebo groups, regardless of a small increase in serum creatinine but not BUN during tolvaptan treatment.[17]

The impact of loop diuretics on renal function as well as the clinical relevance of WRF as a result of loop diuretics in patients with HF is a matter of debate and has not been completely elucidated.[18] Similarly, the jury is still out on the effects of venovenous ultrafiltration (UF). In the UNLOAD (Ultrafiltration versus Intravenous Diuretics for Patients Hospitalized for Acute Decompensated Heart Failure) trial, the efficacy and safety of venovenous UF was compared with standard diuretic therapy. The investigators concluded that UF therapy allowed for greater weight and fluid reduction as well as a reduction in rehospitalization due to HF.[19] To the contrary, the CARESS-HF (Cardiorenal Rescue Study in Acute Decompensated Heart Failure) trial suggested that UF was inferior to diuretics in treating fluid overload and was associated with an increase in SCr levels.[20]

In summary, although there a certain heterogeneity still exists, available evidence supports the notion that a substantial proportion of patients with ADHF experience some degree of renal dysfunction and that AKI complicates the course of ADHF disease. However, until new data become available, the clinical setting in which WRF develops (previous CKD, hemodynamic pattern, and cause of HF) needs to be taken into account to gauge the risk to which a single individual is exposed.

PATHOPHYSIOLOGY OF ACUTE KIDNEY INJURY IN HEART FAILURE
High-Output Versus Low-Output Acute Decompensated Heart Failure Related to Acute Kidney Injury

Traditionally, kidney dysfunction/injury in patients with HF has been perceived as a consequence of impairment of heart systolic and diastolic function that leads to reduced cardiac output, arterial underfilling, constriction of glomerular renal afferent arterioles, and poor renal perfusion (Guyton hypothesis). According to this view, systemic and renal vasoconstriction and activation of neurohormonal pathways can be regarded as an adaptive mechanism that turns into a maladaptive mechanism and contributes to WRF.[21]

Although this is the case with low cardiac output ADHF, reduction in blood pressure and low cardiac output cannot totally explain WRF in high cardiac output ADHF.[22] Indeed, as renal blood flow progressively reduces, an increase in the renal tubular filtration fraction occurs as a compensatory response and GFR is maintained despite renal hemodynamic changes. If this compensatory mechanism confounds the association between systemic and renal hemodynamics, further findings call into question the primary role of intraglomerular hemodynamic changes in patients with ADHF to explain WRF. Blood pressure is often normal or even increased in patients with reduced renal function. Similarly, cardiac systolic function is normal in almost 30% of patients with high cardiac output ADHF. Kidney injury could be related to right heart failure, venous congestion, and increased central venous pressure.[23,24] Indeed, changes in right heart systolic and diastolic function promote changes in kidney tubular function, tubular epithelial cell collapse, and salt and water retention.[25]

Neurohormonal Activation in WRF

In patients with in high-output and low-output ADHF with kidney dysfunction, a clear relationship between kidney damage and neurohormonal activation can be observed. The most studied hormonal pathways involved in CRS are RAAS, SNS, natriuretic peptides, inflammation, and adrenomedullin (**Fig. 1**).

RAAS and SNS hyperactivity could explain water and sodium reabsorption to prevent GFR decline and maintain intraglomerular pressure as well as renal perfusion. However, in the long term, continuous neurohormonal hyperactivity promotes left ventricular hypertrophy, fibrosis,

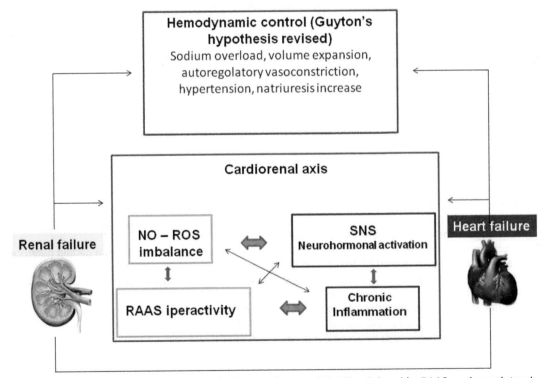

Fig. 1. Guyton hypothesis revised for pathophysiology of type 1 CRS. NO, nitric oxide; RAAS, renin-angiotensin-aldosterone system; ROS, reactive oxygen species; SNS, sympathetic nervous system.

and myocardial cell apoptosis. Prolonged and continuous RAAS and SNS activation induces an increase in both plasma volume and cardiac output as well as hemodynamic changes at kidney level (reduced medullary blood flow, glomerulosclerosis, tubular fibrosis, efferent and afferent arterial vasoconstriction). These mechanisms may compensate for the initial reduction in renal perfusion and prevent a decrease in GFR, but in the long term, intraglomerular constriction is responsible for impaired filtration and loss of effective GFR.[26]

Activation of both SNS and RAAS directly affects intratubular and capillary oncotic and hydrostatic pressure, triggering sodium retention. Indeed, RAAS activation and angiotensin II release promote aldosterone production and water reabsorption. These are responsible for the sodium shift toward the interstitial compartment as well as expansion of the interstitial volume. RAAS and angiotensin II activation also account for endothelial dysfunction, increase in production of oxygen reactive species, and inflammation.[27]

Inflammation, in turn, fosters systemic vascular damage by accelerating atherosclerosis, plaque instability, calcification development together with overproduction of pro-inflammatory cytokines directly affecting both heart and kidney.[27]

As in acute coronary syndrome, arginine vasopressin (AVP) can also contribute to fluid overload by activating both V2 (so-called aquaporins) and vascular smooth muscle cell V1a receptors, causing coronary constriction and cardiomyocytes proliferation. The final result of AVP synthesis is a negative inotropic effect further fostering left ventricular systolic dysfunction[28] (**Fig. 2**).

Finally, an expanding body of evidence suggests that adrenomedullin also plays a role in CRS. This hormone is physiologically secreted by the adrenal gland, heart, and kidneys to counteract fluid overload and RAAS activation by promoting diuresis and natriuresis. Recent findings show that in patients with ADHF with kidney derangement, adrenomedullin could be ineffective.[1]

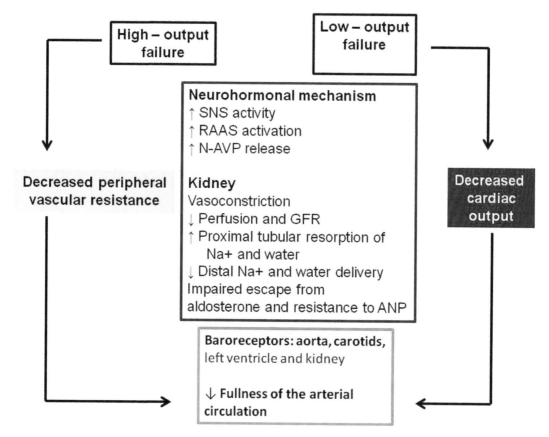

Fig. 2. Pathophysiology of type 1 CRS according to different scenarios of both high-output and low-output heart failure. AVP, arginine vasopressin peptide; GFR, glomerular filtration rate; RAAS, renin-angiotensin-aldosterone system; SNS, sympathetic nervous system.

Right Heart Dysfunction and Central Venous Hypertension

Central venous pressure (CVP) is a key pathophysiologic factor of AKI in patients with ADHF. Renal function is strictly related to CVP because renal perfusion pressure is dependent on the correct balance between mean arterial pressure and CVP. Venous congestion and kidney dysfunction may be related to right heart failure and severe tricuspid regurgitation (with low tricuspid annular plane systolic excursion and high pulmonary arterial pressure on trans-thoracic echocardiography).[23] Low cardiac output and increased CVP lead to tubular capillary distention, renal venous congestion, tubular capillary distention, and increased renal interstitial pressure with consequent hypoxia that stimulates both SNS and RAAS.[27] Furthermore, CVP hypertension is linked with increased intra-abdominal and interstitial pressure, resulting in tubular collapse, further exacerbating tissue hypoxia, and establishing a vicious pathologic cycle.[28]

In a large trial enrolling more than 1900 patients with chronic HF, GFR and New York Heart Association (NYHA) class were the most powerful predictors of mortality. Although left ventricular ejection fraction was not predictive, advanced CKD stages portended both cardiovascular and all-cause mortality. GFR and SCr were related to N-terminal atrial natriuretic peptide, showing a linear relationship between renal function and CVP.[1]

RENAL DYSFUNCTION IN PATIENTS WITH ACUTE DECOMPENSATED HEART FAILURE: CLINICAL SCENARIO

Kidney dysfunction is the result of several mechanisms primarily associated with venous congestion and hemodynamic changes leading to tubular damage (and secondary glomerular injury), salt and water retention (with consequent fluid overload), renal congestion, sclerosis, and fibrosis. RAAS activation also contributes to water and sodium retention together with efferent and afferent arterial constriction[29] (**Figs. 3** and **4**). Comorbidities can also worsen renal function; hypertension and diabetes also lead to glomerular injury.[29]

Kidney dysfunction can be more evident in sicker or older patients with ADHF who have lost intrarenal vascular autoregulation. In this setting, inappropriate diuretic administration can lead to extracellular volume contraction and renin incretion, accountable for further parenchymal injury. Loop diuretics could also reduce renal blood flow

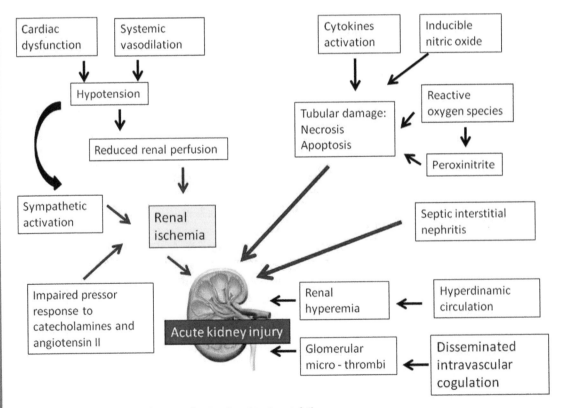

Fig. 3. Pathophysiologic pathways of AKI related to heart failure.

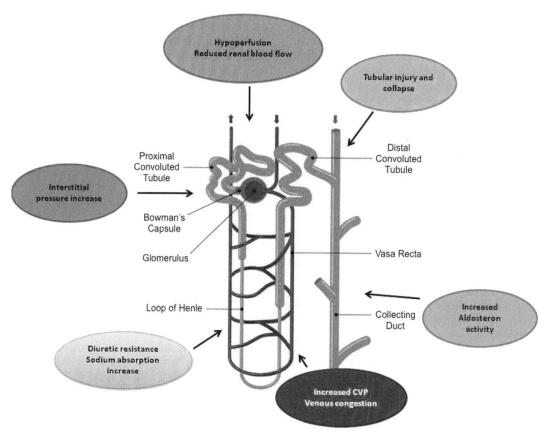

Fig. 4. Kidney damage in patients with heart failure patients. CVP, central venous pressure.

and increase proximal tubular sodium retention, delivering a large amount of sodium to distal nephrons and leading to WRF.[29]

The prevalence of WRF/AKI in ADHF ranges from 25% to 70% according to diverse sources. However, differences in the case mix among studies and WRF/AKI definitions may account for some of this variability.[30] There is no agreement concerning biomarkers to be used to identify kidney injury; AKI in the ADHF setting may have various causes, such as acute tubular necrosis, interstitial nephritis, or glomerular nephropathy, and comorbidities (hypertension, diabetes, dyslipidemia) have to be taken into account because they may contribute to type 1 CRS.[31]

At the present time, none of the available biomarkers in serum or urine have been validated to define WRF in ADHF. SCr is not sensitive and it cannot be used to determine tubular injury if GFR is preserved. Equations to estimates GFR depend on multiple variables, such as the method of calculation, age, gender, ethnicity, and are yet to be validated in patients with AKI.[18] Aside from renal function, BUN levels reflect nutrition and are influenced by the renal effects of different hormones

such as vasopressin as well as arterial underfilling or increased diuresis.[32]

In the recent past, several other biomarkers have been proposed and investigated to detect early onset of AKI. Among these, neutrophil gelatinase-associated lipocalin (N-GAL), kidney injury molecule-1 (KIM-1), interleukin 18 (IL-18), cystatin C, liver-type fatty acid-binding protein (L-FABP), tissue inhibitor of metalloproteinases (TIMP-2), IGF-binding protein 7 (IGFBP7), angiotensinogen are the most comprehensively studied.[33,34]

In a prospective study, the combination of cystatin C and KIM-1 effectively predicted AKI and subclinical renal dysfunction in more than 100 patients with ADHF.[35]

Liver-type fatty acid-binding protein (L-FABP) levels are upregulated in the proximal tubules after renal ischemia and, in a population study, the baseline urinary L-FABP (uL-FABP) level was an independent predictor of AKI in patients with ADHF.[36] Notably, uL-FABP was also a predictor of survival in hospitalized patients with ADHF who developed AKI during the first week.[37] Furthermore, L-FABP may also be effective in distinguishing patients with cardiogenic shock and

AKI at high risk for renal replacement therapy.[38] N-GAL is a member of the lipocalin family and is expressed by the renal tubular epithelium, released into urine and blood in response to tubular injury, and associated with adverse clinical outcomes in patients with ADHF.[39]

Several studies have tried to demonstrate the power and strength of N-GAL dosage to detect early onset of AKI, but results are conflicting.[39] However, plasma N-GAL in combination with creatinine was superior to creatinine only in the diagnosis of AKI in patients with ADHF.[40] In this study, early treatment of AKI was also associated with better outcome and decreased hospitalization period.[41] In the PROTECT study and AKINESIS (Acute Kidney Injury Neutrophil Gelatinase-Associated Lipocalin Evaluation of Symptomatic Heart Failure Study), involving more than 2000 patients with ADHF, WRF was diagnosed in almost 20% of patients, and N-GAL levels were independently associated with its development. Higher N-GAL levels were also associated with all-cause death and renal/cardiovascular hospitalization.[42] In a retrospective study, levels of urinary N-GAL in combination with eGFR were associated with improvement in prediction of AKI and all-cause and cardiovascular death.[42]

In another prospective multicenter study, several kidney injury biomarkers were tested. Higher tertiles of urinary N-GAL, IL-18, and angiotensinogen were associated with AKI progression.[43] Notably, plasma N-GAL was not associated with renal outcome, likely because N-GAL is not a marker of tubular injury but is related to GFR and to the immune system response to AKI as suggested by its correlation with C-reactive protein and hepcidin.[43]

Because RAAS hyperactivity has been postulated as 1 of the most important risk factor for the development of type 1 CRS, serum levels of pro-inflammatory cytokines, such as transforming growth factor alpha(TGF-α) and TNF-α, and urinary levels of angiotensinogen (uAGT) have been tested as a biomarker of RAAS activity predictors of AKI.[33] Some recently published data have documented an association between uAGT levels and increased risk of developing AKI in patients hospitalized for ADHF, both with CKD as well as normal kidney function at admission.[44] Also, uAGT was found to be an independent predictor of 1-year mortality and risk of rehospitalization.[44]

TREATMENT APPROACHES
Pharmacologic Options

Patients with HF are a heterogeneous population that encompasses different acute and chronic diseases, preserved (HFpEF), or reduced (HFrEF) ejection fraction. Hence, treatment is multifaceted and depends on the underlying disease. Nonetheless, the common primary goal is to provide relief from symptoms (ie, dyspnea, peripheral edema), improve cardiac function and quality of life, and, ultimately, decrease hospitalization and mortality rates.

The 2016 European Society of Cardiology (ESC) guidelines on the management of HF provide class I recommendations for use of maximum-tolerated evidence-based doses of angiotensin converting enzyme (ACE) inhibition and β-blockers to relieve symptoms of HFrEF. The addition of a mineralocorticoid receptor antagonist (MRA) is also recommended in those individuals who remain symptomatic after titration of other medications. Substitution of ACE inhibitors with angiotensin receptor blocker (ARB) is acceptable in patients who are not compliant with ACE inhibitors. Diuretic therapy is the basis for treating volume overload (reducing edema) and congestion. In selected patients, ACE inhibitors can be exchanged with angiotensin receptor neprilysin inhibitor (ARNI), whereas replacement therapies (such as UF) have to be addressed for patients unresponsive to medical therapies. Finally, in selected patients with HFrEF, cardioverter defibrillator implantation and other therapeutic approaches (ivabradine, digoxin, hydralazine/isosorbide dinitrate, mechanical support) may be considered until heart transplant is indicated.[45]

Because individuals with advanced CKD have been excluded in most of clinical HF trials, evidence to support the use of these drugs in CRS is less conclusive. However, in the SOLVD (Studies of Left Ventricular Dysfunction Treatment), and SAVE (Survival and Ventricular Enlargement) trials, more than 4500 patients with HFrEF (>50% with eGFR <60 mL/min) have been enrolled.[46,47] In both trials, ACE inhibitors significantly reduced hospitalization for HF and cardiovascular events also patients with in CKD stage 3B (eGFR <60 and >30 mL/min/1.73 m^2).[46,47] The Cooperative North Scandinavian Enalapril Survival (CONSENSUS) study, randomized 253 patients with HF NHYA class IV to enalapril (ranging from 2.5 mg daily to20 mg twice daily) or matching placebo. The study was terminated early because of a compelling difference in the 180-day mortality rates (44% versus 26% in the placebo and enalapril group, respectively) and significant improvement in symptoms associated with ACE inhibitors.[48] Similarly, in the Val-HeFT (Valsartan in Heart Failure) trial, almost 5000 patients with HF NYHA class II to IV (of these about 60% had eGFR <60 mL/min/m^2 and 8% had proteinuria) were randomly assigned to valsartan or placebo in addition to optimal therapy for HF. Although valsartan did not decrease the overall all-cause and cardiovascular mortality, it improved the occurrence of first morbid event (death, hospitalization for HF) in patients with CKD.[49]

The use of β-blockers in patients with is also supported by evidence derived from large clinical trials. In MERIT-HF (Metoprolol CR/XL Randomized Intervention Trial in Chronic HF), patients with eGFR <45 mL/min/m² experienced the same favorable outcomes (reduced death and hospitalization rates) as those with eGFR >60 mL/min/m².[41] In the SENIORS (Effects of Nebivolol Intervention on Outcomes and Rehospitalization in Seniors With Heart Failure) trial, the primary outcome (composite of all-cause mortality and cardiovascular hospital admission) was significantly reduced in patients with CKD treated with nebivolol.[50]

The relatively recent availability of a sacubitril (neprilysin inhibitor)-valsartan combination (LCZ696) has led the ESC to recommend its use in patients with symptomatic HFrEF with left ventricular ejection fraction ≤35% despite maximal therapy with ACE inhibitors (or ARBs), β-blockers, and MRAs. Indeed, the PARADIGM-HF (Prospective Comparison of ARNI with ACE Inhibitor to Determine Impact on Global Mortality and Morbidity in Heart Failure Trial) trial, which included more than 8000 patients with HFrEF randomly assigned to enalapril or sacubitril/valsartan, was stopped early as a result of an overwhelming benefit of LCZ696 in terms of overall and cardiovascular mortality, hospitalizations, and HF symptoms. Unfortunately, the study excluded patients with baseline eGFRs less than 30 mL/min/1.73 m², and all patients who experienced a decrease in eGFR less than 30 mL/min/1.73 m² or had a >35% decrease in eGFR from baseline or potassium concentration ≥5.5 mEq/L during follow-up.[51] Thus, further investigations are required to provide more information about the use of LCZ696 in patients with HF with moderate to advanced CKD.

Congestion relief is another essential therapeutic target in patients with ADHF, because it has an impact on hospitalization, morbidity, and mortality. Achieving patient "dry weight" represents an undiscussed marker of successful treatment. Currently available treatment options include high doses or continuous infusion of intravenous diuretics, parenteral inotropes, and UF.[20,52]

Diuretics are fundamental to induce salt and water venous refill from the interstitial space. They act on different and specific targets along the nephron (**Fig. 5**), and often a combination of these compounds is needed to achieve an adequate urinary volume output. Diuretics are bound to albumin and, because they are not filtered by the nephron, they have to be secreted by proximal tubule (S2 segment) to be effective. Hypoalbuminemia results in an increased volume of distribution of diuretics and less delivery to the kidneys and may influence diuretic responsiveness. Loop diuretics (eg, furosemide, bumetanide, torsemide, ethacrynic acid) are the most widely prescribed diuretic class because they are accountable for the excretion of 20% to 25% of filtrated sodium load.[53] Furosemide is catabolized by the kidneys and can accumulate in the presence of CKD or AKI, whereas bumetanide and torasemide are cleared by the liver.[53] Loop diuretics can be effectively administered both as bolus or continuous infusion. However, bolus administration is associated with lower rates of hyponatremia and hypotension.[54]

Thiazide diuretics act in the distal convoluted tubules and inhibit sodium reuptake from the lumen. Chlorothiazide intravenously and metolazone orally are the most commonly used thiazide diuretics in HF. This class of diuretics is often associated with hypokalemia because they triggers aldosterone secretion.[53]

In patients with ADHF, loop diuretics, thiazides, and MRAs are often used together to better control congestion and electrolyte imbalances, engaging what is called the sequential nephron blockade.[55] However, in patients treated with high doses of diuretics, ACE inhibitors, ARBs, ARNI, and MRAs, hyperkalemia may develop irrespective of sequential nephron blockade.[56] Novel strategies using agents to enable chronic hyperkalemia control (patiromer calcium, sodium zirconium cyclosilicate) may be needed to allow for optimal RAAS blockage.[56]

Inotropic agents can improve cardiac function especially in low-output HF to provide better renal perfusion and diuretic response in patients with type 1 CRS, but published results are controversial.[57] In a retrospective study, the incidence of CRS was higher in patients treated with dobutamine rather than levosimendan (levosimendan also has diuretic effects), and those on levosimendan experienced more favorable cardiovascular outcomes.[57] Compared with milrinone, dobutamine was also shown to be associated with higher short-term out-of-hospital mortality in the first 180 days from hospital discharge after an episode of ADHF.[58] Hence, based on these conflicting pieces of evidence, the Working Group on AKI Prevention of the European Society of Intensive Care Medicine recommended against the use of low-dose dopamine for AKI protection (grade 1A).[59]

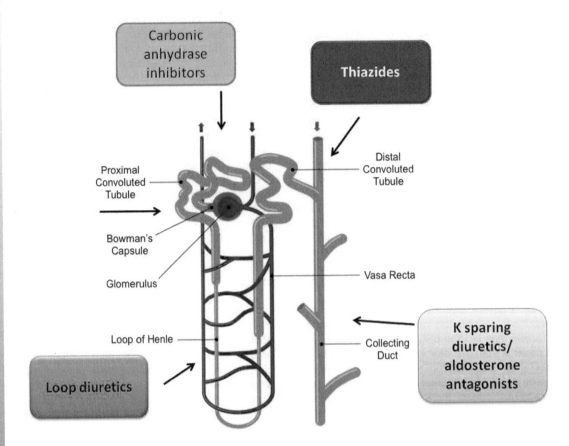

Fig. 5. Sites of action of diuretics in the nephron.

Tolvaptan is a novel aquaretic agent that inhibits vasopressin V2 receptors in the renal collecting ducts. Added to standard diuretic therapy, tolvaptan improves the signs and symptoms of congestion without serious adverse events in ADHF.[60] In 2016, the ESC guidelines for HF management suggested (class IIb) its use in patients with signs of volume overload and resistant hyponatremia mainly based on the results of the EVEREST trial.[17]

Serelaxin is a human recombinant form of relaxin-2 that mediates vasodilation by increasing the production of nitric oxide. The RELAX-AHF trial showed that serelaxin improved dyspnea and reduced both WRF (by 47%) and cardiovascular mortality in a mid-range period after hospital discharge.[61] However, some preliminary reports from RELAX-AHF 2, a multicenter, randomized, double-blind, placebo-controlled, event-driven, phase 3 trial, enrolling approximately 6600 patients hospitalized for ADHF with dyspnea, congestion on chest radiographs suggested that serelaxin failed to reduce the occurrence of the primary endpoints (180-day cardiovascular death and occurrence of worsening HF through day 5) but data have not actually been published.

When pharmacologic treatment fails and diuretic resistance (despite sequential nephron blockage) and severe renal failure ensue, renal replacement therapy (RRT) has to be considered. The primary goal of RRT is to compensate for the abrupt loss of renal function and prevent further fluid overload or electrolyte metabolic imbalances.

Isolated venovenous UF can be used as an alternative to loop diuretics.[62,63] UF has been made feasible with the advent of simplified devices that permit volume removal with peripheral venous access, adjustable blood flow, and small extracorporeal blood volumes.[62] In isolated venovenous UF, plasma water is produced from whole blood across a semipermeable membrane (hemofilter) in response to a transmembrane pressure gradient that is driven by hydrostatic forces generated by extracorporeal pumps. These hydrostatic forces can be adjusted manually, allowing for tightly controlled UF fluid removal rates. The solute concentration in the ultrafiltrate is equal to that in the water component of the plasma, allowing for effective removal of isotonic sodium from the patient.[63] The SAFE trial was the first to show that, in 21 congested patients with ADHF, the removal of an average of 2600 mL of ultrafiltrate during an 8-hour treatment period resulted in a mean weight loss of approximately 3 kg without changes in heart rate, blood pressure, SCr, electrolytes, or the occurrence of major adverse events.[62] In the Relief of Acutely Fluid-Overloaded Patients with Decompensated Congestive Heart Failure (RAPID-CHF) trial, 40 patients were randomized to either a single 8-hour course of UF plus usual care or to usual care alone.[63] Compared with the usual care group, UF-treated patients had greater net fluid loss at 24 and 48 hours as well as greater 48-hour improvement in dyspnea. Usual care and UF were similar in terms of renal function, electrolytes, heart rate, systolic blood pressure, and duration of the index hospitalization.[63] Notably, effective decongestion and clinical improvement were observed with early initiation of UF, before the increase in SCr levels as a result of loop diuretic administration.[63]

The goal of the UNLOAD trial was to compare the safety and efficacy of an early strategy of UF versus standard intravenous diuretic therapy in patients with ADHF with signs of congestion. At 90 days, the UF group had less episodes of rehospitalization or worsening HF. Hypokalemia occurred in only 1% of UF patients versus 12% of the diuretic-treated group.[19,64] The Cardiorenal Rescue Study in Acute Decompensated Heart Failure (CARRESS-HF) trial compared the effects of a fixed dose of 200 mL/h UF with a stepped pharmacologic therapy (SPT; inclusive of adjustable doses of intravenous loop diuretics, thiazide diuretics, vasodilators, and inotropes) in patients with ADHF with evidence of increased SCr between 12 weeks before and 7 days after hospital admission despite escalating doses of diuretics.[20] In this patient population, patients treated with UF versus SPT experienced a significant 96-hour increase in SCr levels without any improvement in body weight.[20]

Based on the available body of evidence, current guidelines on HF management suggest that an inadequate response to an initial dose of intravenous loop diuretic can be treated with an increased dose of the same drug.[65] If this measure is not effective, invasive hemodynamic assessment is recommended. Persistent congestion can then be treated with the addition of a thiazide diuretic, an aldosterone antagonist, or the use of continuous intravenous infusion of a loop diuretic. If all of these measures fail, then mechanical fluid removal can be considered.[65] However, these recommendations are in stark contrast to clinical trial data on the efficacy of early intervention with UF therapies and are alarmingly similar to the enrollment criteria

required for patient entry in the CARRESS-HF trial. Based on the UNLOAD study results,[19] UF should be considered in patients with ADHF before they fail high-dose intravenous diuretics, taking into account the potential complications and cost of UF therapy.

To be safe and effective, all decongestive therapies, including UF, have to remove fluid avoiding hemodynamic instability or WRF/AKI. The rate and amount of fluid removal must be initially established according to the hemodynamic and clinical status of the patient to be treated with careful attention to refilling pressures once euvolemic targets are approaching. In patients with ADHF, UF rates greater than 250 mL/h have to be avoided, especially in those with right heart failure or preserved ejection fraction with restrictive pattern at echocardiographic evaluation (in these patients UF rates <150 mL/h are recommended).[66] Extracorporeal fluid removal seems to be better tolerated when conducted with low UF rates over prolonged periods of time (more than 8 hours and up to 72 hours) and discontinued as soon as signs of congestion subside. In this regard, bioimpedance vector analysis can be used to noninvasively evaluate the total body water content[67,68] and integrate anthropometric and biomarker pieces of information, such as body weight, blood pressure, or natriuretic peptide levels.[68,69]

SUMMARY

Kidney injury presents a difficult challenge in patients with both acute and chronic HF. Clinicians have to pay attention to early onset of kidney dysfunction to avoid the occurrence of WRF or AKI. Early diagnosis and immediate therapeutic approaches could lead to favorable clinical outcomes and avoid the risk of CKD or end-stage renal disease. Both pharmacologic and mechanical support could be suitable for treating congestion in patients with HF, although further trials are needed to provide ultimate guidelines for treating patients with type 1 CRS.

REFERENCES

1. Hillege HL, Girbes ARJ, de Kam PJ, et al. Renal function, neurohormonal activation, and survival in patients with chronic heart failure. Circulation 2000; 102(2):203–10.
2. Ronco C, Bellasi A, Di Lullo L. Cardiorenal syndrome: an overview. Adv Chronic Kidney Dis 2018; 25(5):382–90.
3. Agrawal V, Krause KR, Chengelis DL, et al. Relation between degree of weight loss after bariatric

surgery and reduction in albuminuria and C-reactive protein. Surg Obes Relat Dis 2008;5(1):20–6.

4. Russo R, Di Iorio B, Di Lullo L, et al. Epicardial adipose tissue: new parameter for cardiovascular risk assessment in high risk populations. J Nephrol 2018;31(6):847–53.

5. Kooman JP, Kotanko P, Schols AM, et al. Chronic kidney disease and premature ageing. Nat Rev Nephrol 2014;10(12):732–42.

6. Ravera M, Rosa GM, Fontanive P, et al. Impaired left ventricular global longitudinal strain among patients with chronic kidney disease and end-stage renal disease and renal transplant recipients. Cardiorenal Med 2019;9(1):61–8.

7. Kato A. Increased hepcidin-25 and erythropoietin responsiveness in patients with cardio-renal anemia syndrome. Future Cardiol 2010;6(6):769–71.

8. Alam ML, Katz R, Bellovich KA, et al. Soluble ST2 and galectin-3 and progression of CKD. Kidney Int Rep 2018;4(1):103–11.

9. Heywood JT, Fonarow GC, Costanzo MR, et al. High prevalence of renal dysfunction and its impact on outcome in 118,465 patients hospitalized with acute decompensated heart failure: a report from the ADHERE database. J Card Fail 2007;13(6):422–30.

10. Nohria A, Hasselblad V, Stebbins A, et al. Cardiorenal interactions: insights from the ESCAPE trial. J Am Coll Cardiol 2008;51(13):1268–74.

11. Damman K, Jaarsma T, Voors AA, et al. Both in- and out-hospital worsening of renal function predict outcome in patients with heart failure: results from the Coordinating Study Evaluating Outcome of Advising and Counseling in Heart Failure (COACH). Eur J Heart Fail 2009;11(9):847–54.

12. Hata N, Yokoyama S, Shinada T, et al. Acute kidney injury and outcomes in acute decompensated heart failure: evaluation of the RIFLE criteria in an acutely ill heart failure population. Eur J Heart Fail 2009; 12(1):32–7.

13. Gotsman I, Zwas D, Planer D, et al. The significance of serum urea and renal function in patients with heart failure. Medicine 2010;89(4):197–203.

14. van Deursen VM, Hernandez AF, Stebbins A, et al. Nesiritide, renal function, and associated outcomes during hospitalization for acute decompensated heart failure: results from the acute study of clinical effectiveness of nesiritide and decompensated heart failure (ASCEND-HF). Circulation 2014; 130(12):958–65.

15. Shirakabe A, Hata N, Kobayashi N, et al. Prognostic impact of acute kidney injury in patients with acute decompensated heart failure. Circ J 2013;77(3):687–96.

16. Cleland JGF, Teerlink JR, Davison BA, et al. Measurement of troponin and natriuretic peptides shortly after admission in patients with heart failure—does it add useful prognostic information? An analysis of the Value of Endothelin Receptor Inhibition with Tezosentan in Acute heart failure Studies (VERITAS). Eur J Heart Fail 2017;19(6):739–47.

17. Blair JE, Pang PS, Schrier RW, et al. Changes in renal function during hospitalization and soon after discharge in patients admitted for worsening heart failure in the placebo group of the EVEREST trial. Eur Heart J 2011;32(20):2563–72.

18. Di Lullo L, Di Iorio BR, Ronco C, et al. Search for a reliable biomarker of acute kidney injury: to the heart of the problem. Ann Transl Med 2018;6(Suppl 1):S5.

19. Costanzo MR, Saltzberg MT, Jessup M, et al, Ultrafiltration Versus Intravenous Diuretics for Patients Hospitalized for Acute Decompensated Heart Failure (UNLOAD) Investigators. Ultrafiltration is associated with fewer re - hospitalizations than continuous diuretic infusion in patients with decompensated heart failure: results from UNLOAD. J Card Fail 2010;16(4):277–84.

20. Bart BA, Goldsmith SR, Lee KL, et al. Ultrafiltration in decompensated heart failure with cardiorenal syndrome. N Engl J Med 2012;367(24):2296–304.

21. Ronco C, Cicoira M, McCullough PA. Cardiorenal syndrome type 1: pathophysiological crosstalk leading to combined heart and kidney dysfunction in the setting of acutely decompensated heart failure. J Am Coll Cardiol 2012;60(12):1031–42.

22. Testani JM, Coca SG, McCauley BD, et al. Impact of changes in blood pressure during the treatment of acute decompensated heart failure on renal and clinical outcomes. Eur J Heart Fail 2011;13(8):877–84.

23. Di Lullo L, Floccari F, Rivera R, et al. Pulmonary hypertension and right heart failure in chronic kidney disease: new challenge for 21st-century cardionephrologists. Cardiorenal Med 2013;3(2):96–103.

24. Di Lullo L, Floccari F, Polito P. Right ventricular diastolic function in dialysis patients could be affected by vascular access. Nephron Clin Pract 2011; 118(3):c257–61.

25. Mullens W, Abrahams Z, Francis GS, et al. Importance of venous congestion for worsening of renal function in advanced decompensated heart failure. J Am Coll Cardiol 2009;53(7):589–96.

26. Ruggenenti P, Remuzzi G. Worsening kidney function in decompensated heart failure: treat the heart, don't mind the kidney. Eur Heart J 2011;32(20):2476–8.

27. Schrier RW, Abraham WT. Hormones and hemodynamics in heart failure. N Engl J Med 1999;341(8):577–85.

28. Sinkeler SJ, Damman K, van Veldhuisen DJ, et al. A reappraisal of volume status and renal function impairment in chronic heart failure: combined effects of pre-renal failure and venous congestion on renal function. Heart Fail Rev 2011;17(2):263–70.

29. Brewster UC, Perazella MA, Setaro JF. The renin-angiotensin-aldosterone system: cardiorenal effects

and implications for renal and cardiovascular disease states. Am J Med Sci 2003;326(1):15–24.

30. Gottlieb SS, Abraham W, Butler J, et al. The prognostic importance of different definitions of worsening renal function in congestive heart failure. J Card Fail 2002;8(3):136–41.

31. Palazzuoli A, Ronco C. Cardio-renal syndrome: an entity cardiologists and nephrologists should be dealing with collegially. Heart Fail Rev 2011;16(6):503–8.

32. Kazory A. Emergence of blood urea nitrogen as a biomarker of neurohormonal activation in heart failure. Am J Cardiol 2010;106(5):694–700.

33. Devarajan P. Neutrophil gelatinase-associated lipocalin: a troponin-like biomarker for human acute kidney injury. Nephrology (Carlton). 2010;15:419–28.

34. Ba Aqeel SH, Sanchez A, Batlle D. Angiotensinogen as a biomarker of acute kidney injury. Clin Kidney J 2017;10(6):759–68.

35. Yang CH, Chang CH, Chen TH, et al. Combination of urinary biomarkers improves early detection of acute kidney injury in patients with heart failure. Circ J 2016;80(4):1017–23.

36. Hishikari K, Hikita H, Nakamura S, et al. Urinary liver-type fatty acid-binding protein level as a predictive biomarker of acute kidney injury in patients with acute decompensated heart failure. Cardiorenal Med 2017;7(4):267–75.

37. Shirakabe A, Hata N, Kobayashi N, et al. Clinical usefulness of urinary liver fatty acid binding protein excretion for predicting acute kidney injury during the first 7 days and the short-term prognosis in acute heart failure patients with non-chronic kidney disease. Cardiorenal Med 2017;7(4):301–15.

38. Van Veldhuisen DJ, Ruilope LM, Maisel AS, et al. Biomarkers of renal injury and function: diagnostic, prognostic and therapeutic implications in heart failure. Eur Heart J 2016;37:2577–85.

39. Alvelos M, Lourenco P, Dias C, et al. Prognostic value of neutrophil gelatinase-associated Lipocalin in acute heart failure. Int J Cardiol 2013;165:51–5.

40. Angeletti S, Fogolari M, Morolla D, et al. Role of neutrophil gelatinase-associated lipocalin in the diagnosis and early treatment of acute kidney injury in a case series of patients with acute decompensated heart failure: a case series. Cardiol Res Pract 2016;2016:3708210.

41. Ghali JK, Wikstrand J, Van Veldhuisen DJ, et al. The influence of renal function on clinical outcome and response to beta-blockade in systolic heart failure: insights from Metoprolol CR/XL Randomized Intervention Trial in Chronic HF (MERIT-HF). J Card Fail 2009;15(4):310–8.

42. Maisel AS, Wettersten N, van Veldhuisen DJ, et al. Neutrophil gelatinase-associated lipocalin for acute kidney injury during acute heart failure hospitalizations: the AKINESIS study. J Am Coll Cardiol 2016; 68:1420–31.

43. Schmidt-Ott KM, Mori K, Li JY, et al. Dual action of neutrophil gelatinase-associated lipocalin. J Am Soc Nephrol 2007;18:407–13.

44. Yang X, Chen C, Tian J, et al. Urinary angiotensinogen level predicts AKI in acute decompensated heart failure: a prospective, two-stage study. J Am Soc Nephrol 2015;26:2032–41.

45. Ponikowski P, Voors AA, Anker SD, et al, Authors/ Task Force Members, Document Reviewers. 2016 ESC guidelines for the diagnosis and treatment of acute and chronic heart failure: The Task Force for the diagnosis and treatment of acute and chronic heart failure of the European Society of Cardiology (ESC). Developed with the special contribution of the Heart Failure Association (HFA) of the ESC. Eur J Heart Fail 2016;18(8):891–975.

46. Bowling CB, Sanders PW, Allman RM, et al. Effects of enalapril in systolic heart failure patients with and without chronic kidney disease: insights from the SOLVD Treatment trial. Int J Cardiol 2013; 167(1):151–6.

47. Anand IS, Bishu K, Rector TS, et al. Proteinuria, chronic kidney disease, and the effect of an angiotensin receptor blocker in addition to an angiotensin-converting enzyme inhibitor in patients with moderate to severe heart failure. Circulation 2009;120(16):1577–84.

48. CONSENSUS Trial Study Group. Effects of enalapril on mortality in severe congestive heart failure. Results of the Cooperative North Scandinavian Enalapril Survival Study (CONSENSUS). N Engl J Med 1987;316(23):1429–35.

49. Florea VG, Rector TS, Anand IS, et al. Heart failure with improved ejection fraction: clinical characteristics, correlates of recovery, and survival: results from the Valsartan Heart Failure Trial. Circ Heart Fail 2016;9(7) [pii:e003123].

50. Cohen-Solal A, Kotecha D, van Veldhuisen DJ, et al. Efficacy and safety of nebivolol in elderly heart failure patients with impaired renal function: insights from the SENIORS trial. Eur J Heart Fail 2009; 11(9):872–80.

51. McMurray JJ, Packer M, Desai AS, et al. Angiotensin-neprilysin inhibition versus enalapril in heart failure. N Engl J Med 2014;371(11):993–1004.

52. Lafrenière G, Béliveau P, Bégin JY, et al. Effects of hypertonic saline solution on body weight and serum creatinine in patients with acute decompensated heart failure. World J Cardiol 2017;9(8):685–92.

53. Puschett JB. Pharmacological classification and renal actions of diuretics. Cardiology 1994; 84(suppl 2):4–13.

54. Palazzuoli A, Ruocco G, Ronco C, et al. Loop diuretics in acute heart failure: beyond the decongestive relief for the kidney. Crit Care 2015;19:296.

55. McCullough PA, Beaver TM, Bennett-Guerrero E, et al. Acute and chronic cardiovascular effects of

hyperkalemia: new insights into prevention and clinical management. Rev Cardiovasc Med 2014;15(1): 11–23.

56. Di Lullo L, Ronco C, Granata A, et al. Chronic hyperkalemia in cardiorenal patients: risk factors, diagnosis, and new treatment options. Cardiorenal Med 2019;9(1):8–21.

57. Madeira M, Caetano F, Almeida I, et al. Inotropes and cardiorenal syndrome in acute heart failure—a retrospective comparative analysis. Rev Port Cardiol 2017;36(9):619–25.

58. King JB, Shah RU, Sainski-Nguyen A, et al. Effect of inpatient dobutamine versus milrinone on out-of-hospital mortality in patients with acute decompensated heart failure. Pharmacotherapy 2017;37(6): 662–72.

59. Joannidis M, Druml W, Forni LG, et al. Prevention of acute kidney injury and protection of renal function in the intensive care unit: update 2017: expert opinion of the working group on prevention, AKI section, European Society of Intensive Care Medicine. Intensive Care Med 2017;43(6):730–49.

60. Gheorghiade M, Gattis WA, O'Connor CM, et al. Effects of tolvaptan, a vasopressin antagonist, in patients hospitalized with worsening heart failure: a randomized controlled trial. JAMA 2004;291(16): 1963–71.

61. Teerlink JR, Cotter G, Davison BA, et al. RELAXin in acute heart failure (RELAXAHF) investigators. Serelaxin, recombinant human relaxin-2, for treatment of acute heart failure (RELAX-AHF): a randomised, placebo-controlled trial. Lancet 2013;81(9860): 29–39.

62. Costanzo MR, Ronco C. Isolated ultrafiltration in heart failure patients. Curr Cardiol Rep 2012;14(3): 254–64.

63. Bart BA, Boyle A, Bank AJ, et al. Ultrafiltration versus usual care for hospitalized patients with heart failure: the Relief for Acutely Fluid-Overloaded Patients With Decompensated Congestive Heart Failure (RAPID-CHF) trial. J Am Coll Cardiol 2005;46(11):2043–6.

64. Costanzo MR, Guglin ME, Saltzberg MT, et al. Ultrafiltration versus intravenous diuretics for patients hospitalized for acute decompensated heart failure. J Am Coll Cardiol 2007;49(6):675–83.

65. Jessup M, Abraham WT, Casey DE, et al. 2009 focused update: ACCF/AHA Guidelines for the Diagnosis and Management of Heart Failure in Adults: a report of the American College of Cardiology Foundation/American Heart Association Task Force on Practice Guidelines: developed in collaboration with the International Society for Heart and Lung Transplantation. Circulation 2009;119(14): 1977–2016.

66. Gheorghiade M, Follath F, Ponikowski P, et al, European Society of Cardiology, European Society of Intensive Care Medicine. Assessing and grading congestion in acute heart failure: a scientific statement from the acute heart failure committee of the heart failure association of the European Society of Cardiology and endorsed by the European Society of Intensive Care Medicine. Eur J Heart Fail 2010; 12(5):423–33.

67. Larsen TR, Singh G, Velocci V, et al. Frequency of fluid overload and usefulness of bioimpedance in patients requiring intensive care for sepsis syndromes. Proc (Bayl Univ Med Cent) 2016;29(1): 12–5.

68. Ronco C, Kaushik M, Valle R, et al. Diagnosis and management of fluid overload in heart failure and cardio-renal syndrome: the "5B" approach. Semin Nephrol 2012;32(1):129–41.

69. Costanzo MR, Cozzolino M, Aspromonte N, et al. Extracorporeal ultrafiltration in heart failure and cardio-renal syndromes. Semin Nephrol 2012; 32(1):100–11.

Special Populations

Hypertensive Heart Failure in the Very Old

Gmerice Hammond, MD, MPH, Michael W. Rich, MD*

KEYWORDS

- Hypertension • Hypertensive heart failure • Elderly • Aged • Hypertensive cardiomyopathy

KEY POINTS

- Age-related changes in the cardiovascular system predispose the development of hypertension and heart failure in older adults.
- The clinical features of heart failure in older adults often are atypical, and a high index of suspicion must be maintained.
- Management of hypertensive heart failure in older adults must be patient centered, with due consideration given to prevalent comorbidities and each patient's goals and preferences.
- Prevention of hypertension and of progression from hypertension to heart failure holds the greatest promise for reducing the personal and societal impact of hypertensive heart failure.

INTRODUCTION

The incidence and prevalence of both hypertension (HTN) and heart failure (HF) increase progressively with age.[1] As a result, hypertensive HF (HHF) is highly prevalent among older adults and it is one of the most common phenotypes of HF in the very old, herein defined as greater than or equal to 80 years of age. This article provides an overview of the epidemiology, pathophysiology, clinical features, diagnosis, management, prognosis, and prevention of HHF in the elderly population.

EPIDEMIOLOGY

The prevalence of HTN increases inexorably with age, exceeding 70% in men and 80% in women 75 years of age or older in the United States.[2] Because these estimates predate the revised criteria for diagnosing HTN published in 2017,[3] the current prevalence of HTN among older adults is likely even higher. The prevalence of HF also increases progressively with age, reaching 12.8% in men and 12.0% in women greater than or equal to 80 years of age Fig. 1.[1] Similarly, the incidence of HF increases with age. In the Atherosclerosis Risk in Communities Study, the annual incidence of acute decompensated HF in individuals greater than or equal to 75 years of age was 2.6% in white women, 3.1% in black women, 3.2% in white men, and 3.5% in black men Fig. 2.[1] Due to the rising incidence and prevalence of HF with age, HF is predominantly a disorder of older adults, with approximately 50% of all HF cases in the United States occurring in the 6% of the population greater than or equal to 75 years of age. Importantly, although the incidence and prevalence rates of HF are higher in older men than in older women, there are more older women living with HF due to the longer life expectancy of women and somewhat better prognosis of HF in women compared with men. Furthermore, because HTN is more common in older women compared with men and also is a stronger risk factor for HF in women, women comprise a majority of older adults with HHF. Additional risk factors for the development of HF in older adults with HTN include obesity, smoking, preexisting

Disclosures: Dr. G. Hammond is supported by the National Heart, Lung, and Blood Institute of the National Institutes of Health under award number T32HL007081.
Cardiovascular Division, Washington University School of Medicine, 660 South Euclid Avenue, Campus Box 8086, St Louis, MO 63110, USA
* Corresponding author.
E-mail address: mrich@wustl.edu

Heart Failure Clin 15 (2019) 477–485
https://doi.org/10.1016/j.hfc.2019.06.001
1551-7136/19/© 2019 Elsevier Inc. All rights reserved.

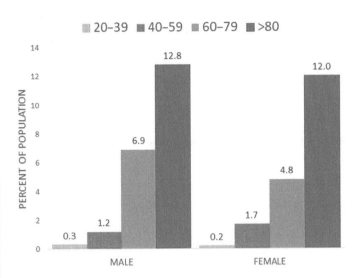

Fig. 1. Prevalence of heart failure by gender and age (*National Health and Nutrition Examination Survey,* 2013–2016). (*Data from* Center for Disease Control, National Center for Health Statistics. National Health and Nutrition Examination Survey 2013 to 2016 (NHANES). Available at: https://www.cdc.gov/nchs/nhanes/index.htm.)

cardiovascular disease, and visit-to-visit variability in systolic blood pressure.[4]

HF in older adults is almost always multifactorial, reflecting various combinations of physiologic aging, HTN, ischemic heart disease, valve disease, amyloid, and a host of other factors. It is, therefore, difficult to provide precise estimates of the incidence and prevalence of HHF per se. Several studies, however, have identified HTN as associated with a high population attributable risk for HF in older adults. In the Framingham Heart Study, 39% of HF in men and 59% of HF in women were attributable to HTN.[5,6] In the Cardiovascular Health Study, 12.8% of incident HF was attributed to HTN, and only ischemic heart disease was associated with a higher population attributable risk at 13.1%.[7]

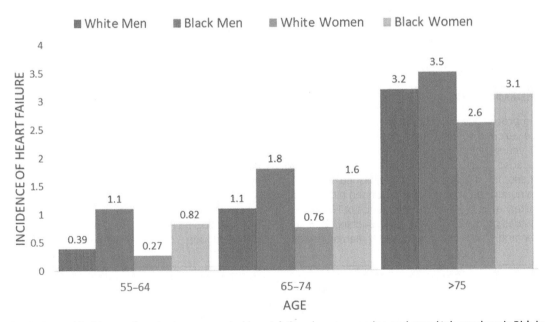

Fig. 2. Annual incidence of acute decompensated heart failure by age, gender, and race (Atherosclerosis Risk in Communities Study, 2005–2014). (*Data from* National Institute of Health, National Heart, Lung, and Blood Institute. The Atherosclerosis Risk in Communities Study (ARIC) 2005-2014. Available at: https://www.nhlbi.nih.gov/research/resources/obesity/population/aric.htm.)

PATHOPHYSIOLOGY

Normal aging is associated with fundamental changes in the cardiovascular system that foster the development of both HTN and HF.[8] Increased stiffness of the great vessels and large arteries is a hallmark of aging that is due primarily to increased collagen deposition and cross-linking in the vessel walls in conjunction with degeneration of nonregenerative elastin fibers.[9,10] This leads to increased impedance to left ventricular ejection, higher systolic blood pressure due to loss of resiliency and buffering capacity of the large arteries, and increased rate of transmission of the arterial pulse wave (ie, increased pulse wave velocity). Conversely, there is a more rapid decline in pressure during diastole. As a result of these changes, systolic blood pressure gradually increases with age, diastolic blood pressure tends to peak and plateau in late middle age and gradually decline thereafter, and pulse pressure (ie, the difference between systolic and diastolic pressure) increases with age.[11,12] Note that due to directionally opposite changes in systolic and diastolic blood pressure, the mean arterial pressure remains relatively constant in the context of normal aging.

The increased impedance to left ventricular ejection imposed by increased arterial stiffness and systolic blood pressure leads to compensatory myocardial hypertrophy in order to reduce wall stress (afterload).[13] This is accompanied by increased deposition of collagen, lipofuscin, and other moieties in the myocardial interstitium, with the net effect of increased passive myocardial stiffness.[14] In addition, aging is associated with impairment in active myocardial relaxation during the early phase of diastole due in part to delayed release of calcium from the contractile proteins, in effect leaving the heart in a state of partial contraction.[15] Taken together, these changes lead to characteristic age-associated alterations in the pattern of diastolic filling, with a reduced rate of filling during early diastole (manifested by a blunted E-wave on echocardiography) and compensatory augmentation of filling during atrial contraction (increased A-wave on echocardiography) to preserve left ventricular end-diastolic volume (preload) and stroke volume. Although these changes may be properly viewed as the effects of normal aging, they nonetheless predispose older adults to the development of HF with preserved ejection fraction (HFpEF) as well as to atrial fibrillation. Furthermore, elevated blood pressure to levels beyond those associated with normal aging exacerbates diastolic dysfunction, thereby accelerating the progression to HF.

Apart from the direct interactions between aging, HTN, and HF, aging is associated with numerous other cardiac and noncardiac alterations that predispose to these conditions. In the cardiovascular domain, aging is associated with impaired responsiveness to β-adrenergic stimulation, which results in a near-linear decline in maximum heart rate with increasing age, often approximated by the formula: 220-age.[16] Peak myocardial contractility declines with age, and there is impaired peripheral vasodilation mediated by β_2-receptors.[17] Endothelium-dependent coronary vasodilation, mediated primarily by nitric oxide, also declines with age, resulting in a decline in peak coronary blood flow and increased risk for myocardial ischemia due to supply/demand mismatch, even in the absence of obstructive coronary artery disease.[18] Taken together, these changes lead to a marked and progressive decline in cardiovascular reserve capacity with increasing age, predisposing to the development of acute and chronic HF in response to stressors that might be well tolerated in younger individuals.

Among noncardiac changes, age-related declines in renal function contribute to the development of both HTN and HF at older age as well as to difficulties in managing these conditions.[19] The glomerular filtration rate declines with age, as reflected in all equations for estimating glomerular filtration rate, and there is also a progressive decline in renal tubular concentrating and diluting capacity. These factors impair the capacity of the kidneys to handle sodium and fluid loads, diminish the efficacy of diuretics, and increase the risk for adverse effects related to medications commonly used to treat HTN and HF.

Pulmonary aging reduces the capacity of the lungs to compensate for cardiac abnormalities, including HF,[20] whereas age-related changes in the hemostatic system increase risk for both thrombosis (arterial and venous) and bleeding.[21] Age-associated alterations in neurohumoral regulation also contribute to the pathophysiology of HF in older adults.

Although mechanisms have not been fully elucidated, gender and racial differences in the cardiac response to HTN and left ventricular pressure overload have been described. In turn, these differences may have an impact on the likelihood of progression from HTN to HF. In an analysis of older participants in the Framingham Heart Study with isolated systolic HTN, both men and women developed left ventricular hypertrophy and increased left ventricular mass.[22] The magnitude of the response was greater in women, however, and whereas women developed increased wall thickness without left ventricular chamber enlargement (ie, concentric remodeling), men had less increase in wall thickness with greater increase in chamber size (ie, eccentric remodeling). Similarly, in the Hypertension Genetic Epidemiology Network study, black patients with HTN developed substantially greater left ventricular mass and relative wall thickness than white patients, and the differences persisted after adjustment for potentially confounding clinical and hemodynamic variables.[23,24] These differences in response to HTN as a function of gender and race contribute to HFpEF being the dominant form of HHF in the very old, especially among women and African Americans. These complex interactions between gender, race, HTN, and HF are reviewed in detail elsewhere in this monograph.

CLINICAL FEATURES
Symptoms and Signs

The symptoms and signs of HHF in the very old generally are similar to those of HF in the general population and HHF in younger patients. Exertional shortness of breath and effort intolerance are the dominant symptoms in all forms of HF in adults of all ages. Additional symptoms commonly include orthopnea, lower extremity swelling, and fatigue. Due to sedentary lifestyle and prevalent comorbidities, however, such as arthritis and neurologic disorders, older patients with HF are less likely than younger patients to report exertional symptoms. In addition, even when present, exertional symptoms may be attributed by both patients and clinicians, sometimes appropriately, to deconditioning, obesity, chronic lung disease, depression, or normal aging. Conversely, older patients with HF are more likely than younger patients to present with atypical symptoms, including altered mental status, irritability, sleep disorders, gastrointestinal disturbances, and other nonspecific complaints.

Cardinal signs of HF, including an S_3 (HF with reduced ejection fraction [HFrEF]) or S_4 (HFpEF) gallop, moist pulmonary rales, elevated jugular venous pressure, and lower extremity edema, when present, provide support for a diagnosis of HF. An S_4 gallop, however, is common in older adults without HF; pulmonary crackles may be due to pulmonary disease or atelectasis; and lower extremity swelling may be due to venous insufficiency, medications (especially calcium channel blockers), or other conditions. In older adults with acute decompensated HF due to HHF, a substantially elevated systolic blood pressure is almost invariably present at the time of presentation.

Diagnostic Testing

Because the sensitivity and specificity of classical symptoms and signs of HF decline with age, in most cases it is necessary to perform additional evaluation to establish a diagnosis and guide therapy. Aging is associated, however, with limitations in most of the standard diagnostic tests for HF. The quality of chest radiographs may be limited by altered chest geometry (eg, kyphosis) or inability of a patient to comply with breathing instructions. Additionally, pulmonary infiltrates may be due to chronic lung disease, pneumonia (including aspiration pneumonia), or noncardiogenic pulmonary edema. Natriuretic peptide levels (B-type natriuretic peptide and N-terminal pro-B type natriuretic peptide), increase slightly with age (more so in women) and in the presence of renal insufficiency; as a result, the specificity of these biomarkers declines with age. Soluble ST2 receptor and galactin-3 have been shown to have diagnostic and prognostic utility in younger patients, but their validity in older patients has not been established.[25] Cardiac troponin is commonly elevated in ambulatory older adults without HF,[26] so its role in diagnosing myocardial ischemia in older patients with acute or chronic HF requires further study.

Aging and age-associated comorbidities may introduce technical challenges to performing and interpreting noninvasive diagnostic imaging procedures, including echocardiography, myocardial perfusion imaging, cardiac computed tomography, and magnetic resonance imaging. Increased anterior-posterior diameter, kyphosis/scoliosis, and chronic lung disease may reduce image quality. Cognitive impairment and chronic pain may impair older patients' ability to comply with imaging protocols, for example, breath-holding during image acquisition. Atrial fibrillation, which increases in prevalence with age, may confound the echocardiographic assessment of diastolic function, an important component of the evaluation of patients with HHF.

Hypertensive Hypertrophic Cardiomyopathy

In 1985, Topol and colleagues[27] described a syndrome characterized by marked concentric left ventricular hypertrophy, small left ventricular cavity with hyperdynamic systolic function, impaired diastolic function, and left atrial enlargement. Cavity obliteration during systole, systolic anterior motion of the mitral valve, and mitral annular calcification were additional features in some patients. Patients were older (mean age 73 years), predominantly women (76%), and mostly black (71%). All patients had longstanding systolic

HTN, none had a history of ischemic heart disease, and a majority presented with symptoms of dyspnea and/or chest pain. This syndrome, termed, *hypertensive hypertrophic cardiomyopathy of the elderly*, has been increasingly recognized since it was first described. Because it often presents with symptoms and signs of HF, it represents an early description of HHF. In addition, it shares features with classical hypertrophic cardiomyopathy with systolic anterior motion of the mitral valve and dynamic obstruction of the left ventricular outflow tract that may be exacerbated by intravascular volume contraction and vasodilators, occasionally leading to hypotension and/or syncope.

DIAGNOSIS

With the caveats discussed previously, the diagnosis of HHF rests on the constellation of typical symptoms and signs of HF in conjunction with a diagnosis of HTN and evidence for left ventricular hypertrophy on electrocardiogram or echocardiography. Among elderly patients with poor functional status or cognitive impairment, the classical symptoms of HF may be obfuscated, and a high index of suspicion must be maintained in order to avoid under-diagnosis, under-treatment, and poorer outcomes.

The differential diagnosis of HHF includes other etiologies of HF, such as ischemic heart disease, valvular heart disease, and HF attributable to medications (eg, trastuzumab, thiazolinediones, and some antiarrhythmic drugs). In addition, HF due to amyloid cardiomyopathy, which becomes increasingly common at older age, may be difficult to distinguish from HHF, yet the distinction is important as new agents become available to treat subtypes of amyloid heart disease.[28]

MANAGEMENT

HHF in the very old typically occurs in the context of 1 or more coexisting chronic conditions and, in many cases, concomitant geriatric syndromes, such as cognitive, functional, and sensory impairments (especially visual and hearing deficits), polypharmacy, falls, incontinence, and frailty, all of which complicate the management of HF.[29] It is, therefore, essential that the approach to management be patient centered rather than focused on any specific disease. Optimal treatment thus begins with a holistic assessment of a patient's health care goals and preferences—that is, what is important to the patient and what does the patient hope to accomplish—and what are the principal barriers that must be overcome to achieve those goals? For example, many older patients identify maintaining independence and avoiding being a burden as major goals. Potential health barriers to achieving these goals may include HF but also may include arthritis, chronic obstructive pulmonary disease (COPD), and Parkinson disease. Arthritis and Parkinson disease may impose more limitations to a sedentary older adult than HF or COPD. Therefore, therapy should be directed primarily at a patient's arthritis and Parkinson disease, with HF and COPD taking a back seat. Because nonsteroidal anti-inflammatory drugs are a first-line treatment of arthritis, they become a rational therapy to achieve a patient's goals, even though they are anathema to conventional HF management.

Embedded in patient-centered care is the precept of shared decision making—a process whereby patients, family/significant others, and health care providers work together to decide the most desirable course of action for achieving a patient's personal goals. This often involves trade-offs, both for patients and providers. For older patients with HF and multimorbidity, it usually is not possible to maximize both length of life and quality of life, so patients have to make some compromises. For the provider, optimizing disease-centered care of HHF through aggressive control of blood pressure and volume status may lead to significant side effects (eg, orthostatic hypotension and urinary incontinence) that substantially diminish quality of life, thus mandating a less aggressive approach.

With this background, the management of HHF in the very old is similar to the management of this condition in younger individuals and to the management of HF in general, with particular attention to effective blood pressure control. Other comorbidities and behaviors, such as obesity, obstructive sleep apnea, smoking, and sedentary lifestyle, should be addressed in accordance with current guidelines.

Because HFpEF is the predominant phenotype of HHF in the elderly, especially in women and blacks, pharmacotherapeutic options of proved benefit are limited. Despite multiple clinical trials testing a wide range of medications with diverse mechanisms of action in patients with HFpEF, to date no agents have been shown to reduce mortality (**Table 1**), and the effect of these therapies on other outcomes, including hospitalizations, quality of life, and exercise tolerance, has been modest. In the TOPCAT trial, however, spironolactone was associated with a significant 17% reduction in hospitalizations for HF (P = .04).[30] Moreover, in a post hoc analysis of patients enrolled in North and South America, spironolactone was associated with an

Table 1
Major trials for heart failure with preserved ejection fraction

	Agent	N	Age(y)	Mortality
CHARM-Preserved	Candesartan	3023	67 ± 11	No effect
I-PRESERVE	Irbesartan	4128	72 ± 7	No effect
PEP-CHF	Perindopril	850	75 (72–79)	No effect
SENIORS	Nebivolol	2128	76 ± 5	No effect
DIG-Ancillary	Digoxin	988	67 ± 10	No effect
RELAX	Sildenafil	216	69 (62–77)	No effect
Aldo-DHF	Spironolactone	422	67 ± 8	No effect
TOPCAT	Spironolactone	3445	69 (61–76)	No effect
ESS-DHF	Sitaxsentan	192	65 ± 10	No effect

Abbreviations: Aldo-DHF, Effect of Spironolactone on Diastolic Function and Exercise Capacity in Patients with Heart Failure With Preserved Ejection Fraction; CHARM-Preserved, Effects of Candesartan in Patients with Chronic Heart Failure and Preserved Left-Ventricular Ejection Fraction; DIG-Ancillary, Effects of Digoxin on Morbidity and Mortality in Diastolic Heart Failure: The Ancillary Digitalis Investigation Group Trial; ESS-DHF, Effectiveness of Sitaxsentan Sodium in Patients with Diastolic HF; I-PRESERVE, Irbesartan in Patients with Heart Failure and Preserved Ejection Fraction; PEP-CHF, Perindopril in Elderly People with Chronic Heart Failure; RELAX, Phosphdiesterase-5 Inhibition to Improve Clinical Status and Exercise Capacity in diastolic Heart Failure; SENIORS, Randomized Trial to Determine the Effect of Nebivolol on Mortality and Cardiovascular Hospital Admission in Elderly Patients with Heart Failure; TOPCAT, Treatment of Preserved Cardiac Function Heart Failure With an Aldosterone Antagonist.

18% reduction in the primary outcome (cardiovascular death, aborted cardiac arrest, hospitalization for HF; $P = .026$), a 26% reduction in cardiovascular mortality ($P = .027$), and a nonsignificant 17% reduction in all-cause mortality ($P = .08$).[31] Thus, in the absence of other proved therapies, spironolactone is a reasonable choice for appropriately selected patients with HFpEF and by extension older adults with HHF. Older patients treated with mineralocorticoid antagonists are at increased risk for worsening renal function and hyperkalemia; therefore, close monitoring of serum creatinine and potassium is advised, especially during initiation and dose titration. In addition, dosage reduction is recommended in patients with creatinine clearance 30 mL/min to 50 mL/min, and these agents are contraindicated in patients with creatinine clearance less than 30 mL/min.

The combination of sacubitril, a neprolysin inhibitor, and valsartan, an angiotensin receptor blocker has been shown to reduce mortality and hospitalizations and improve quality of life in patients with HFrEF.[32] The Efficacy and Safety of LCZ696 Compared to Valsartan, on Morbidity and Mortality in Heart Failure Patients with Preserved Ejection Fraction (PARAGON-HF) trial is testing sacubitril-valsartan in patients with HFpEF, and results of this trial are anticipated in late 2019.[33]

PROGNOSIS

Overall 5-year mortality among patients with HF approaches 50%, but it exceeds 75% in those over 85 years of age.[34,35] Data on outcomes and prognosis of HHF in older adults are unavailable. Age is a strong independent predictor, however, of decreased survival in patients with either HFrEF or HFpEF. This reflects both the inherent decline in life expectancy with age and the impact of cardiac and noncardiac comorbidity. Coronary artery disease, atrial fibrillation, peripheral arterial disease, diabetes mellitus, chronic kidney disease, cognitive dysfunction, and frailty all increase in prevalence with age and are associated with increased mortality in patients with HF. Women with HF tend to have better survival than men, in part due to lower prevalence of ischemic heart disease, but women tend to have more symptoms and greater impairment in exercise tolerance and quality of life. Mortality rates for HFpEF are somewhat lower than those for HFrEF, but symptoms, quality of life, and hospitalization rates do not differ between the 2 phenotypes. Among patients with HFrEF, however, a majority of deaths and hospitalizations are due to cardiac causes, whereas in patients with HFpEF, most deaths and hospitalizations are unrelated to HF. Thus, a majority of elderly patients with HHF do not die from HF.

PREVENTION

Prevention of HHF centers on prevention of HTN (ie, primordial prevention) and on primary prevention of progression from stage A HF (risk factors for HF, such as HTN) to stage B HF (asymptomatic structural abnormalities, such as left ventricular

Table 2
Major hypertension trials in older adults—risk reduction percentages

Trials	N	Age(y)	CVA (%)	CAD (%)	CHF (%)	All CVD (%)
Australian	582	60–69	33	18	NR	31
EWPHE	840	>60	36	20	22	29
Coope	884	60–79	42	−3	32	24
STOP-HTN	1627	70–84	47	13	51	40
MRC	4396	65–74	25	19	NR	17
HDFP	2374	60–69	44	15	NR	16
SHEP	4736	≥60	33	27	55	32
SYST-Eur	4695	≥60	42	26	36	31
STONE	1632	60–79	57	6	68	60
SYST-China	2394	≥60	38	33	38	37
HYVET	3845	≥80	30	28	64	34
SPRINT	9361	≥50	11	12	33	25

Abbreviations: CAD, coronary artery disease; CHF, congestive HF; CVA, cerebrovascular accident; CVD, cardiovascular disease; EWPHE, European Working Party on High Blood Pressure in Elderly; HDFP, Hypertension Detection and Follow-Up Program; MRC, Medical Research Council; NR, No reduction; SHEP, Systolic Hypertension in the Elderly Program; STONE, Shanghai Trial if Nifedipine in the Elderly; STOP-HTN, Swedish Trial in Old Patients with Hypertension; SYST-China, Systolic Hypertension in China; SYST-Eur, Systolic Hypertension in Europe.

hypertrophy), and from stage B HF to stage C HF (symptomatic HF). These issues are discussed in detail elsewhere in this monograph and briefly summarized in this article. Primordial prevention of HTN involves maintaining healthy behaviors throughout life, including a healthy diet low in sodium, regular aerobic exercise, optimal body weight, and avoiding tobacco products and excess sedentary activity. Although these behaviors do not prevent cardiovascular aging, there is evidence that regular exercise attenuates the effects of aging on vascular stiffness,[36] which plays

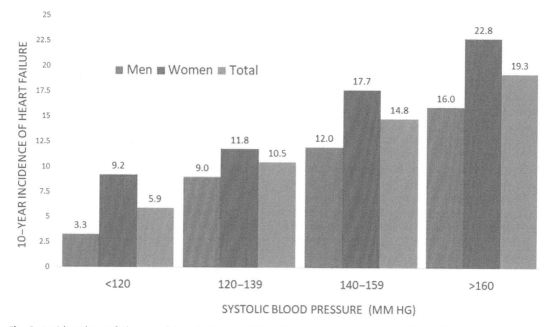

Fig. 3. Incident heart failure in older adults by systolic blood pressure and gender. (*Data from* Butler J, Kalogeropoulos AP, Georgiopoulou VV, et al. Systolic blood pressure and incident heart failure in the elderly. The Cardiovascular Health Study and the Health, Ageing and Body Composition Study. Heart 2011;97(16):1304-11.)

a fundamental role in the age-dependent rise in systolic blood pressure.

Primary prevention of progression from stage A HHF and stage B HHF to stage C HHF is predicated on effective treatment of HTN. As shown in **Table 2**, numerous randomized trials provide compelling evidence that even modest reductions in blood pressure substantially reduce the incidence of HF over relatively short-term follow-up. Similarly, **Fig. 3** illustrates a stepwise increase in incident HF with increasing systolic blood pressure among older adults in the Cardiovascular Health Study.[37,38] In the Hypertension in the Very Elderly Trial (HYVET), which enrolled 3845 patients greater than or equal to 80 years of age, treatment with indapamide and perindopril (if needed) was associated with a 64% reduction in new HF events relative to placebo.[39] More recently, in the Systolic Blood Pressure Intervention Trial (SPRINT), more intensive treatment of HTN, to a target of 120 mm Hg, was associated with a 33% reduction in incident HF overall and a 38% reduction among the 2636 patients greater than or equal to 75 years of age, relative to the conventional treatment target of 140 mm Hg.[40] Although the potential benefit of even more aggressive treatment of HTN is unknown, in older adults enrolled in SPRINT, more intensive treatment was associated with increased risk for hypotension, syncope, worsening renal function, and electrolyte abnormalities but not injurious falls. Thus, the benefits of aggressive reduction of blood pressure in older adults must be weighed against the potential for serious adverse events.

SUMMARY

Age-related vascular stiffness fosters a rise in systolic blood pressure with age, which in turn contributes to the rising prevalence of HTN and HHF in older adults. The presentation of HHF is the very old often is atypical and may be confounded by the presence of multimorbidity and geriatric syndromes. Similarly, aging has an impact on the sensitivity and specificity of most diagnostic tests for HF, as a result of which HF is both over-diagnosed and under-diagnosed in elderly individuals. Management of HHF in older adults is similar to that in younger patients but must be patient centered and consider a patient's clinical milieu and personal health care goals and preferences. Because most patients with HHF have HFpEF, there is a paucity of proved therapies, and treatment is directed primarily at control of blood pressure and management of other comorbidities (eg, coronary artery disease and atrial fibrillation). The prognosis for all forms of HF declines with age but is somewhat better in women than in men and in patients with HFpEF compared with HFrEF. Although it is likely that more effective therapies for the treatment of HHF will be developed, prevention of HHF by reducing the prevalence of HTN and ameliorating the progression from HTN to HF holds the greatest promise for limiting the impact of HHF on the health and well-being of older adults as well as its societal costs.

REFERENCES

1. Benjamin EJ, Muntner P, Alonso A, et al. Heart disease and stroke statistics-2019 update: a report from the American Heart Association. Circulation 2019;139(10):e56–528.
2. Fryar CD, Ostchega Y, Hales CM, et al. Hypertension prevalence and control among adults: United States, 2015-2016. NCHS Data Brief 2017;(289):1–8.
3. Whelton PK, Carey RM, Aronow WS, et al. 2017 ACC/AHA/AAPA/ABC/ACPM/AGS/APhA/ASH/ASPC/NMA/PCNA guideline for the prevention, detection, evaluation, and management of high blood pressure in adults: executive summary: A Report of the American College of Cardiology/American Heart Association Task Force on Clinical Practice Guidelines. Circulation 2018;138(17):e426–83.
4. Sahle BW, Owen AJ, Wing LM, et al. Prediction of 10-year risk of incident heart failure in elderly hypertensive population: the ANBP2 study. Am J Hypertens 2017;30(1):88–94.
5. Kenchaiah S, Vasan RS. Heart failure in women–insights from the Framingham Heart Study. Cardiovasc Drugs Ther 2015;29(4):377–90.
6. Levy D, Larson MG, Vasan RS, et al. The progression from hypertension to congestive heart failure. JAMA 1996;275(20):1557–62.
7. Gottdiener JS, Arnold AM, Aurigemma GP, et al. Predictors of congestive heart failure in the elderly: the Cardiovascular Health Study. J Am Coll Cardiol 2000;35(6):1628–37.
8. Paneni F, Diaz Cañestro C, Libby P, et al. The aging cardiovascular system: understanding it at the cellular and clinical levels. J Am Coll Cardiol 2017;69(15):1952–67.
9. Zieman SJ, Melenovsky V, Kass DA. Mechanisms, pathophysiology, and therapy of arterial stiffness. Arterioscler Thromb Vasc Biol 2005;25(5):932–43.
10. Dao HH, Essalihi R, Bouvet C, et al. Evolution and modulation of age-related medial elastocalcinosis: impact on large artery stiffness and isolated systolic hypertension. Cardiovasc Res 2005;66(2):307–17.
11. McEniery CM, Wilkinson IB, Avolio AP. Age, hypertension and arterial function. Clin Exp Pharmacol Physiol 2007;34(7):665–71.
12. Franklin SS, Gustin W 4th, Wong ND, et al. Hemodynamic patterns of age-related changes in blood

pressure. The Framingham Heart Study. Circulation 1997;96(1):308–15.

13. Viau DM, Sala-Mercado JA, Spranger MD, et al. The pathophysiology of hypertensive acute heart failure. Heart 2015;101(23):1861–7.

14. Eckhouse SR, Spinale FG. Changes in the myocardial interstitium and contribution to the progression of heart failure. Heart Fail Clin 2012;8(1):7–20.

15. Lakatta EG. Myocardial adaptations in advanced age. Basic Res Cardiol 1993;88(Suppl 2):125–33.

16. Ferrara N, Komici K, Corbi G, et al. β-adrenergic receptor responsiveness in aging heart and clinical implications. Front Physiol 2014;4:396.

17. Wolsk E, Bakkestrøm R, Thomsen JH, et al. The influence of age on hemodynamic parameters during rest and exercise in healthy individuals. JACC Heart Fail 2017;5(5):337–46.

18. Feher A, Broskova Z, Bagi Z. Age-related impairment of conducted dilation in human coronary arterioles. Am J Physiol Heart Circ Physiol 2014;306(12): H1595–601.

19. Bowling CB, Feller MA, Mujib M, et al. Relationship between stage of kidney disease and incident heart failure in older adults. Am J Nephrol 2011;34(2): 135–41.

20. Georgiopoulou VV, Kalogeropoulos AP, Psaty BM, et al. Lung function and risk for heart failure among older adults: the Health ABC Study. Am J Med 2011; 124(4):334–41.

21. Franchini M. Hemostasis and aging. Crit Rev Oncol Hematol 2006;60(2):144–51.

22. Krumholz HM, Larson M, Levy D. Sex differences in cardiac adaptation to isolated systolic hypertension. Am J Cardiol 1993;72(3):310–3.

23. de Simone G, Palmieri V, Bella JN, et al. Association of left ventricular hypertrophy with metabolic risk factors: the HyperGEN study. J Hypertens 2002; 20(2):323–31.

24. Kizer JR, Arnett DK, Bella JN, et al. Differences in left ventricular structure between black and white hypertensive adults: the Hypertension Genetic Epidemiology Network study. Hypertension 2004;43(6): 1182–8.

25. Bayes-Genis A, de Antonio M, Vila J, et al. Head-to-head comparison of 2 myocardial fibrosis biomarkers for long- term heart failure risk stratification: ST2 versus galectin-3. J Am Coll Cardiol 2014;63(2): 158–66.

26. deFilippi CR, de Lemos JA, Christenson RH, et al. Association of serial measures of cardiac troponin T using a sensitive assay with incident heart failure and cardiovascular mortality in older adults. JAMA 2010;304(22):2494–502.

27. Topol EJ, Traill TA, Fortuin NJ. Hypertensive hypertrophic cardiomyopathy of the elderly. N Engl J Med 1985;312(5):277–83.

28. Maurer MS, Schwartz JH, Gundapaneni B, et al. Tafamidis treatment for patients with transthyretin amyloid cardiomyopathy. N Engl J Med 2018;379(11): 1007–16.

29. Joseph SM, Rich MW. Targeting frailty in heart failure. Curr Treat Options Cardiovasc Med 2017; 19(4):31.

30. Pitt B, Pfeffer MA, Assmann SF, et al. Spironolactone for heart failure with preserved ejection fraction. N Engl J Med 2014;370(15):1383–92.

31. Pfeffer MA, Claggett B, Assmann SF, et al. Regional variation in patients and outcomes in the Treatment of Preserved Cardiac Function Heart Failure With an Aldosterone Antagonist (TOPCAT) trial. Circulation 2015;131(1):34–42.

32. McMurray JJ, Packer M, Desai AS, et al. Angiotensin-neprilysin inhibition versus enalapril in heart failure. N Engl J Med 2014;371(11):993–1004.

33. Solomon SD, Rizkala AR, Gong J, et al. Angiotensin receptor neprilysin inhibition in heart failure with preserved ejection fraction: rationale and design of the PARAGON-HF trial. JACC Heart Fail 2017;5(7): 471–82.

34. Levy D, Kenchaiah S, Larson MG, et al. Long-term trends in the incidence of and survival with heart failure. N Engl J Med 2002;347(18):1397–402.

35. Croft JB, Giles WH, Pollard RA, et al. Heart failure survival among older adults in the United States: a poor prognosis for an emerging epidemic in the Medicare population. Arch Intern Med 1999;159(5): 505–10.

36. Endes S, Schaffner E, Caviezel S, et al. Long-term physical activity is associated with reduced arterial stiffness in older adults: longitudinal results of the SAPALDIA cohort study. Age Ageing 2016;45(1): 110–5.

37. Iyer AS, Ahmed MI, Filippatos GS, et al. Uncontrolled hypertension and increased risk for incident heart failure in older adults with hypertension: findings from a propensity-matched prospective population study. J Am Soc Hypertens 2010;4(1):22–31.

38. Butler J, Kalogeropoulos AP, Georgiopoulou VV, et al. Systolic blood pressure and incident heart failure in the elderly. The Cardiovascular Health Study and the Health, Ageing and Body Composition Study. Heart 2011;97(16):1304–11.

39. Beckett NS, Peters R, Fletcher AE, et al. Treatment of hypertension in patients 80 years of age or older. N Engl J Med 2008;358(18):1887–98.

40. Williamson JD, Supiano MA, Applegate WB, et al. Intensive vs standard blood pressure control and cardiovascular disease outcomes in adults aged >=75 years: a randomized clinical trial. JAMA 2016;315(24):2673–82.

Hypertension in the Cardio-Oncology Clinic

Lauren J. Hassen, MD, MPH[a],*, Daniel J. Lenihan, MD, FESC[b],
Ragavendra R. Baliga, MD, MBA, FRCP[c]

KEYWORDS

- Hypertension • Cardio-oncology • Cardiotoxicity • Heart failure
- Vascular endothelial growth factor signaling pathway inhibitor

KEY POINTS

- Hypertension is common in patients with cancer and survivors, and it contributes to their elevated long term risk of cardiovascular disease.
- Patients with cancer should undergo pretreatment risk assessment to identify preexisting hypertension and to help predict the risk of developing of hypertension with therapy.
- Hypertension in patients with cancer and survivors should be defined and managed similarly to its management in the general population to reduce risk of ventricular dysfunction and other forms of cardiovascular disease.

INTRODUCTION

Mortality rates from cancer have steadily decreased over the last 25 years, owed largely to both earlier detection and improvements in efficacy and specificity of cancer therapies.[1] As of 2012, there were 13.7 million survivors of cancer living in the United States, and that number is projected to increase to 18 million by 2022.[2] Prolonged survival from malignancies has led to increased scrutiny of the downstream effects of these cancer therapeutics. Cardiovascular toxicity is widely recognized as a possible consequence of many pharmacologic agents used to treat cancers, and cardiovascular disease (CVD) is the

leading nonmalignant cause of morbidity and mortality in survivors of cancer.[3] Patients may experience exacerbation of underlying CVD or may develop new disease as a result of their treatment, even decades later. Additionally, the use of multiple therapeutic agents in combination may create additive or synergistic toxic effects on the cardiovascular system. As a result, pediatric and adult patients with cancer require risk factor assessment in advance of their therapy, as well as close monitoring throughout the course of treatment and survivorship.

Cardiovascular toxicity related to cancer therapies can arise in many different forms. Reported effects include hypertension, left ventricular

Disclosure Statement: Dr L.J. Hassen has nothing to disclose. Dr D.J. Lenihan reports relationships with Pfizer, Roche, and Prothena and has received research funding from Myocardial Solutions. Dr R.R. Baliga reports relationships with the following: American College of Cardiology, Elsevier Publishing, Oxford University Press, Springer Publishing Company, MasterMedFacts.com, Wolters Kluwer, and McGraw Hill Education.
[a] Department of Internal Medicine, The Ohio State University Wexner Medical Center, 395 West 12th Avenue, 3rd Floor, Columbus, OH 43210-1267, USA; [b] Cardiovascular Division, John T. Milliken Department of Internal Medicine, Cardio-Oncology Center of Excellence, Washington University School of Medicine in St. Louis, 660 South Euclid Avenue, Campus Box 8086, St Louis, MO 63110, USA; [c] Division of Cardiovascular Medicine, Department of Internal Medicine, The Ohio State University College of Medicine, Cardio-Oncology Center of Excellence, The Ohio State University Wexner Medical Center, 473 West 12th Avenue, 200 DHLRI, Columbus, OH 43210-1267, USA
* Corresponding author.
E-mail address: lauren.hassen@osumc.edu

Heart Failure Clin 15 (2019) 487–495
https://doi.org/10.1016/j.hfc.2019.06.010
1551-7136/19/© 2019 Elsevier Inc. All rights reserved.

dysfunction, ischemia caused by vasospastic and thromboembolic etiologies, Q-T interval prolongation, and a variety of arrhythmias. Toxicities can occur acutely, develop subclinically over time, or present themselves decades later. Hypertension is the common comorbidity in reported cancer registries[4,5] and in fact may be higher in survivors of cancer than in the general population, in part as a result of the shared pathways to CVD and cancer[6] (**Fig. 1**).

DEFINITIONS AND EPIDEMIOLOGY

The 2017 guidelines from the American College of Cardiology and American Heart Association (AHA) define hypertension as a systolic blood pressure (SBP) of greater than 130 and/or a diastolic BP of greater than 80. More specifically, an SBP of 130 to 139 mm Hg and/or a diastolic BP of 80 to 89 mm Hg is defined as stage 1 hypertension, whereas an SBP greater than 140 mm Hg and/or a diastolic BP greater than 90 mm Hg is defined as stage 2 hypertension.[7] The BP should be checked in both arms (unless contraindicated by lymphedema or other impairments), given that unilateral subclavian steal can be seen in patients treated with mediastinal or neck irradiation.[8] The guidelines encourage the use of ambulatory BP monitoring as a means to avoid a diagnosis of hypertension that is merely related to the medical setting.

The National Cancer Institute also publishes Common Terminology Criteria for Adverse Events.[9] **Table 1** grades the severity of hypertension occurring as an effect of antineoplastic therapies; pediatric and adolescent criteria are defined also, but excluded here. The grading system is primarily used by oncologists to streamline the documentation of adverse events in the literature for novel therapies.

The incidence and prevalence of hypertension in adolescent and adult survivors of cancer is increased compared with the general population.[10,11] In a retrospective study of more than 5600 adolescent and young adult survivors of cancer, Chao and colleagues[12] identified hypertension in 11.4% of patients, significantly higher than the 7.4% of patients with hypertension in the comparison group. Gibson and colleagues[13] characterized the BP status of more than 3000 adult survivors of childhood cancers who were at least 10 years from diagnosis. The prevalence of hypertension in the study population was 2.6-fold higher among childhood survivors of cancer than expected, based on age-, sex-, race, and body mass index-specific rates in the general population, per National Health and Nutrition Examination Survey data. It should be noted that studies predating the 2017 American College of Cardiology/AHA BP guidelines may underestimate the number of patients with hypertension, because the recent guidelines include a more liberal definition of hypertension than has been previously used.

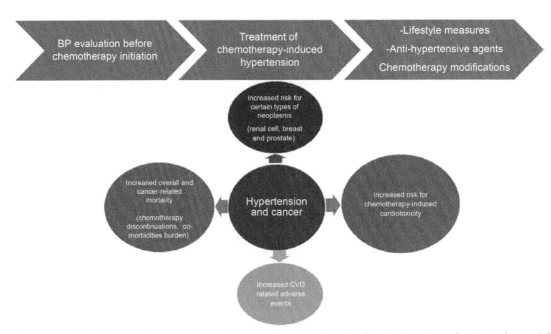

Fig. 1. Association between hypertension and cancer. (*From* Katsi V, Magkas N, Georgiopoulos G, et al. Arterial hypertension in patients under antineoplastic therapy: a systematic review. J Hypertens. 2019;37(5):887; with permission.)

Table 1
Severity of hypertension in adults, occurring as an effect of antineoplastic therapies, per the common terminology criteria for adverse events

Grade 1	Grade 2	Grade 3	Grade 4	Grade 5
Systolic BP 120–139 mm Hg or diastolic BP 80–89 mm Hg	Systolic BP 140–159 mm Hg or diastolic BP 90–99 mm Hg if previously within normal limits; change in baseline medical intervention indicated; recurrent or persistent (≥24 h); symptomatic increase by >20 mm Hg (diastolic) or to >140/90 mm Hg; monotherapy indicated initiated	Systolic BP ≥160 mm Hg or diastolic BP ≥100 mm Hg; medical intervention indicated; more than one drug or more intensive therapy than previously used indicated	Life threatening consequences (eg, malignant hypertension, transient or permanent neurologic deficit, hypertensive crisis); urgent intervention indicated	Death

From National Cancer Institute. Common terminology criteria for adverse events. Available at: https://ctep.cancer.gov/protocolDevelopment/electronic_applications/docs/CTCAE_v5_Quick_Reference_8.5x11.pdf.

CAUSATIVE AGENTS

Several different classes of antineoplastic agents have been linked to the development of hypertension in patients with cancer and survivors.

Vascular Endothelial Growth Factor Signaling Pathway Inhibitors

Angiogenesis, the formation of new blood vessels, is a necessary part of tumor growth; therefore, angiogenesis inhibition is an attractive target for the treatment of a variety of solid tumor malignancies. Therapeutics in this class exert their effect through inhibition of a component of the vascular endothelial growth factor (VEGF) signaling pathway (VSP). For example, the monoclonal antibodies bevacizumab and ramucirumab directly inhibit the attachment of VEGF to its target receptor via its ligand. By contrast, tyrosine kinase inhibitors hinder angiogenesis by inhibiting small molecules that would typically be activated by the attachment of VEGF to its receptor. Tyrosine kinase inhibitors include sunitinib, sorafenib, and pazopanib, among many others.

VSP inhibitors likely cause cardiovascular injury through a number of different mechanisms. One such proposed mechanism is the suppression of the nitric oxide pathway. VEGF activation induces the expression of nitric oxide synthase in endothelial cells, which promotes vasodilation; the inhibition of this pathway thus suppresses the nitric oxide pathway and induces hypertension. Increases in circulating levels of endothelin-1, a potent vasoconstrictor, is thought to contribute. Parallel losses of capillary circulation in both tumor and nontumor tissue likely play a role as well.[14–17]

Angiogenesis inhibitors are perhaps the class of antineoplastic agents for which an adverse effect of hypertension is most well-established. Hypertension has been reported as an adverse effect for every available agent, in addition to thromboembolic events, myocardial ischemia, left ventricular dysfunction, heart failure, and Q-T interval prolongation.[14,15,18,19] Abdel-Qadir and colleagues[19] performed a review and meta-analysis of 77 phase III and IV clinical trials of 11 VSP inhibitors, and using adverse event data, found that they were significantly associated with a high risk of hypertension (odds ratio, 5.28). Underscoring the relationship, VSP inhibitors were also associated with a high risk of the development of severe hypertension, defined by the authors as grade 3 or higher (see **Table 1**), with an odds ratio of 5.59.[19] A recent study reported that preexisting hypertension, age, and body mass index identify patients at risk for significant anti-VEGF therapy-induced BP elevation.[20] It has been suggested that elevated BP may be a clinical biomarker of efficacy of anti-VEGF therapies in malignancy.[20]

Hypertension is a common adverse effect in patients who are treated with bevacizumab, sorafenib, and sunitinib.[21] The reported incidence of hypertension ranges from 25% with sunitinib,[22] sorafenib,[23] and vandetanib[24] to 40% with axitinib[25] and pazopanib.[24] Also, several case reports have described acute hypertensive complications of therapy, including malignant hypertension[26] and posterior reversible encephalopathy syndrome, with anti-VEGF therapies.

The Cardiovascular Toxicities Panel of the National Cancer Institute recommends pretreatment risk assessment for patients for whom VSP inhibitors are a potential treatment option. Risk assessment should include repeated BP measurements as well as a history and physical examination, and laboratory testing as indicated for specific risk factors that put the patient at higher risk for adverse outcomes from elevated BP (**Box 1**). Identifying individuals at higher risk allows for a risk-benefit discussion between the patient and the provider, as well as careful monitoring after starting the drug. Patients who are already hypertensive before starting therapy should have antihypertensives initiated, ideally achieving target BPs before VSP inhibitors are prescribed.[15]

Vinca Alkaloids

Vinca alkaloids alone or in combination with other drugs may cause hypertension.[27] It has been suggested that these effects are due to the caspase-mediated apoptosis and inhibition of endothelial cell proliferation.[28]

Platinum Agents

Platinum-based agents such as cisplatin have been linked with hypertension, arising during treatment and decades afterward.[29] A Norwegian study of survivors of testicular cancer found that patients treated with cisplatin had significantly higher rates of hypertension (50%) than both controls and those treated with surgery and/or radiation alone. There seemed to be a dose–response relationship as well, with a trend toward higher rates of hypertension (53%) in those treated with cumulative doses greater than 850 mg/m$_2$.[30] The mechanism of toxicity is not well-described, but may be related to the well-described nephrotoxic effects of platinum-based agents[31] and direct toxicity on vascular

---

Box 1
Risk factors for adverse consequences of high BP in patients prescribed VSP inhibitors

Systolic BP $\geq$ 160 mm Hg or diastolic BP $\geq$ 100 mm Hg

Diabetes mellitus

Established CV disease including any history of:

  Ischemic stroke, cerebral hemorrhage, or transient ischemic attack

  Myocardial infarction, angina, coronary revascularization, or heart failure

  Peripheral artery disease

  Retinal hemorrhages or exudates and papilledema

Established or subclinical renal disease, including:

  Microalbuminuria or proteinuria (>30 mg/24 h)

  Serum creatinine in men of greater than 1.5 mg/dL, women of greater than 1.4 mg/dL

  Calculated or estimated glomerular filtration rate of less than 60 mL/min/1.73 m^2

Subclinical organ damage previously documented by:

  ECG or echocardiogram revealing left ventricular hypertrophy

  Carotid ultrasound study revealing wall thickening or plaque

Three or more of the following CV risk factors:

  Age (men >55 y, women >65 y)

  Cigarette smoking

  Dyslipidemia as measured by:

    Total cholesterol of greater than 190 mg/dL or

    Low-density lipoprotein cholesterol of greater than 130 mg/dL or

    High-density lipoprotein cholesterol (men <40 mg/dL; women <46 mg/dL) or Triglyceride of greater than 150 mg/dL

  Fasting plasma glucose of greater than 100 mg/d

  Family history of premature CV disease (first-degree male relative age <55 y or first-degree female relative <65 y)

  Abdominal obesity male waist circumference greater than 40 in; female greater than 35 in (in persons of East Asian ancestry: male waist circumference >35 in and for women >31 in)

From Maitland ML, Bakris GL, Black HR, et al. Initial assessment, surveillance, and management of blood pressure in patients receiving vascular endothelial growth factor signaling pathway inhibitors. J Natl Cancer Inst. 2010;102(9):599; with permission.

---

endothelial cells[32,33] possibly through an anti-VEGF–mediated mechanism.[34]

Anthracyclines

Anthracyclines such as doxorubicin and daunorubicin are well-known to cause CVD, most commonly left ventricular dysfunction, with varying chronicity.[35–40] The available data do not overwhelmingly suggest that anthracyclines cause hypertension. However, hypertension seems to have a synergistic effect with anthracycline-induced cardiotoxicity, producing a higher risk of heart failure. Data from elderly individuals with diffuse large B-cell lymphoma suggested the presence of a synergistic effect

between hypertension and doxorubicin therapy.[41] A report from the Childhood Cancer Survivor Study showed that although both cardiotoxic treatments and hypertension were independently associated with an increased risk of coronary artery disease or heart failure, the combination of these factors resulted in an additive effect that yielded an 86-fold increased risk of heart failure in survivors exposed to both anthracyclines and hypertension, compared with neither factor.[11] Therefore, hypertension should be aggressively managed in these patients before, during, and after their treatment with anthracyclines to help mitigate any additional risk of the development of left ventricular dysfunction.

IMPACT OF HYPERTENSION ON CARDIOVASCULAR DISEASE RISK

As stated, survivors of cancer are at a high risk for CVD, and studies have shown that both adolescents and adult survivors are at a higher risk than comparison groups without cancer.[10,42] Available data suggest that the presence of hypertension in survivors of cancer further increases this risk,[12] as does the presence of additional CVD risk factors, in an additive fashion.[11] Armenian and colleagues[42] showed that the presence of 2 or more conventional cardiovascular risk factors (diabetes mellitus, hypertension, or dyslipidemia) in survivors of adult-onset cancers portended the highest risk of CVD when compared with those with fewer risk factors and/or without cancer diagnoses.

It is well-established that uncontrolled hypertension contributes to the development of heart failure over time, and similarly that the control of hypertension can decrease this risk.[43–46] The importance of adequate antihypertensive therapy is even greater in patients who have a history of treatment with cardiotoxic antineoplastic agents or who have received them in the past, because the combined effects of hypertension and cardiotoxicity have been reported to exponentially increase the risk of CVD.[11,41]

MANAGEMENT
Blood Pressure Targets

Given that patients with cancer and survivors of cancer are more likely than control subjects[42] to have hypertension (65.9% vs 59.5%, respectively; P<.01) and that this risk extends to more than 10 years after diagnosis, the management of hypertension requires a long-term approach. The Systolic Blood Pressure Intervention Trial (SPRINT) investigators found that treating to a target SBP of 120 resulted in reduced mortality and major cardiovascular events[45] when compared with a target of less than 140 mm Hg, in patients greater than 50 years of age with an increased cardiovascular risk (as defined by the presence of clinical or subclinical CVD, chronic kidney disease, a 10-year risk of CVD of ≥15% based on the Framingham risk score, or an age of ≥75 years). As a result, a recent AHA scientific statement[8] suggested that aggressive BP targets endorsed by the AHA/American College of Cardiology BP guidelines[7] should be considered in survivors of cancer, particularly when left ventricular function is impaired or in patients on VSP inhibitors.

There are also existing recommendations for patients with hypertension specifically resulting from VSP inhibitors. The Cardiovascular Toxicities Panel of the National Cancer Institute recommends a BP target of 140/90 mm Hg for hypertensive patients on VSP inhibitors, and also suggests an aggressive goal of 130/80 mm Hg in patients with chronic kidney disease or diabetes mellitus.[15] The Canadian Cardiovascular Society Guidelines for Evaluation and Management of Cardiovascular Complications of Cancer Therapy has issued similar recommendations.[47] Patients with BPs of 140/90 mm Hg or higher or with increases in diastolic BP of 20 mm Hg and higher from baseline should either be initiated on antihypertensive therapy, have current therapy titrated to better control, or have another agent added.[15] In general, the hypertensive effect of VSP inhibitors dissipates after the agent is discontinued, although this effect varies by the half-life of the drug.

Because survivors of cancer are known to be at higher risk of CVD, it may be prudent to consider a treatment target more in line with the SPRINT findings (<120/80 mm Hg) for some patients. However, treatment goals will ultimately depend on the individual patient's comorbid conditions, tolerance of therapy including propensity to hypotension, and other considerations, and are best determined on a case-by-case basis.

Antihypertensive Agent Selection

No specific recommendations exist for antihypertensive treatment class selection. Standard choices such as angiotensin-converting enzyme inhibitors, angiotensin II receptor blockers, calcium channel blockers, beta-blockers, and diuretics have been used. Drug selection is typically guided by the patient's comorbid conditions, such as chronic kidney disease, diabetes, or preexisting CVD such as coronary artery disease or ventricular dysfunction. Success has been reported treating VSP inhibitor-induced hypertension using calcium channel blocker as single-agent therapy.[48,49] **Fig. 2** depicts strategies for the management of hypertension before and during VSP inhibitor therapy, as suggested by Spallarossa and colleagues.

Medication interactions and compatibility deserve special consideration in this population as well, particularly for those still undergoing antineoplastic therapy regimens. Of note, nondihydropyridine calcium channel blockers inhibit CYP3A4, and should thus be avoided in patients receiving tyrosine kinase inhibitors, such as sunitinib and sorafenib.[47,50] Because sunitinib therapy is associated with left ventricular dysfunction,[51,52] it is best that angiotensin-converting enzyme inhibitors,[53] beta-blockers, or aldosterone receptor blockers be considered for management of

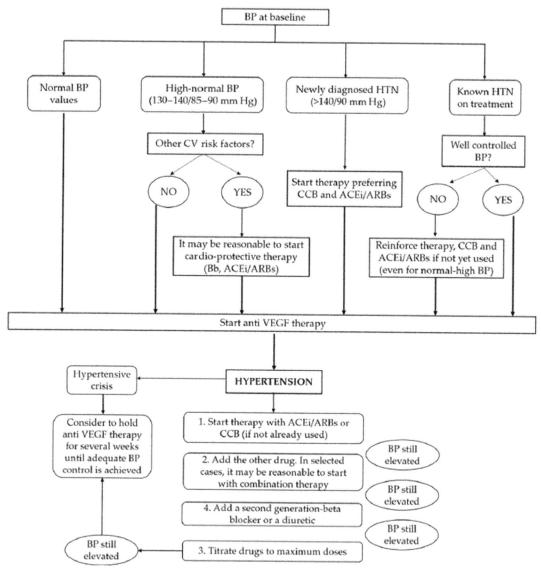

Fig. 2. Algorithm for BP management in patients receiving anti-VEGF agents. ACEi, angiotensin converting enzyme inhibitors; ARBs, angiotensin receptor blockers; Bb, beta blockers; CCB, calcium-channel blockers; CV, cardiovascular; HTN, arterial hypertension. (*From* Spallarossa P, Tini G, Lenihan D. Arterial hypertension. In: Russo A, Novo G, Lancellotti A, et al, editors. Cardiovascular complications in cancer therapy. Cham, Switzerland: Humana Press; 2019. p. 108; with permission.)

hypertension in these patients. One hypothesis-generating study[54] suggested that statin use may be associated with improved survival in patients with metastatic renal carcinoma treated in the targeted therapy era and that statins could represent an adjunct therapy for such patients.

SUMMARY

Hypertension is common in patients being treated for cancer, particularly with VSP inhibitors, and it

contributes to their increased long-term risk of CVD.[55] Therefore, patients should undergo pretreatment risk assessment to identify preexisting hypertension, and to help predict the risk of developing of hypertension with therapy. All patients, and particularly those at higher risk, warrant careful monitoring of BP throughout their therapy and after its conclusion. Incident hypertension and dyslipidemia[54] should be defined and managed similarly to its management in the general population (or one could argue, more aggressively[8]), to decrease risk of ventricular dysfunction and other forms of CVD.

REFERENCES

1. U.S. Cancer Statistics data visualizations tool. U.S. Department of Health and Human Services, Centers for Disease Control and Prevention and National Cancer Institute; 1999-2015. http://www.cdc.gov/cancer/dataviz. Accessed February 1, 2019.

2. Siegel R, DeSantis C, Virgo K, et al. Cancer treatment and survivorship statistics, 2012. CA Cancer J Clin 2012;62(4):220–41.

3. Shelburne N, Adhikari B, Brell J, et al. Cancer treatment-related cardiotoxicity: current state of knowledge and future research priorities. J Natl Cancer Inst 2014;106(9) [pii:dju232].

4. Watson GJ, Kugel MR, Shih H, et al. Cardiac comorbidities in women with metastatic breast cancer treated with doxorubicin-based and non-doxorubicin-based chemotherapy. J Clin Oncol 2009;27(15_suppl):1052.

5. Jain M, Townsend RR. Chemotherapy agents and hypertension: a focus on angiogenesis blockade. Curr Hypertens Rep 2007;9(4):320–8.

6. Koene RJ, Prizment AE, Blaes A, et al. Shared risk factors in cardiovascular disease and cancer. Circulation 2016;133(11):1104–14.

7. Whelton PK, Carey RM, Aronow WS, et al. 2017 ACC/AHA/AAPA/ABC/ACPM/AGS/APhA/ASH/ASPC/NMA/PCNA guideline for the prevention, detection, evaluation, and management of high blood pressure in adults: executive summary: a report of the American College of Cardiology/American Heart Association Task Force on Clinical Practice Guidelines. Circulation 2018;138(17):e426–83.

8. Gilchrist SC, Barac A, Ades PA, et al. Cardio-oncology rehabilitation to manage cardiovascular outcomes in cancer patients and survivors: a scientific statement from the American Heart Association. Circulation 2019;139(21):e997–1012.

9. Program NCICTE. Common terminology criteria for adverse events 2017. 5.0 ed. Available at: https://ctep.cancer.gov/protocolDevelopment/electronic_applications/ctc.htm#ctc_50.

10. Tai E, Buchanan N, Townsend J, et al. Health status of adolescent and young adult cancer survivors. Cancer 2012;118(19):4884–91.

11. Armstrong GT, Oeffinger KC, Chen Y, et al. Modifiable risk factors and major cardiac events among adult survivors of childhood cancer. J Clin Oncol 2013;31(29):3673–80.

12. Chao C, Xu L, Bhatia S, et al. Cardiovascular disease risk profiles in survivors of Adolescent and Young Adult (AYA) cancer: the Kaiser Permanente AYA cancer survivors study. J Clin Oncol 2016;34(14):1626–33.

13. Gibson TM, Li Z, Green DM, et al. Blood pressure status in adult survivors of childhood cancer: a report from the St. Jude Lifetime Cohort Study. Cancer Epidemiol Biomarkers Prev 2017;26(12):1705–13.

14. Nazer B, Humphreys BD, Moslehi J. Effects of novel angiogenesis inhibitors for the treatment of cancer on the cardiovascular system: focus on hypertension. Circulation 2011;124(15):1687–91.

15. Maitland ML, Bakris GL, Black HR, et al. Initial assessment, surveillance, and management of blood pressure in patients receiving vascular endothelial growth factor signaling pathway inhibitors. J Natl Cancer Inst 2010;102(9):596–604.

16. Hahn VS, Lenihan DJ, Ky B. Cancer therapy-induced cardiotoxicity: basic mechanisms and potential cardioprotective therapies. J Am Heart Assoc 2014;3(2):e000665.

17. de Jesus-Gonzalez N, Robinson E, Moslehi J, et al. Management of antiangiogenic therapy-induced hypertension. Hypertension 2012;60(3):607–15.

18. Steingart RM, Bakris GL, Chen HX, et al. Management of cardiac toxicity in patients receiving vascular endothelial growth factor signaling pathway inhibitors. Am Heart J 2012;163(2):156–63.

19. Abdel-Qadir H, Ethier JL, Lee DS, et al. Cardiovascular toxicity of angiogenesis inhibitors in treatment of malignancy: a systematic review and meta-analysis. Cancer Treat Rev 2017;53:120–7.

20. Hamnvik OP, Choueiri TK, Turchin A, et al. Clinical risk factors for the development of hypertension in patients treated with inhibitors of the VEGF signaling pathway. Cancer 2015;121(2):311–9.

21. Yeh ET, Bickford CL. Cardiovascular complications of cancer therapy: incidence, pathogenesis, diagnosis, and management. J Am Coll Cardiol 2009;53(24):2231–47.

22. Zhu X, Stergiopoulos K, Wu S. Risk of hypertension and renal dysfunction with an angiogenesis inhibitor sunitinib: systematic review and meta-analysis. Acta Oncol 2009;48(1):9–17.

23. Wu S, Chen JJ, Kudelka A, et al. Incidence and risk of hypertension with sorafenib in patients with cancer: a systematic review and meta-analysis. Lancet Oncol 2008;9(2):117–23.

24. Qi WX, Shen Z, Lin F, et al. Incidence and risk of hypertension with vandetanib in cancer patients: a systematic review and meta-analysis of clinical trials. Br J Clin Pharmacol 2013;75(4):919–30.

25. Qi WX, He AN, Shen Z, et al. Incidence and risk of hypertension with a novel multi-targeted kinase inhibitor axitinib in cancer patients: a systematic review and meta-analysis. Br J Clin Pharmacol 2013;76(3):348–57.

26. Caro J, Morales E, Gutierrez E, et al. Malignant hypertension in patients treated with vascular endothelial growth factor inhibitors. J Clin Hypertens (Greenwich) 2013;15(3):215–6.

27. Stoter G, Koopman A, Vendrik CP, et al. Ten-year survival and late sequelae in testicular cancer patients treated with cisplatin, vinblastine, and bleomycin. J Clin Oncol 1989;7(8):1099–104.

28. Soultati A, Mountzios G, Avgerinou C, et al. Endothelial vascular toxicity from chemotherapeutic agents: preclinical evidence and clinical implications. Cancer Treat Rev 2012;38(5):473–83.

29. Meinardi MT, Gietema JA, van Veldhuisen DJ, et al. Long-term chemotherapy-related cardiovascular morbidity. Cancer Treat Rev 2000;26(6):429–47.

30. Sagstuen H, Aass N, Fosså SD, et al. Blood pressure and body mass index in long-term survivors of testicular cancer. J Clin Oncol 2005;23(22):4980–90.

31. Manohar S, Leung N. Cisplatin nephrotoxicity: a review of the literature. J Nephrol 2018;31(1):15–25.

32. Nuver J, De Haas EC, Van Zweeden M, et al. Vascular damage in testicular cancer patients: a study on endothelial activation by bleomycin and cisplatin in vitro. Oncol Rep 2010;23(1):247–53.

33. Daher IN, Yeh ET. Vascular complications of selected cancer therapies. Nat Clin Pract Cardiovasc Med 2008;5(12):797–805.

34. Kirchmair R, Walter DH, Ii M, et al. Antiangiogenesis mediates cisplatin-induced peripheral neuropathy: attenuation or reversal by local vascular endothelial growth factor gene therapy without augmenting tumor growth. Circulation 2005;111(20):2662–70.

35. Von Hoff DD, Layard MW, Basa P, et al. Risk factors for doxorubicin-induced congestive heart failure. Ann Intern Med 1979;91(5):710–7.

36. Swain SM, Whaley FS, Ewer MS. Congestive heart failure in patients treated with doxorubicin: a retrospective analysis of three trials. Cancer 2003;97(11):2869–79.

37. Cardinale D, Colombo A, Bacchiani G, et al. Early detection of anthracycline cardiotoxicity and improvement with heart failure therapy. Circulation 2015;131(22):1981–8.

38. Curigliano G, Cardinale D, Dent S, et al. Cardiotoxicity of anticancer treatments: epidemiology, detection, and management. CA Cancer J Clin 2016;66(4):309–25.

39. Domercant J, Polin N, Jahangir E. Cardio-oncology: a focused review of anthracycline-, human epidermal growth factor receptor 2 inhibitor-, and radiation-induced cardiotoxicity and management. Ochsner J 2016;16(3):250–6.

40. Agmon Nardi I, Iakobishvili Z. Cardiovascular risk in cancer survivors. Curr Treat Options Cardiovasc Med 2018;20(6):47.

41. Hershman DL, McBride RB, Eisenberger A, et al. Doxorubicin, cardiac risk factors, and cardiac toxicity in elderly patients with diffuse B-cell non-Hodgkin's lymphoma. J Clin Oncol 2008;26(19):3159–65.

42. Armenian SH, Xu L, Ky B, et al. Cardiovascular disease among survivors of adult-onset cancer: a community-based retrospective cohort study. J Clin Oncol 2016;34(10):1122–30.

43. Beckett NS, Peters R, Fletcher AE, et al. Treatment of hypertension in patients 80 years of age or older. N Engl J Med 2008;358(18):1887–98.

44. Sciarretta S, Palano F, Tocci G, et al. Antihypertensive treatment and development of heart failure in hypertension: a Bayesian network meta-analysis of studies in patients with hypertension and high cardiovascular risk. Arch Intern Med 2011;171(5):384–94.

45. Wright JT, Williamson JD, Whelton PK, et al. A randomized trial of intensive versus standard blood-pressure control. N Engl J Med 2015;373(22):2103–16.

46. Han X, Zhou Y, Liu W. Precision cardio-oncology: understanding the cardiotoxicity of cancer therapy. NPJ Precis Oncol 2017;1(1):31.

47. Virani SA, Dent S, Brezden-Masley C, et al. Canadian cardiovascular society guidelines for evaluation and management of cardiovascular complications of cancer therapy. Can J Cardiol 2016;32(7):831–41.

48. Fukumura D, Gohongi T, Kadambi A, et al. Predominant role of endothelial nitric oxide synthase in vascular endothelial growth factor-induced angiogenesis and vascular permeability. Proc Natl Acad Sci U S A 2001;98(5):2604–9.

49. Mir O, Coriat R, Ropert S, et al. Treatment of bevacizumab-induced hypertension by amlodipine. Invest New Drugs 2012;30(2):702–7.

50. Izzedine H, Derosa L, Le Teuff G, et al. Hypertension and angiotensin system inhibitors: impact on outcome in sunitinib-treated patients for metastatic renal cell carcinoma. Ann Oncol 2015;26(6):1128–33.

51. Narayan V, Keefe S, Haas N, et al. Prospective evaluation of sunitinib-induced cardiotoxicity in patients with metastatic renal cell carcinoma. Clin Cancer Res 2017;23(14):3601–9.

52. Catino AB, Hubbard RA, Chirinos JA, et al. Longitudinal assessment of vascular function with sunitinib in patients with metastatic renal cell carcinoma. Circ Heart Fail 2018;11(3):e004408.

53. McKay RR, Rodriguez GE, Lin X, et al. Angiotensin system inhibitors and survival outcomes in patients with metastatic renal cell carcinoma. Clin Cancer Res 2015;21(11):2471–9.

54. McKay RR, Lin X, Albiges L, et al. Statins and survival outcomes in patients with metastatic renal cell carcinoma. Eur J Cancer 2016;52:155–62.

55. Campia U, Moslehi JJ, Amiri-Kordestani L, et al. Cardio-oncology: vascular and metabolic perspectives: a scientific statement from the American Heart Association. Circulation 2019;139(13):e579–602.

Heart Failure in Women Due to Hypertensive Heart Disease

Jennifer Ballard-Hernandez, DNP, AACC[a], Dipti Itchhaporia, MD, FESC[b],*

KEYWORDS

- Hypertensive heart failure • Heart failure • Women • Heart failure with preserved ejection fraction
- Heart failure with reduced ejection fraction

KEY POINTS

- Heart failure (HF) is a significant cause of cardiovascular morbidity and mortality for women in the United States.
- When comparing men and women with HF, there are clear sex-specific differences in etiology, disease progression, and outcomes.
- Heart failure with preserved ejection fraction accounts for the most common type of HF in women, with hypertensive heart disease playing a pivotal role in its etiology.
- The current Heart Failure Guidelines do not endorse sex-specific recommendations for standard medical therapy of HF management.
- Women are underrepresented in HF clinical trials, leading to a lacking evidence base supporting sex-specific therapy. Further studies are needed to evaluate targeted HF therapies in women.

INTRODUCTION

Heart failure (HF) is a complex, progressive syndrome, resulting from any process that impairs the ability of the ventricles of the heart to fill and/or eject blood.[1,2] Associated with high morbidity and mortality, marked disability, high symptom burden, and poor quality of life, HF is managed by a complex therapeutic regimen of pharmacologic and nonpharmacologic therapies coupled with strict lifestyle adherence.[3–9] A common cause of HF is hypertensive heart disease, which is most notable in women. Hypertensive heart disease encompasses a wide spectrum of cardiac diseases across a continuum from clinically silent structural heart changes to the development of symptomatic HF.[10] It is recognized that untreated hypertensive heart disease ultimately leads to HF, both from diastolic and systolic dysfunction.

This review of the available literature aims to identify factors that contribute to the development of hypertensive heart failure in women and discusses interventions that may reduce morbidity and mortality for women with HF.

EPIDEMIOLOGY

HF is a common cardiovascular disease in industrialized nations, affecting an estimated 6.5 million Americans, of whom 3.6 million are women.[11] There are clear race, age, and sex-specific differences related to the development of hypertensive HF. Black women have a higher prevalence of HF than white or Hispanic women (3.9% vs 2.5% and 2.4%).[11] When compared with their male counterparts, women tend to develop HF later in life.[11] Older women have an increased incidence and prevalence of HF, particularly of HF with preserved

[a] Department of Medicine, Cardiology Division, U.S. Department of Veterans Affairs, VA Long Beach Healthcare System, 1 Hoag Drive, Newport Beach, CA 92663, USA; [b] Department of Medicine, Cardiology Division, Hoag Memorial Hospital, University of California, Irvine, Irvine, CA, USA
* Corresponding author. 520 Superior Avenue, Newport Beach, CA 92663.
E-mail address: drdipti@yahoo.com

Heart Failure Clin 15 (2019) 497–507
https://doi.org/10.1016/j.hfc.2019.06.002
1551-7136/19/© 2019 Elsevier Inc. All rights reserved.

ejection fraction (HFpEF).[11–14] Women with HF tend to have more hypertension than men.[15] A large proportion of women who are admitted to the hospital for acute decompensated HF have HFpEF, nearly twice as often as do men.[16,17]

HEART FAILURE DEFINED

Currently, HF is differentiated into subtypes by left ventricular ejection fraction (EF), functional capacity, and staging based on risk factors and abnormalities of cardiac structure.[8,18] HF with reduced ejection fraction (HFrEF) is defined as the clinical diagnosis of HF and EF ≤40%.[8] HFpEF is defined as the clinical signs or symptoms of HF, a left ventricular (LV) ejection fraction of greater than or equal to 50%, and evidence of abnormal LV diastolic dysfunction.[8] Women are affected by both HFpEF and HFrEF, although HFpEF is more prevalent in women than is HFrEF. It has been postulated that this difference is due to increased prevalence of hypertension and diastolic dysfunction in women with HF as compared with men with HF. Diastolic dysfunction is a much more common sequela of longstanding hypertension than is systolic dysfunction.[10]

RISK FACTORS

Multiple modifiable and nonmodifiable risk factors are associated with an increased risk for HF.

Nonmodifiable risk factors include age, genetics, and race. Modifiable risk factors include hypertension, obesity, diabetes mellitus, coronary artery disease, and cigarette smoking (**Fig. 1**). Interventions targeted at treating modifiable risk factors may be successful in reducing the incidence of HF in women.[19] Risk factors for HFpEF and HFrEF are similar, but because the HFpEF phenotype is heterogeneous, specific risk factors in its development include hypertension, obesity, and atrial fibrillation.[8] Hypertension is the strongest risk factor in the development of HF and precedes the development of HF in 91% of newly diagnosed cases.[20] Given the high prevalence of hypertension as a risk factor, it is an important target for HF prevention.

ETIOLOGY

Ischemic cardiomyopathy caused by occlusive coronary artery disease is widely acknowledged as the most common cause of symptomatic adult HFrEF in the United States, although prevalence data are sparse.[21] The nonischemic cardiomyopathies encompass an abundant list of diverse etiologies and include the following: hypertensive, valvular heart disease, congenital, familial, genetic, endocrine/metabolic, tachycardia-mediated, inflammatory/infectious, peripartum, and stress cardiomyopathy. Interestingly, when sex-specific characteristics are examined, the

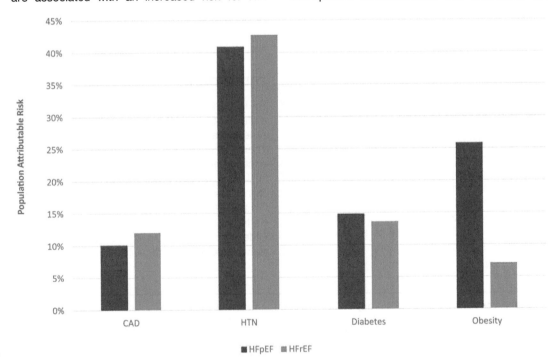

Fig. 1. Population attributable risk of comorbidities for HFrEF and HFpEF in women. (*From* Daubert MA, Douglas PS. Primary Prevention of Heart Failure in Women. JACC Heart Fail 2019;7(3):187; with permission.)

underlying etiology for HF in women is more likely to be hypertension and valvular heart disease and less likely to be coronary artery disease.[12,15,17] In the presence of hemodynamic stress, such as hypertension, the female myocardium has a tendency to remodel in a concentric pattern, whereas men tend to remodel in an eccentric pattern.[22] Another etiology of HF that is more common in women is stress cardiomyopathy.[23] Peripartum cardiomyopathy, a diagnosis that can occur up to 6 months after delivery, is an etiology of HF unique to women.

PATHOPHYSIOLOGY OF HYPERTENSIVE HEART FAILURE

A consequence of longstanding hypertensive heart disease, when left to its natural course, is progression to HF. Chronic hypertension and its associated neurohormonal stimulation ultimately leads to cardiomyocyte dysfunction, an increase in cardiac extracellular matrix causing fibrosis, and disturbance of intramyocardial microvasculature.[10] Hypertensive heart disease can progress to HF from the resultant pressure overload and/or volume overload. Sustained pressure overload results in diastolic dysfunction, where in contrast persistent volume overload results in systolic dysfunction.[24]

DIASTOLIC DYSFUNCTION

Persistent, sustained pressure overload that occurs in chronic hypertension results in the development of diastolic dysfunction and concentric

LV hypertrophy.[24] Diastolic dysfunction is often the early manifestation of many cardiac diseases and is characterized by abnormal ventricular compliance in addition to impaired relaxation.[25] As pressure overload is continual and diastolic dysfunction progresses, the LV decompensates and hypertensive HFpEF results (**Fig. 2**).[24] Diastolic dysfunction is the predominant cause of symptoms in HFpEF.[25]

SYSTOLIC DYSFUNCTION

Persistent, sustained volume overload causes eccentric hypertrophy, progressive LV dilatation, and decompensation, resulting in the development of systolic dysfunction.[24] End-stage hypertensive heart disease is typically a product of both longstanding pressure and volume overload, leading to diastolic dysfunction and reduced EF (see **Fig. 2**).

DIAGNOSIS

The tests to diagnose HF in women and men are similar, although the results may vary. Echocardiographic and other imaging of cardiac structures should take into account body surface area (BSA), as normal values for sizes of cardiac structures can differ depending on age, BSA, and gender.[26] Beale and colleagues[27] evaluated sex differences in central and peripheral factors that contribute to HFpEF pathophysiology using echocardiographic and invasive hemodynamic testing. The investigators found that women with HFpEF

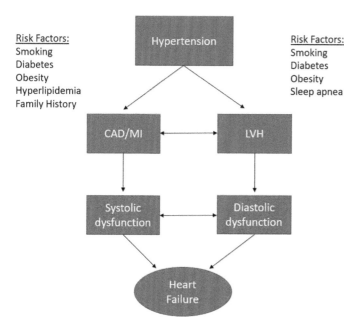

Risk Factors:
Smoking
Diabetes
Obesity
Hyperlipidemia
Family History

Risk Factors:
Smoking
Diabetes
Obesity
Sleep apnea

Fig. 2. Risk factors and progression of hypertensive HF.

demonstrate poorer diastolic reserve, higher LV filling pressures at exercise, accompanied by lower systemic and pulmonary compliance (**Fig. 3**) when compared with their male counterparts.[27] These findings highlight potential mechanisms of impaired exercise tolerance associated with HFpEF in women.

With regard to biomarkers, natriuretic peptides are usually higher in women than in men but can vary by age.[28,29] Peak V_{O_2} is usually lower for women than men.[30] This finding may be related to body weight, not body mass, as women tend to have more body fat than men.[31]

TREATMENT

HF is a deleterious disease process that affects men and women equally, with nearly 50% of patients with HF being women. However, women have been severely underrepresented in randomized clinical trials that explore sex-based differences in the efficacy of HF medication. On average, cohorts in the seminal randomized

controlled trials for HF were only 20% women. As a result, the current HF guidelines do not endorse any sex-specific recommendations with regard to standard HF therapy.

Highlighting sex-based differences is crucial not only in considering the efficacy of these therapies in women, but also because of potential differences in drug tolerance and toxicity; for example, women represent more than 60% of patients with drug-induced torsade-de-pointes. Female sex is a known to be a risk factor in developing long QT syndrome, a ventricular arrhythmia that can be induced by several different classes of drugs, for example, antipsychotics, antiarrhythmics, H1 antagonists, and antibiotics.[32]

Although there are nonpharmacologic therapies for HF that focus on comorbidities like hypertension, such as decreased salt intake and increased exercise, the most common therapeutic modalities for HF currently include renin-angiotensin blockade, beta blockade, mineralocorticoid receptor antagonists, neprilysin inhibitors, digoxin, and device therapy. Of note, these therapies

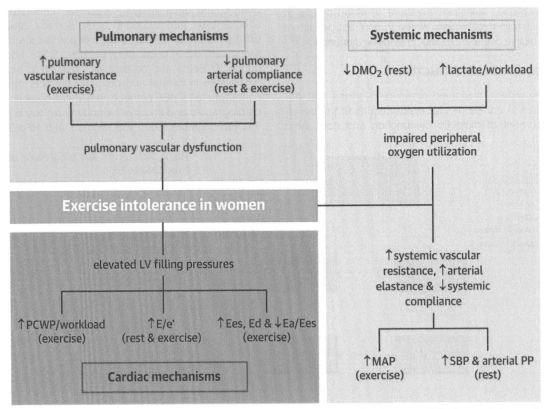

Fig. 3. Mechanisms of impaired exercise tolerance in women. DMO_2, peripheral oxygen diffusion; LV, left ventricular; MAP, mean arterial pressure; PCWP, pulmonary capillary wedge pressure; PP, pulse pressure; SBP, systolic blood pressure. (*From* Beale AL, Nanayakkara S, Segan L, et al. Sex Differences in Heart Failure With Preserved Ejection Fraction Pathophysiology: A Detailed Invasive Hemodynamic and Echocardiographic Analysis. JACC Heart Fail 2019;7(3):246; with permission.)

have been shown to be effective in the treatment of HFrEF; conversely, their efficacy in the treatment of HFpEF has been largely inconclusive.[32]

RENIN-ANGIOTENSIN BLOCKADE

Renin-angiotensin blockades in the form of either angiotensin-converting enzyme inhibitors (ACEI) or angiotensin receptor blockers (ARBs) are both used routinely in HF therapy. In general, there has been no clearly established sex-based difference in the efficacy of either ACEIs or ARBs.

Both the SOLVD (Studies of Left Ventricular Dysfunction) and CONSENSUS trials showed a consistent benefit of ACEIs in both men and women.[33,34] That said, there is evidence that ACEIs tend to be less effective in women than in men. A pooled analysis of more than 30 studies indicated that ACEIs conferred a 37% decrease in mortality for men, in contrast to a 22% decrease in women.[35] Although the etiology of this sex-specific difference is not clear, it has been postulated by Shin and colleagues,[35] that this difference may be due to a natural inhibition of the renin-angiotensin system by estrogen, thus making ACEIs less effective. In a sex-specific analysis of the ATLAS trial, which tested the efficacy of high-dose versus low-dose ACEIs, high-dose lisinopril decreased mortality or hospitalizations only in men.[36] In addition to decreased efficacy in women, ACEI treatment has been linked to increased risk of angioedema that is, especially observed in women.[32] Ultimately, the data suffer from decreased representation of women in the trials, making conclusions about the differences in efficacy and safety challenging; the ATLAS trial for example, enrolled only 20% women.

For subgroups of patients with HF who are intolerant to ACEIs, ARBs are often used. In the Valsartan Heart Failure Trial (Val-HeFT) trial, an ARB was tested against a placebo and was found to have a significant treatment effect in men only.[37] However, ARBs tested against a placebo in 3 different trials of the CHARM program did not find any difference in treatment effect between the 2 sexes.[30,38] Meta-analyses have shown a greater decrease in blood pressure with ACEIs when compared with ARBs. Whether this result translates into better outcomes in women with ACEI versus ARB has not been demonstrated.

ANGIOTENSIN-NEPRILYSIN INHIBITION

There is now evidence that the use of the novel sacubitril/valsartan combination that achieves inhibition of both neprilysin and angiotensin receptors in concert may confer more benefit to patients than does the use of ARBs alone, or even ACEIs, often considered the gold standard in HFrEF treatment. Neprilysin inhibition has been used in the past in combination with angiotensin converting enzyme (ACE) inhibition, and, although it proved superior to inhibition by either neprilysin or ACE alone, its usage was associated with significant angioedema.[39] In 2014, McMurray and colleagues,[40] in the Paradigm-HF trial, examined the efficacy of the sacubitril/valsartan compound, then known as LCZ696, compared with the ACEI enalapril in 8442 patients with New York Heart Association (NHYA) Class 2, 3, or 4 HF with an EF of less than 40% (later amended to ≤35%). The researchers found that LCZ696 outperformed enalapril in reducing the risks of death and hospitalization; compared with enalapril, LCZ696 reduced the risk of hospitalization by 21% ($P<.001$). With these observed benefits to patients with HF, in addition to minimizing the angioedema seen in neprilysin/ACE inhibition, LCZ696, sold today as Entresto, is leading the way for more effective HF treatment.

The presence of a sex-specific difference in its benefit has not yet been ascertained. A prespecified subgroup analysis of the PARADIGM-HF trial showed a beneficial effect of valsartan/sacubitril in both sexes for the composite outcome, but adverse events were not stratified by sex.[40]

BETA BLOCKERS

Underlying the recommendation for β-blocker use in HFrEF are the randomized controlled trials that include the Metoprolol CR/XL Randomized Intervention Trial-HF (MERIT-HF), CIBIS II (Cardiac Insufficiency Bisoprolol Study II), COPERNICUS, and SENIORS. Sex hormones play an important role in the regulation of beta receptors; therefore, it was expected that there may be sex-based differences in the efficacy of beta blockers in the treatment of HF.

However, in clinical trials of beta blockers in patients with HF, similar to clinical trials of other treatment modalities, there is a paucity of data with regard to women. Once again, given the low number of women in these studies, it is challenging to make any meaningful conclusions about sex-based differences. Indeed, the major trials of the efficacy of beta blockades recruited an average of 20% women, with the exception of the Beta Blocker Evaluation of Survival Trial (BEST), which stratified patients on the basis of sex; interestingly, this analysis found that in nonischemic patients, women had significantly better survival rates than did men.[41]

In addition, in the SENIORS study, which examined the effects of beta blockers on mortality and hospitalizations of elderly patients, there was a significant effect on the primary endpoint only in women.[42] However, most of the presently available data from a pooled analysis of these studies, such as the Metropolol CR/XL Randomized Intervention Trial in Heart Failure (MERIT-HF), indicates comparable decreases in mortality among both men and women.[43] However, when these studies are examined independently rather than in a pooled analysis, women often fare worse than do men with beta blockers. This fact, again, highlights the need for increased representation of women in these studies.

MINERALOCORTICOID ANTAGONISM

Mineralocorticoid receptor antagonism, with aldosterone and eplerenone, for example, has also been shown to be effective HF therapy, especially in conjunction with ACEIs or beta blockers in patients with an EF ≤35%. In 1999, Pitt and colleagues[44] found that the blockage of aldosterone receptors by spironolactone, when combined with standard therapy, markedly reduced the risk of both morbidity and death among patients with severe HF.

The basis for the guideline recommendation of treatment with aldosterone antagonists is 2 trials: the Randomized Aldactone Evaluation Study (RALES) and the Eplerenone in Mild Patients Hospitalization And Survival Study-HF (EMPHASIS-HF). Trials on the efficacy of aldosterone antagonism also suffered from underrepresentation of women. For example, RALES tested spironolactone versus placebo in 1663 patients, only 27% of whom were women.[45] Both men and women derived better survival. The EMPHASIS-HF study, which compared the benefit of eplerenone versus placebo in 2743 patients, including 22% women, with systolic HF also found a significant treatment effect on cardiovascular (CV) death or HF hospitalization in both men and women.[46]

Another trial, the Eplerenone Post-Acute Myocardial Infarction (MI) Heart Failure Efficacy and Survival Study (EPHESUS) trial, examined the benefit of eplerenone in patients with LV dysfunction and a myocardial infarction, and found a reduction of all-cause mortality in women only and a reduction of CV death or CV hospitalization in men only.[47]

Merrill and colleagues[48] performed a subgroup analysis of the TOPCAT trial examining the sex differences in outcomes and responses to spironolactone in HFpEF. No significant interaction between sex and the treatment arm in the primary TOPCAT analysis with respect to the primary outcome (death from cardiovascular cause, aborted cardiac arrest of HF hospitalization). When the investigators performed a subgroup analysis evaluating the Americas only, there was signal of possible sex-related differences in treatment response to spironolactone with respect to all-cause mortality. Caution should be applied when interpreting the investigators' findings in this secondary analysis of the TOPCAT data due to lack of statistical power.

DIGOXIN

Digoxin is used in patients with HF to reduce the risk of hospitalization. The basis for this approach was found in a 1997 investigation by the Digitalis Group Investigation, that noted a marked decrease in HF rehospitalization with digoxin.[49] Most of the data for digoxin predates the use of current guideline-directed medical therapy. Given this situation and that there is no mortality benefit with digoxin, its benefits are uncertain and its use for HF treatment has diminished and is limited.

Now, digoxin is often used as adjunct in the treatment of arrhythmias, such as atrial fibrillation and flutter. However, in women, digoxin has been shown to increase toxicity and, in some cases, mortality; the HERS trial suggested an increased cardiovascular event rate in women on digoxin and hormone replacement therapy.[50] This finding has been attributed to increased serum levels of digoxin in women compared with their male counterparts; the reasons are still uncertain. A substudy of the Digitalis Investigation Group trial showed that women with HF randomized to digoxin had a higher death rate than did women randomized to placebo. A follow-up retrospective analysis provided further insight and highlighted that this association may have been attributable to modestly higher digoxin concentrations in women than in men, which have been associated with an increased risk of death.[51] They found that women with digoxin levels of 1.2 to 2.0 ng/mL had an increase in death of 33%.[52]

ISOSORBIDE DINITRATE AND HYDRALAZINE

The efficacy of hydralazine-isosorbide dinitrate (H-ISDN) therapy for HF was established in the first V-HeFT I (Vasodilator-Heart Failure Trial) with post hoc analyses suggesting that African-American patients may particularly benefit from H-ISDN.[53–55] In the subsequent A-HeFT (African-American Heart Failure Trial), the addition of a combination pill of H-ISDN to optimal medical therapy was found to improve quality of life and to reduce HF-related hospitalizations and mortality rates similarly in both men and women.[56]

DEVICES

Advanced HF is characterized by significant impairment of cardiac function and symptom-induced activity limitation, despite optimal medical therapy. Implantable cardioverter defibrillators (ICDs) and cardiac resynchronization therapy (CRT) with a biventricular ICD or pacemaker play an important role in the management of these patients with advanced HF by treating life-threatening arrhythmias, and improving morbidity and survival.

The indications for ICDs do not have any distinctions based on sex, and outcomes are comparable in men and women. One meta-analysis of clinical trials found that mortality with ICD use did not differ significantly between men and women.[57] Despite the demonstrated benefits of these devices, the GWTG-HF registry data show that device therapy is still largely underused in both men and women; furthermore, this underuse is worse for women, who are 40% less likely to receive ICDs than men.[58] But in general, various studies have had conflicting results. For example, one study found that both men and women were equally likely to receive an ICD after referral to an electrophysiologist.[59] However, there was no information regarding the proportion of women who were referred to one.

There is some indication from clinical trials that the survival benefit from ICDs is greater in men, which may be related to the higher incidence of ischemic cardiomyopathy and ventricular tachycardia/ventricular fibrillation (VT/VF) in men. However, women have been underrepresented in clinical trials of ICD therapy, presenting difficulties in establishing any firm conclusions. At the present time, decisions on ICD implantation should not differ in men and women. As with other implantable devices, however, the complication rate is acknowledged to be somewhat higher in women.

In large, prospective, randomized multicenter analyses, CRT has been proven to improve symptoms, functional capacity, and total mortality rates, namely for patients with LVEF less than 35%, in both men and women, with little, if any, difference between the sexes.[60] That said, certain trials have found CRTs to be more effective in women compared with men,[61] even when factoring the decreased rate of usage in women.

Although current guidelines do not have any differences in indications for CRT based on sex, it is clear that, in general, women are more likely to benefit than men. The CARE-HF data indicated that CRT is more beneficial to women with HF than pharmacologic solutions alone.[60] The higher incidence of nonischemic cardiomyopathy in women may contribute to this observation. Although complication rates in women are somewhat higher than in men, the greater expected benefit in women indicates that physicians should be more willing to consider CRT implantation in women.

PROGNOSIS

Although survival after HF has improved, the death rate remains high, as 50% of patients diagnosed with HF die within 5 years.[5] The incidence of HF has declined among women in the past 50 years, but the same is not true for men. Interestingly, survival has improved for both sexes in the same period, although men have had longer survival gains in comparison with women.[5,62]

In general, women with HF tend to survive longer than their male counterparts, which is especially noted when the etiology is nonischemic.[63] When the etiology is ischemic coronary artery disease, men and women have similar survival. This finding is important because women are more likely to develop HF after a MI than in men.[6,62,63] In women with CAD, the prevalence of HF is less than that of men, even with comparable EFs. The clinical manifestation of HF is more severe in women with HFpEF; hospitalizations are not increased in comparison with men and survival is better than men.[64]

SUMMARY

Despite survival rates that have increased in the past 30 years, HF remains a significant health care concern for men and women, as the numbers of HF cases continue to grow in the United States. Given that approximately 50% of patients living with HF are women, it becomes important to understand the role that sex plays in the recognition, diagnosis, and management of HF. Distinct differences in sex hormones and their effects on cardiovascular pathophysiology likely account for the differences between women and men with HF. Women with HF tend to be older and exhibit better LV function compared with men. Women are also more likely to have hypertension, tend to be more symptomatic at presentation, and describe worse quality of life than men with similar HF disease severity. Hypertension is the most prevalent modifiable risk factor for the development of HF. Treatment of hypertension in patients with HF must take into account the type of HF that is present: systolic dysfunction with HFrEF or diastolic dysfunction with HFpEF.

Data are conflicting on whether there is a mortality difference in these 2 broad categories of HF.

Table 1
Female representation in heart failure trials

Trial	% Women Represented	LVEF, %	Therapy Evaluated
A-HeFT[56]	40	≤35	Hydralazine/isosorbide dinitrate
CHARM-Preserved[66]	40	>40	Candesartan
CIBIS II[67]	19	≤35	Bisoprolol
COMET[68]	20	≤35	Carvedilol vs metoprolol
COMPANION[69]	32	≤35	Medical therapy/pacing/defibrillation
CONSENSUS[34]	30	"Severe CHF"	Enalapril
COPERNICUS[70]	20	≤25	Carvedilol
DIG[49]	22	≤45	Digoxin
EMPHASIS-HF[71]	29	≤35	Eplerenone
MADIT II[72]	16	≤30	ICD
MERIT-HF[43]	23	≤40	Metoprolol Cr/Xl
PARADIGM-HF[40]	22	≤40	ARNI vs enalapril
RALES[44]	27	≤35	Spironolactone
SCD HeFT[73]	23	≤35	ICD
SOLVD-treatment[33]	20	≤35	Enalapril
TOPCAT[74]	51	≥45	Spironolactone
Val-HEFT[37]	20	≤40	Valsartan

Abbreviations: ICD, implantable cardioverter defibrillator; LVEF, left ventricular ejection fraction.

There is some evidence that outcomes in HFpEF differ for women and men; the I-PRESERVE trial, which specifically considered HFpEF and had an unusually high enrollment of women at 60%, showed that women are approximately 20% less likely to experience death or hospitalization compared with men, a finding similarly noted in other studies on HFpEF.[65]

The data supporting drug therapy in HFpEF are more limited than for HFrEF. HFpEF deaths are more often non-CV deaths compared with HFrEF deaths. Most treatments given to patients with HFpEF are aimed at symptoms, risk factors, comorbidities, and blood pressure control using ACE inhibitors, ARBs, and beta blockers. Therapeutic treatment for HFrEF has enabled important progress both in terms of disease progression and mortality, whereas an effective treatment for HFpEF remains to be found.

Large HF trials have underrepresented women in their enrollment numbers, often including 30% or fewer women (**Table 1**). One of the reasons for this situation is the entry criteria that put restrictions on women entering randomized controlled trials. For example, excluding women with pregnancy, because of concerns about fetal outcomes, has limited enrollment of younger women.

Nonetheless, increasing the number of women in HF trials at a rate commensurate with the prevalence of HF can help in a systematic assessment of drug safety and efficacy rather than extrapolating from data gathered from the effect on men. In particular, as the therapeutic options for HF expand, sex-based differences in treatment need to be considered.

The National Institutes of Health has tried to address this issue by adding a sex/gender requirement to all applications for funding. Researchers will need to attract and maintain women in clinical trials. In addition, to provide the necessary sex-sensitive evidence for treatment efficacy, future studies should establish predetermined target female ratios. As health care evolves to personalized medicine, there will be a greater need for sex-specific medicine.

REFERENCES

1. Lundberg GP, Bossone E, Mehta LS. Heart failure in women: an increasing health concern. Heart Fail Clin 2019;15(1):xiii–xiv.
2. Hunt SA, Abraham WT, Chin MH, et al. ACC/AHA 2005 Guideline Update for the Diagnosis and Management of Chronic Heart Failure in the Adult: a

report of the American College of Cardiology/American Heart Association Task Force on Practice Guidelines (Writing Committee to Update the 2001 Guidelines for the Evaluation and Management of Heart Failure): developed in collaboration with the American College of Chest Physicians and the International Society for Heart and Lung Transplantation: endorsed by the Heart Rhythm Society. Circulation 2005;112(12):e154–235.

3. Go AS, Mozaffarian D, Roger VL, et al. Executive summary: heart disease and stroke statistics–2013 update: a report from the American Heart Association. Circulation 2013;127(1):143–52.

4. Heo S, Doering LV, Widener J, et al. Predictors and effect of physical symptom status on health-related quality of life in patients with heart failure. Am J Crit Care 2008;17(2):124–32.

5. Roger VL, Weston SA, Redfield MM, et al. Trends in heart failure incidence and survival in a community-based population. JAMA 2004;292(3):344–50.

6. Levy D, Kenchaiah S, Larson MG, et al. Long-term trends in the incidence of and survival with heart failure. N Engl J Med 2002;347(18):1397–402.

7. Lesman-Leegte I, Jaarsma T, Coyne JC, et al. Quality of life and depressive symptoms in the elderly: a comparison between patients with heart failure and age- and gender-matched community controls. J Card Fail 2009;15(1):17–23.

8. Yancy CW, Jessup M, Bozkurt B, et al. 2013 ACCF/AHA guideline for the management of heart failure: a report of the American College of Cardiology Foundation/American Heart Association Task Force on Practice Guidelines. J Am Coll Cardiol 2013;62(16):e147–239.

9. Gure TR, Kabeto MU, Blaum CS, et al. Degree of disability and patterns of caregiving among older Americans with congestive heart failure. J Gen Intern Med 2008;23(1):70–6.

10. Mann DL, Felker GM. Heart failure : a companion to Braunwald's heart disease. 3rd edition. Philadelphia: Elsevier-Saunders; 2016.

11. Benjamin EJ, Virani SS, Callaway CW, et al. Heart disease and stroke statistics-2018 update: a report from the American Heart Association. Circulation 2018;137(12):e67–492.

12. Eaton CB, Pettinger M, Rossouw J, et al. Risk factors for incident hospitalized heart failure with preserved versus reduced ejection fraction in a multiracial cohort of postmenopausal women. Circ Heart Fail 2016;9(10) [pii:e002883].

13. Ho JE, Enserro D, Brouwers FP, et al. Predicting heart failure with preserved and reduced ejection fraction: the international collaboration on heart failure subtypes. Circ Heart Fail 2016;9(6) [pii: e003116].

14. Pandey A, Omar W, Ayers C, et al. Sex and race differences in lifetime risk of heart failure with preserved ejection fraction and heart failure with reduced ejection fraction. Circulation 2018;137(17): 1814–23.

15. O'Meara E, Clayton T, McEntegart MB, et al. Sex differences in clinical characteristics and prognosis in a broad spectrum of patients with heart failure: results of the Candesartan in Heart failure: assessment of reduction in mortality and morbidity (CHARM) program. Circulation 2007;115(24):3111–20.

16. Adams KF Jr, Fonarow GC, Emerman CL, et al. Characteristics and outcomes of patients hospitalized for heart failure in the United States: rationale, design, and preliminary observations from the first 100,000 cases in the Acute Decompensated Heart Failure National Registry (ADHERE). Am Heart J 2005;149(2):209–16.

17. Galvao M, Kalman J, DeMarco T, et al. Gender differences in in-hospital management and outcomes in patients with decompensated heart failure: analysis from the Acute Decompensated Heart Failure National Registry (ADHERE). J Card Fail 2006;12(2): 100–7.

18. Ponikowski P, Voors AA, Anker SD, et al. 2016 ESC Guidelines for the diagnosis and treatment of acute and chronic heart failure: The Task Force for the diagnosis and treatment of acute and chronic heart failure of the European Society of Cardiology (ESC). Developed with the special contribution of the Heart Failure Association (HFA) of the ESC. Eur J Heart Fail 2016;18(8):891–975.

19. Daubert MA, Douglas PS. Primary prevention of heart failure in women. JACC Heart Fail 2019;7(3): 181–91.

20. Levy D, Larson MG, Vasan RS, et al. The progression from hypertension to congestive heart failure. JAMA 1996;275(20):1557–62.

21. Johnson FL. Pathophysiology and etiology of heart failure. Cardiol Clin 2014;32(1):9–19, vii.

22. Stock EO, Redberg R. Cardiovascular disease in women. Curr Probl Cardiol 2012;37(11):450–526.

23. Sharkey SW, Windenburg DC, Lesser JR, et al. Natural history and expansive clinical profile of stress (tako-tsubo) cardiomyopathy. J Am Coll Cardiol 2010;55(4):333–41.

24. Messerli FH, Rimoldi SF, Bangalore S. The transition from hypertension to heart failure: contemporary update. JACC Heart Fail 2017;5(8):543–51.

25. Otto CM. Textbook of clinical echocardiography. In: 6th edition. ed.: Available at: https://www.clinicalkey.com/dura/browse/bookChapter/3-s2.0-C20160001997. Accessed April 5, 2019.

26. Lang RM, Badano LP, Mor-Avi V, et al. Recommendations for cardiac chamber quantification by echocardiography in adults: an update from the American Society of Echocardiography and the European Association of Cardiovascular Imaging. J Am Soc Echocardiogr 2015;28(1):1–39.e14.

27. Beale AL, Nanayakkara S, Segan L, et al. Sex differences in heart failure with preserved ejection fraction pathophysiology: a detailed invasive hemodynamic and echocardiographic analysis. JACC Heart Fail 2019;7(3):239–49.

28. Keyzer JM, Hoffmann JJ, Ringoir L, et al. Age- and gender-specific brain natriuretic peptide (BNP) reference ranges in primary care. Clin Chem Lab Med 2014;52(9):1341–6.

29. Redfield MM, Rodeheffer RJ, Jacobsen SJ, et al. Plasma brain natriuretic peptide concentration: impact of age and gender. J Am Coll Cardiol 2002;40(5):976–82.

30. Wang TJ, Larson MG, Levy D, et al. Impact of age and sex on plasma natriuretic peptide levels in healthy adults. Am J Cardiol 2002;90(3):254–8.

31. Richards DR, Mehra MR, Ventura HO, et al. Usefulness of peak oxygen consumption in predicting outcome of heart failure in women versus men. Am J Cardiol 1997;80(9):1236–8.

32. Levinsson A, Dube MP, Tardif JC, et al. Sex, drugs, and heart failure: a sex-sensitive review of the evidence base behind current heart failure clinical guidelines. ESC Heart Fail 2018;5(5):745–54.

33. Investigators SOLVD, Yusuf S, Pitt B, Davis CE, et al. Effect of enalapril on survival in patients with reduced left ventricular ejection fractions and congestive heart failure. N Engl J Med 1991;325(5):293–302.

34. CONSENSUS Trial Study Group. Effects of enalapril on mortality in severe congestive heart failure. Results of the Cooperative North Scandinavian Enalapril Survival Study (CONSENSUS). N Engl J Med 1987;316(23):1429–35.

35. Shin JJ, Hamad E, Murthy S, et al. Heart failure in women. Clin Cardiol 2012;35(3):172–7.

36. Packer M, Poole-Wilson PA, Armstrong PW, et al. Comparative effects of low and high doses of the angiotensin-converting enzyme inhibitor, lisinopril, on morbidity and mortality in chronic heart failure. ATLAS Study Group. Circulation 1999;100(23):2312–8.

37. Cohn JN, Tognoni G, Valsartan Heart Failure Trial Investigators. A randomized trial of the angiotensin-receptor blocker valsartan in chronic heart failure. N Engl J Med 2001;345(23):1667–75.

38. Pfeffer MA, Swedberg K, Granger CB, et al. Effects of candesartan on mortality and morbidity in patients with chronic heart failure: the CHARM-Overall programme. Lancet 2003;362(9386):759–66.

39. Kostis JB, Packer M, Black HR, et al. Omapatrilat and enalapril in patients with hypertension: the Omapatrilat Cardiovascular Treatment vs. Enalapril (OCTAVE) trial. Am J Hypertens 2004;17(2):103–11.

40. McMurray JJ, Packer M, Desai AS, et al. Angiotensin-neprilysin inhibition versus enalapril in heart failure. N Engl J Med 2014;371(11):993–1004.

41. Ghali JK, Krause-Steinrauf HJ, Adams KF, et al. Gender differences in advanced heart failure: insights from the BEST study. J Am Coll Cardiol 2003;42(12):2128–34.

42. Flather MD, Shibata MC, Coats AJ, et al. Randomized trial to determine the effect of nebivolol on mortality and cardiovascular hospital admission in elderly patients with heart failure (SENIORS). Eur Heart J 2005;26(3):215–25.

43. Effect of metoprolol CR/XL in chronic heart failure: metoprolol CR/XL randomised intervention trial in congestive heart failure (MERIT-HF). Lancet 1999;353(9169):2001–7.

44. Pitt B, Zannad F, Remme WJ, et al. The effect of spironolactone on morbidity and mortality in patients with severe heart failure. Randomized Aldactone Evaluation Study Investigators. N Engl J Med 1999;341(10):709–17.

45. de Denus S, O'Meara E, Desai AS, et al. Spironolactone metabolites in TOPCAT—new insights into regional variation. N Engl J Med 2017;376(17):1690–2.

46. Collier TJ, Pocock SJ, McMurray JJ, et al. The impact of eplerenone at different levels of risk in patients with systolic heart failure and mild symptoms: insight from a novel risk score for prognosis derived from the EMPHASIS-HF trial. Eur Heart J 2013;34(36):2823–9.

47. Pitt B, Remme W, Zannad F, et al. Eplerenone, a selective aldosterone blocker, in patients with left ventricular dysfunction after myocardial infarction. N Engl J Med 2003;348(14):1309–21.

48. Merrill M, Sweitzer NK, Lindenfeld J, et al. Sex differences in outcomes and responses to spironolactone in heart failure with preserved ejection fraction: a secondary analysis of TOPCAT trial. JACC Heart Fail 2019;7(3):228–38.

49. Digitalis Investigation G. The effect of digoxin on mortality and morbidity in patients with heart failure. N Engl J Med 1997;336(8):525–33.

50. Hulley S, Grady D, Bush T, et al. Randomized trial of estrogen plus progestin for secondary prevention of coronary heart disease in postmenopausal women. Heart and Estrogen/progestin Replacement Study (HERS) Research Group. JAMA 1998;280(7):605–13.

51. Adams KF Jr, Patterson JH, Gattis WA, et al. Relationship of serum digoxin concentration to mortality and morbidity in women in the digitalis investigation group trial: a retrospective analysis. J Am Coll Cardiol 2005;46(3):497–504.

52. Rathore SS, Curtis JP, Wang Y, et al. Association of serum digoxin concentration and outcomes in patients with heart failure. JAMA 2003;289(7):871–8.

53. Cohn JN, Archibald DG, Ziesche S, et al. Effect of vasodilator therapy on mortality in chronic congestive heart failure. Results of a Veterans

Administration Cooperative Study. N Engl J Med 1986;314(24):1547–52.

54. Cole RT, Kalogeropoulos AP, Georgiopoulou VV, et al. Hydralazine and isosorbide dinitrate in heart failure: historical perspective, mechanisms, and future directions. Circulation 2011;123(21):2414–22.

55. Carson P, Ziesche S, Johnson G, et al. Racial differences in response to therapy for heart failure: analysis of the vasodilator-heart failure trials. Vasodilator-Heart Failure Trial Study Group. J Card Fail 1999;5(3):178–87.

56. Taylor AL, Ziesche S, Yancy C, et al. Combination of isosorbide dinitrate and hydralazine in blacks with heart failure. N Engl J Med 2004;351(20):2049–57.

57. Zareba W, Moss AJ, Jackson Hall W, et al. Clinical course and implantable cardioverter defibrillator therapy in postinfarction women with severe left ventricular dysfunction. J Cardiovasc Electrophysiol 2005;16(12):1265–70.

58. Klein L, Grau-Sepulveda MV, Bonow RO, et al. Quality of care and outcomes in women hospitalized for heart failure. Circ Heart Fail 2011;4(5):589–98.

59. MacFadden DR, Crystal E, Krahn AD, et al. Sex differences in implantable cardioverter-defibrillator outcomes: findings from a prospective defibrillator database. Ann Intern Med 2012;156(3):195–203.

60. Cleland JG, Daubert JC, Erdmann E, et al. The effect of cardiac resynchronization on morbidity and mortality in heart failure. N Engl J Med 2005;352(15):1539–49.

61. Arshad A, Moss AJ, Foster E, et al. Cardiac resynchronization therapy is more effective in women than in men: the MADIT-CRT (Multicenter Automatic Defibrillator Implantation Trial with Cardiac Resynchronization Therapy) trial. J Am Coll Cardiol 2011;57(7):813–20.

62. Bozkurt B, Khalaf S. Heart failure in women. Methodist Debakey Cardiovasc J 2017;13(4):216–23.

63. Vasan RS, Larson MG, Benjamin EJ, et al. Congestive heart failure in subjects with normal versus reduced left ventricular ejection fraction: prevalence and mortality in a population-based cohort. J Am Coll Cardiol 1999;33(7):1948–55.

64. Deswal A, Bozkurt B. Comparison of morbidity in women versus men with heart failure and preserved ejection fraction. Am J Cardiol 2006;97(8):1228–31.

65. Massie BM, Carson PE, McMurray JJ, et al. Irbesartan in patients with heart failure and preserved ejection fraction. N Engl J Med 2008;359(23):2456–67.

66. Yusuf S, Pfeffer MA, Swedberg K, et al. Effects of candesartan in patients with chronic heart failure and preserved left-ventricular ejection fraction: the CHARM-Preserved Trial. Lancet 2003;362(9386):777–81.

67. The Cardiac Insufficiency Bisoprolol Study II (CIBIS-II): a randomised trial. Lancet 1999;353(9146):9–13.

68. Poole-Wilson PA, Swedberg K, Cleland JG, et al. Comparison of carvedilol and metoprolol on clinical outcomes in patients with chronic heart failure in the Carvedilol Or Metoprolol European Trial (COMET): randomised controlled trial. Lancet 2003;362(9377):7–13.

69. Bristow MR, Saxon LA, Boehmer J, et al. Cardiac-resynchronization therapy with or without an implantable defibrillator in advanced chronic heart failure. N Engl J Med 2004;350(21):2140–50.

70. Packer M, Coats AJ, Fowler MB, et al. Effect of carvedilol on survival in severe chronic heart failure. N Engl J Med 2001;344(22):1651–8.

71. Zannad F, McMurray JJ, Krum H, et al. Eplerenone in patients with systolic heart failure and mild symptoms. N Engl J Med 2011;364(1):11–21.

72. Moss AJ, Zareba W, Hall WJ, et al. Prophylactic implantation of a defibrillator in patients with myocardial infarction and reduced ejection fraction. N Engl J Med 2002;346(12):877–83.

73. Bardy GH, Lee KL, Mark DB, et al. Amiodarone or an implantable cardioverter-defibrillator for congestive heart failure. N Engl J Med 2005;352(3):225–37.

74. Pitt B, Pfeffer MA, Assmann SF, et al. Spironolactone for heart failure with preserved ejection fraction. N Engl J Med 2014;370(15):1383–92.

Hypertensive Heart Disease and Obesity
A Review

L. Joseph Saliba, MD[a],*, Scott Maffett, MD[b]

KEYWORDS

- Hypertensive heart disease • Obesity • Adiposity • Inflammation • Metabolic syndrome
- Cardiac natriuretic peptide system • RAAS

KEY POINTS

- Hypertensive heart disease is characterized by myocardial fibrosis, which portends higher risk of developing reduced ejection fraction, diastolic dysfunction, ischemia, and arrhythmias.
- Hypertensive heart disease is caused by local and systemic factors, which involves the renin-angiotensin-aldosterone system and cardiac natriuretic peptide system, neurohormonal influences, and increased hemodynamic stress.
- Angiotensin-converting enzyme inhibitors and angiotensin receptor blockers have been shown to prevent and reverse abnormal anatomy, namely concentric myocardial hypertrophy.
- Obesity causes sympathetic dysregulation, local hypoxia, increased formation of reactive oxygen species, and release of inflammatory cytokines.
- Visceral adiposity increases the likelihood of developing long-standing hypertension, as well as cardiovascular events.

INTRODUCTION

The effects of hypertension and obesity on the human body are paramount to developing frameworks for understanding the results of metabolic syndrome on the cardiovascular system. This review aims to highlight mechanisms of development of obesity and hypertension, their interdependent relationship, and their effect on morbidity and mortality in patient populations. The complex nature of obesity development, as well as certain factors that increase morbidity in obese patients are of particular importance due to its span across most fields of medicine and its rising prevalence in the global population. Although hypertensive heart disease (HHD) pathophysiology has been well-elucidated, the multifactorial mechanisms for developing obesity and metabolic syndrome play paramount roles in the development of HHD.

HYPERTENSIVE HEART DISEASE

Key points:
- Cellular changes distinguish HHD from hypertension, including remodeling and increased extracellular volume: the hallmarks of myocardial fibrosis.
- The causes of systemic HHD are multifaceted, and include hemodynamic factors, inflammation, and oxidative stress via the renin-angiotensin-aldosterone system (RAAS).
- HHD is often caused by a myriad of lung disease and obstructive sleep apnea (OSA).
- Treatment of HHD is aimed at controlling hypertension, preventing/reversing structural

Disclosure Statement: The authors have nothing to disclose.
[a] Department of Internal Medicine, Ohio State University-Wexner Medical Center, 395 West 12th Avenue, Columbus, OH 43210, USA; [b] Ohio State University-Wexner Medical Center, 452 West 10th Avenue, Columbus, OH 43210, USA
* Corresponding author. 4106 Spring Flower Ct, Columbus, OH 43230.
E-mail address: Lawrence.Saliba@osumc.edu

and electrical remodeling, and minimizing risk of arrhythmia and sudden cardiac death.

Hypertension is a common cause of morbidity and mortality, and affects a third of the adult population in the United States.[1] HHD can affect the left or right side of the heart. More commonly, increase in systemic vascular resistance causes anomalous intracardiac pressures in the left heart, leading to left ventricle (LV) damage. The constant overload causes myocyte hypertrophy and interstitial fibrosis, which has been shown to cause concentric LV hypertrophy (LVH). Concentric LVH leads to impaired diastolic filling, resulting in left atrium dilation, and causes increased risk of cardiovascular events compared with other hypertrophy subtypes.[2] Further, LVH portends higher all-cause mortality, and stronger risk for heart failure, stroke, and coronary artery disease than blood pressure, tobacco use, or cholesterol.[3] Left untreated, this pathophysiology causes LV dilation and failure and is a frequent cause of nonischemic cardiomyopathy. Likewise, increased pressures can affect the right ventricle (RV) and cause *cor pulmonale*. Often separate, but similar in hemodynamic results, right-sided HHD is commonly caused by OSA, which highlights a main repercussion of growing obesity trends on cardiovascular disease.[4]

Systemic Hypertensive Heart Disease

Systemic HHD refers to the anatomic response to increased hemodynamic load, sympathetic upregulation, natriuretic peptide system dysregulation, inflammation, and oxidative stress on the left heart, and can be characterized as compensated or decompensated. Compensated HHD describes subclinical changes of the pathophysiology, and is more commonly due to the frequently asymptomatic nature of hypertension. Silent hypertension causes these compensatory anatomic changes to remain untreated for years in some, and repetitive insult of suboptimal control of hypertension may lead to decompensated disease. Cellular changes distinguish HHD from hypertension alone. Specifically, diffuse myocardial fibrosis causes increased extracellular volume and remodeling, and is thought to be the underlying mechanism leading to increased cardiovascular risk in these patients. The pathogenesis of this remodeling is incompletely understood, but is certainly multifactorial. These include not only the simple duration and severity of hypertension, but also inflammatory cytokine (including adipokine) pathways, neurohormonal factors, and genetic predilection.[5] The RAAS is particularly implicated in the development of fibrosis, as angiotensin II (AT2) causes potent induction of inflammation and formation of reactive oxygen species (ROS). Activation of this system induces myofibroblasts to increase collagen formation and deposition, and leads to structural changes in the cardiac vascular bed.[6] The results of myocardial fibrosis portend higher risk for reduced ejection fraction, diastolic dysfunction, ischemia, and arrhythmias.[7] Indeed, even in patients with heart failure with preserved ejection fraction, diffuse fibrosis is associated with increased cardiac events.[8] Although increased fibrosis results in this increased risk, reversal of the pathophysiology improves HHD, and is associated with reduced incidence of sudden cardiac death.[9] As mentioned, inadequate control of these factors results in decompensated HHD, characterized by ischemic heart disease, renal damage, and/or stroke as a result of inadequately controlled hypertension.

Pulmonary Hypertensive Heart Disease

Although most cases are complications of left-sided heart disease, pulmonary HHD has a multitude of alternate causes, commonly from airway disease (eg, chronic obstructive pulmonary disease, bronchiectasis) or parenchymal disease (eg, fibrosis). In addition, diseases of the pulmonary vasculature often contribute to pulmonary HHD. These include recurrent Pulmonary Embolism, primary pulmonary hypertension, pulmonary arteritis, or vascular obstruction. Of note, disorders that affect chest wall movement (eg, obesity, OSA, kyphoscoliosis) contribute to the aberrant physiology. In the absence of increased left heart pressures, isolated pulmonary HHD is termed *cor pulmonale*, and is characterized by RV hypertrophy and dilation. Acute development of *cor pulmonale* commonly suggests the presence of pulmonary embolism.[4]

Obstructive Sleep Apnea and Hypertensive Heart Disease

OSA is a major risk factor for cardiovascular disease, and changes hemodynamic and nonhemodynamic factors that contribute to morbidity and mortality. Namely, intermittent hypoxia and intrathoracic pressure changes lead to physiologic disturbances that contribute to HHD. The oxidative stress from hypoxia in OSA leads to formation of ROS. Subsequent rapid reoxygenation parallels reperfusion injury, leading to cell and tissue damage. In addition, frequent arousals lead to upregulation of sympathetic drive.[10] Altogether, the perturbation of hemodynamic and nonhemodynamic factors in OSA contribute to the development of hypertension, and its treatment is essential to preventing the development of end-organ damage.

Treatment of Hypertensive Heart Disease

As discussed, myocardial fibrosis resulting from long-standing hypertension significantly increases risk for other cardiovascular comorbidities, making its early detection and treatment valuable. RAAS blockade with angiotensin-converting enzyme (ACE) inhibitors and angiotensin receptor blockers (ARBs) have been traditionally used as first-line hypertension agents in many patients. However, unlike many antihypertensive choices including beta-adrenoceptor blockers, calcium channel blockers, and diuretics, these have particular utility in preventing and reversing cardiac myocyte remodeling. Recent studies have validated the use of losartan to reduce collagen deposition in myocytes and reduce LV stiffness.[11] Although all of the first-line drug choices reduce LVH by improving blood pressure, beta blockers appear to have the least effect on LV mass than the other antihypertensive classes, possibly due to less effect on central aortic blood pressure. Compared with ARBs, beta blockers change geometric pattern of LVH from concentric to eccentric, rather than restoring native LV geometry.[12] In addition, angiotensin receptor blockade has been shown to reduce and reverse electrical remodeling (by measure of QT-dispersion), an important contributing factor to sudden cardiac death.[13] Due to effects on reducing left atrial size, ACE inhibitors and ARBs also have been shown to reduce incidence of atrial fibrillation in patients with HHD compared with beta blocker therapy.[9,14] Therefore, current recommendations suggest evaluation (usually electrocardiogram [ECG], but echocardiography is used if ECG is indeterminant) for structural heart disease when hypertension is diagnosed, as its presence can inform treatment choice. In patients with end-organ damage from hypertension, a 2-drug regimen, including ACE inhibitors or ARB with calcium channel blocker or thiazide diuretic is recommended. Based on risk for further morbidity and mortality, stringent blood pressure control targets, 120 to 130/80 mm Hg, are recommended for most patients with HHD.[15]

OBESITY

Key points:

- Development of obesity is multifactorial, with genetic, hormonal, behavioral, and metabolic influences.
- Adiposity distribution carries significant influence on risk for developing obesity-related heart disease. Visceral obesity is closely linked with hypertension, diabetes, and dyslipidemia development.
- Obesity treatment requires comprehensive lifestyle modification, with goal weight loss of 5% to 10% within 6 months for most individuals.

A body of evidence suggests obesity is a predominant risk factor for atherosclerosis, heart failure, and stroke.[16] In fact, approximately 40% of US adults are obese, with highest rates in the fifth and sixth decades of life.[17] The World Health Organization classification of obesity based on body mass index (BMI) is the most widely used system to categorize obesity. As seen in **Table 1**, patients are characterized as normal weight, overweight/pre-obese, or obese, with 3 subclasses for obesity. This classification is of importance because of the increasing effect on development of comorbid conditions with increases in body mass. Further, the distribution of body mass (ie, the location of adiposity) has been shown to affect morbidity.

Causes of Obesity

The causes of obesity are many, and multiple factors contribute to the development and worsening of excess weight in most patients with the disease. Genetic factors may predispose patients to its development, whereas obesogenic environmental influences often play a role. Likewise, complex biological mechanisms inform ingestive behavior by altering hormonal pathways that are centrally controlled. Namely, leptin and ghrelin act in competing pathways via receptors in the hypothalamus to signal hunger and satiety. Altogether, the complex picture contributes to net positive energy balance that leads to excess triglyceride storage, the hallmark of obesity.[18]

Distribution of Adiposity

As mentioned, the distribution of abdominal adiposity carries significant influence on the terminal effect of obesity. It is widely accepted that increased abdominal adiposity, even without obesity or overweight, increases risk for cardiovascular events. Visceral adiposity is strongly associated with aberrations of glucose and lipid metabolism as well as increases in blood pressure.[18] Conversely, subcutaneous obesity, which comprises most cases and has female predominance, carries much lower risk of cardiovascular events.[19]

Table 1
World Health Organization classification of obesity

Body Mass Index, kg/m²	Classification
<18.5	Underweight
18.5–24.9	Normal weight
25.0–29.9	Pre-obesity
30.0–34.9	Obesity class I
35.0–39.9	Obesity class II
>40	Obesity class II (morbid obesity)

Adapted from World Health Organization (WHO). Body mass index – BMI. Available at: http://www.euro.who.int/en/health-topics/disease-prevention/nutrition/a-healthy-lifestyle/body-mass-index-bmi/. Accessed Jan 1 2019; with permission.

Obesity Treatment

In 2013, the American College of Cardiology/American Heart Association Task Force on Practice Guidelines released a review of the state of evidence from observational studies, randomized controlled trials, and meta-analyses.[20] The report strongly recommends a comprehensive lifestyle intervention with prescription of a hypocaloric diet for obese or overweight individuals. Although many strategies to achieve weight loss exist, the central tenet and underlying principle for effective weight loss is a negative energy balance. The specified goal of intervention includes weight loss of 5% to 10% of baseline weight within 6 months for patients with BMI ≥30 kg/m² or BMI between 25.0 and 29.9 kg/m² with additional risk factors. Caloric intake recommendations are presented as a few strategies, including prescribed intake, prescribed energy deficit, or ad libitum approach (ie, elimination of a particular food group). For initial weight loss, physical activity recommendations include ≥150 min/wk of aerobic exercise, then between 200 and 300 min/wk for weight maintenance over 1 year. The review also recommends prescription of a structured program to assist with behavioral therapy strategies with at least 14 face-to-face sessions over a period of 6 months. Although pharmacotherapy may be helpful for achieving the initial weight loss, it should be used as an adjunct to the comprehensive lifestyle intervention. Bariatric surgery is also an option for treatment of obesity, but is traditionally reserved for patients with BMI ≥40 kg/m² or ≥35 kg/m² with obesity-related comorbid conditions who have not responded well to lifestyle modification. Of note, lack of prescribed pharmacotherapy generally does not preclude surgical options in patients with obesity.[20,21]

OBESITY AND HYPERTENSIVE HEART DISEASE

Key points:

- Obesity and sympathetic dysregulation are closely linked because of the production of leptin by adipose cells, causing renin secretion and development of hypertension.
- High caloric intake induces angiotensinogen production, which upregulates systemic RAAS activation.
- Increased sympathetic tone from obesity limits compensation for increased plasma volume due to inappropriately elevated renin and aldosterone levels. High aldosterone levels induce endothelial dysfunction and cardiac fibrosis.
- The cardiac natriuretic peptide system counteracts RAAS activity, but is dysfunctional in obesity, leaving the RAAS system poorly regulated.
- Whether by cause or effect, obesity and HHD are proinflammatory disease states.
- Visceral adiposity causes chronic hypoxia, formation of ROS, and promotes systemic inflammation. This inflammation contributes to myocardial stress, and ultimately HHD.
- Treatment of HHD should focus on RAAS blockade, especially in the overweight/obese population.

Although the mechanisms by which development of obesity and HHD have been independently elucidated, the relationship between these common diseases is more complex. Prevalence of hypertension rises with increased adiposity. Indeed, 56% of the overweight group had hypertension, with a 2.5-fold increase in class I/II obesity and a 4.5-fold increase in morbid obesity.[22] The concomitant development of these diseases occurs through local and systemic pathways, including hormonal, neuronal, and hemodynamic factors.

Obesity and the Sympathetic Nervous System

Adipose cells directly produce leptin and increase angiotensin II levels, and the latter leads to increased sympathetic tone.[23,24] Indeed, the urinary norepinephrine increases with adiposity, and is independently related to abdominal girth and BMI.[25] Catecholamines from the increased sympathetic tone act on renin regulatory centers in the kidney, leading to increased renin secretion. Thus, increased adiposity increases activity of the sympathetic nervous system and induces hypertension. Further, positive feedback loop of the RAAS on adipocytes worsens the synergistic effect of adiposity on hypertension, which is discussed later. Inflammatory cytokines, endothelial dysfunction, and dysregulation of the natriuretic peptide system also significantly contribute to the development of HHD.

Sympathetic Dysregulation

The RAAS influence on the development of concomitant obesity and HHD cannot be understated. A dysregulated RAAS confers local and systemic effects and alters natriuretic peptide downstream blood pressure control. Locally, AT2 serves as a growth factor for adipocytes. These cells excrete angiotensinogen (AGT), thereby increasing local AT2 concentration. This increase in local levels cause systemic effects by increasing systemic RAAS activation.[26,27] The upregulated sympathetic nervous system increases systemic cAMP levels, which further stimulates AGT expression.[28] Because visceral obesity increases levels of AGT and AT2, renin and aldosterone levels are inappropriately normal or even elevated in response to electrolyte and hemodynamic factors. Sodium intake and water retention increase plasma volume. In a normal RAAS, levels of renin and aldosterone decrease to accommodate the hemodynamic changes. However, when these hormone levels are inappropriately elevated (secondary to visceral obesity), the compensatory mechanisms are either absent or unable to overcome the increased plasma volume. Conversely, weight loss results in reduction in blood pressure by allowing the RAAS to appropriately respond to increased sodium intake or plasma volume.[29–31] Namely, increased plasma volume would reduce renin concentration and activity, AGT levels, aldosterone concentration, and blood pressure.[30,32] Diet also contributes to alterations in gene expression. In mouse models, the AGT gene expression increases with increased caloric intake.[27,33] Further, this increased expression is reversible with weight loss and body habitus changes. Even a 5% decrease in weight lowers AGT levels, but interestingly, the decrease in AGT is correlated with waist circumference, independent of body weight and BMI.[31]

Effects on Cardiac Myocytes

Adipocytes also release factors, including leptin, that stimulate aldosterone secretion, thereby increasing sympathetic tone.[34,35] This secretion acts directly on the heart as well, causing endothelial dysfunction and cardiac fibrosis.[36–38] Leptin contributes to the overall effect of systemic factors on HHD by upregulating cellular adhesion molecules (CAMs) and tissue factor (TF) expression in cardiac endothelial cells. CAMs and TF increase leukocyte rolling, leading to increased local proinflammatory cells. Ultimately, this inflammation, in addition to cardiac myocyte shear stress, leads to apoptosis. Myocyte cell death causes increased extracellular volume of the remaining cells, promotes collagen production, and leads to fibrin deposition, which is the mechanism by which cardiac remodeling occurs. In a mechanism analogous to insulin resistance in diabetes, leptin overproduction in obese patients leads to leptin resistance by target organs, compounding the effects of leptin on the cardiac endothelium, as well as further aberrations at the local level.[39–41] Ultimately RAAS deregulation results from increased production of AGT, AT2, and renin, as well as alterations in other regulatory mechanisms, including the cardiac natriuretic peptide system (CNPS), and results in cardiac remodeling.

The Cardiac Natriuretic Peptide System

The CNPS is an important antagonist of AGT and AT2 production and therefore contributes to adequate control of blood pressure if unencumbered. Adipose tissue lowers circulating plasma natriuretic peptide levels. Increase in BMI or waist circumference, or the presence of metabolic syndrome are independent causes of decreased plasma A-type natriuretic peptide (ANP) and B-type natriuretic peptide (BNP).[42] This is consequential because of CNPS regulation of RAAS, as well as the direct action of natriuretic peptides on the cardiovascular system. Both atrial and ventricular natriuretic peptides directly inhibit renin and aldosterone secretion, thereby decreasing sympathetic tone. In addition, both ANP and BNP limit vasopressin secretion. Dysfunction in this system leaves the RAAS unregulated, increases sympathetic activity, and increases hypertension. On the local level, ANP and BNP induce the synthesis of cyclic guanosine monophosphate, which causes potent vasodilation of the peripheral vasculature. In addition, they cause direct effects on cardiac myocytes by signaling pathways that reduce hypertrophy, fibrosis, and arrhythmogenic factors.[43–45] Based on its effect on the CNPS, neprilysin has become an important target for antihypertensive and heart failure therapies, especially in the obese population. This compound is involved in the catabolism of natriuretic peptides. Thus, inhibition of neprilysin and its clearance receptor leads to higher levels of circulating ANP and BNP, causes vasodilation, and reduces blood pressure. The novel angiotensin receptor-neprilysin inhibitor sacubitril/valsartan has been shown to increase insulin sensitivity in patients with hypertension and obesity.[46] Neprilysin levels decrease following Roux-en-Y gastric bypass and associated weight loss, suggesting adiposity has a direct role in the signaling and production of the endopeptidase as well as an inverse relationship with circulating natriuretic peptide levels.[47] Although the benefit has been shown to not be related to increased exercise-induced lipolysis in this population, the mechanisms of benefit are a current area of study.[30]

The Role of Inflammation on Hypertensive Heart Disease

The association of obesity with hypertension and resulting organ damage can also be explained by the production of inflammatory cytokines and endothelial dysfunction.[48–50] Interferon (IFN)- γ plays a role in the activation of macrophages, which are implicated in the development of atherosclerosis and hypertension. A recent study suggested IFN- γ, a proinflammatory cytokine, is increased in patients with comorbid diabetes and hypertension, compared with diabetes alone. This suggests IFN- γ is implicated as either a biomarker for hypertensive disease or a catalyst for its development.[51] In addition, dietary sodium intake increases gene expression of adipogenesis (eg, PPAR-γ), reduces gene expression in lipolysis (eg, AMPK), which results in net fat accumulation. Independent of salt intake, investigation of serum inflammatory adipokines in obese patients shows a shift toward inflammation, with elevations in inflammatory cytokines, as well as resistin, and interelukin-18.[52] Altogether, the specific inflammatory profiles of different disease states such as obesity and HHD are being investigated, but higher levels of proinflammatory cytokines have been consistently shown.

Visceral Adiposity and Inflammation

In addition, visceral adipose cells increase in size threefold to fourfold with fat accumulation, which prohibits oxygen diffusion locally. Chronic hypoxia has been seen in expanded visceral adipose tissue, and leads to formation of ROS locally, which reduces adiponectin production, increases leptin release, and promotes systemic inflammation.[53] This upregulates endothelial adhesion molecules in the microcirculation. This results in sequestration of inflammatory cells by the tissues and ultimately tissue damage.[54,55] As discussed, visceral adiposity represents a smaller proportion of patients compared with subcutaneous adiposity, but its presence portends higher risk of cardiovascular morbidity and mortality.

Hemodynamic Disturbance

As mentioned, in states with increased RAAS and lower natriuretic peptide receptor-C regulation, a higher output state is created. Increased plasma volume and stroke volume drive increased cardiac output, but the lack of systemic vessel response to these changes (inappropriately normal systemic vascular resistance) causes hypertension.[23,56] The hemodynamic changes resulting from severe OSA also contribute to masked hypertension. These lead to increased shear stress and creation of a mild inflammatory state, which trigger cardiac myocytes to produce collagen, and ultimately result in concentric LVH.[57,58] Even in early stages of metabolic syndrome, gross loss of elasticity is seen, the degree of which increases with the number of comorbidities of metabolic syndrome.[59] Increased sympathetic activity, RAAS, inflammatory cytokines, ROS, and reduction of nitric oxide (NO) availability all contribute to arterial stiffening.[60] ROS decrease NO availability and cause endothelial dysfunction, which increases arterial stiffness.[61] In addition, increased serum leptin and decreased serum adiponectin levels, as seen in visceral obesity, promote smooth muscle proliferation and increases collagen deposition.[62] Interestingly, these local changes are reversible with aerobic training, and as little as 6 months of interval training reduces arterial stiffness and microvascular dysfunction.[63–66]

Coronary Perfusion

In addition to changes in skeletal muscle and systemic factors, coronary microvascular function is also altered in obesity. In healthy cardiac microvasculature, myocardial perfusion is "coupled" to cardiac metabolism. However, obesity and hypercholesterolemia lead to alterations in the coupling of coronary blood flow and myocardial metabolic demand.[67] The effect of this uncoupling has been proven with dobutamine stress echo, which has shown impaired coronary flow velocity in obese patients, an aberrancy that also increases with each comorbid component of metabolic syndrome.[68] The repercussions of this uncoupling explain, in part, the pathophysiology of increased cardiovascular risk in metabolic syndrome.

Effect of Treating Obesity and Hypertensive Heart Disease

The treatment of HHD and obesity independently are outlined previously and are critical in reducing morbidity and mortality of metabolic syndrome and its effects, but how does treating one condition affect the other? Recent investigation has evaluated control of overweight and obesity and its reduction of LVH. Compared with patients with normal weight, the regression of LVH is greater with weight loss in the obese population, even with less improvement of blood pressure.[69] This suggests the reduction of weight has a greater effect on LV mass than hemodynamic factors alone. Recent analysis suggests RAAS inhibitors are more effective in reducing LV mass in the overweight/obese hypertensive patients than beta blockers, calcium channel blockers, or diuretics.[70]

DISCUSSION

As the populations with obesity and hypertension continue to grow, it is essential for providers to understand the complex mechanisms that characterize the disease processes and their development in order to inform practice patterns and treatment choices. Although increasingly complex, the constellation of diseases that define metabolic syndrome span the many disciplines of medicine. The relationship between HHD and obesity plays a significant role in increased risk of cardiovascular events and mortality. Their development has a myriad of contributing factors, which involve local and systemic influences. The myocyte geometry (hypertrophy) that characterizes HHD is a direct result of hemodynamic and nonhemodynamic factors. Increased sympathetic drive with RAAS and CNPS dysregulation, oxidative stress, and production of proinflammatory cytokines and adipokines are among the key nonhemodynamic components that define metabolic syndrome. RAAS inhibition has proven effective in preventing and reversing eccentric LVH. Given the increasing prevalence of obesity and its role in HHD, prevention and early treatment of both is of growing importance, and the study of effective novel therapeutic targets is ongoing.

REFERENCES

1. Go AS, Mozaffarian D, Roger VL, et al. Heart disease and stroke statistics—2013 update: a report from the American Heart Association. Circulation 2013;127:e6–245.
2. Cuspidi C, Giudici V, Negri F, et al. Left ventricular geometry, ambulatory blood pressure and extracardiac organ damage in untreated essential hypertension. Blood Press Monit 2010;15:124–31.
3. Vakili BA, Okin PM, Devereux RB. Prognostic implications of left ventricular hypertrophy. Am Heart J 2001;141(3):334–41.
4. Schoen FJ, Mitchell RN. The heart. In: Kumar V, Abbas A, Aster J, editors. Robbins and Cotran pathologic basis of disease, vol. 12, 9th edition. Philadelphia: Elsevier; 2015. p. 523–78.
5. Hill JA, Olson EN. Cardiac plasticity. N Engl J Med 2008;358:1370–80.
6. Weber KT, Sun Y, Gerling IC, et al. Regression of established cardiac fibrosis in hypertensive heart disease. Am J Hypertens 2017;30(11):1049–52.
7. McLenachan JM, Dargie HJ. Ventricular arrhythmias in hypertensive left ventricular hypertrophy. Relationship to coronary artery disease, left ventricular dysfunction, and myocardial fibrosis. Am J Hypertens 1990;3:735–40.
8. Mascherbauer J, Marzluf BA, Tufaro C, et al. Cardiac magnetic resonance postcontrast t1 time is associated with outcome in patients with heart failure and preserved ejection fraction. Circ Cardiovasc Imaging 2013;6:1056–65.
9. Wachtell K, Lehto M, Gerdts E, et al. Angiotensin II receptor blockade reduces new-onset atrial fibrillation and subsequent stroke compared to atenolol: the Losartan Intervention For End Point Reduction in Hypertension (LIFE) study. J Am Coll Cardiol 2005;45(5):712–9.
10. Eltzschig HK, Eckle T. Ischemia and reperfusion–from mechanism to translation. Nat Med 2011;17:1391–401.
11. Kuruvilla S, Janardhanan R, Antkowiak P, et al. Increased extracellular volume and altered mechanics are associated with LVH in hypertensive heart disease, not hypertension alone. JACC Cardiovasc Imaging 2015;8(2):172–80.
12. Malmqvist K, Kahan T, Edner M, et al. Regression of left ventricular hypertrophy in human hypertension with irbesartan. J Hypertens 2001;19(6):1167–76.
13. Lindholm LH, Dahlöf B, Edelman JM, et al. Effect of losartan on sudden cardiac death in people with diabetes: data from the LIFE study. Lancet 2003;362(9384):619–20.
14. Schneider MP, Hua TA, Böhm M, et al. Prevention of atrial fibrillation by renin angiotensin system inhibition a meta-analysis. J Am Coll Cardiol 2010;55(21):2299–307.
15. Jekell A, Nilsson P, Kahan T. Treatment of hypertensive left ventricular hypertrophy. Curr Pharm Des 2019;25:1. Available at: http://www.eurekaselect.com/167972/article/. Accessed February 1, 2019.
16. Kim SH, Despres JP, Koh KK. Obesity and cardiovascular disease: friend or foe? Eur Heart J 2016;37:3560–8.
17. Hales CM, Carroll MD, Fryar CD, et al. Centers for Disease Control and Prevention National Center for Health Statistics Prevalence of Obesity Among Adults and Youth: United States, 2015–2016. NCHS Data Brief 2017;(288):1–8.

18. Lam TK, Carpentier A, Lewis GF, et al. Mechanisms of the free fatty acid-induced increase in hepatic glucose production. Am J Physiol Endocrinol Metab 2003;284:E863–73.

19. Iberti KG, Zimmet P, Shaw J, IDF Epidemiology Task Force Consensus Group. The metabolic syndrome – a new worldwide definition. Lancet 2005; 366:1059–62.

20. Jensen MD, Ryan DH, Apovian CM, et al. 2013 AHA/ACC/TOS guideline for the management of overweight and obesity in adults: a report of the American College of Cardiology/American Heart Association Task Force on Practice Guidelines and The Obesity Society. Circulation 2014;129:S102–38.

21. Yannakoulia M, Poulimeneas D, Mamalaki E, et al. Dietary modifications for weight loss and weight loss maintenance. Metabolism 2019;92:153–62. Available at: http://www.sciencedirect.com/science/article/pii/S0026049519300083/. Accessed February 1, 2019.

22. Sampson UK, Edwards TL, Jahangir E, et al. Factors associated with the prevalence of hypertension in the southeastern United States: insights from 69,211 blacks and whites in the Southern Community Cohort Study. Circ Cardiovasc Qual Outcomes 2014;7(1):33–54.

23. Aneja A, El-Atat F, McFarlane SI, et al. Hypertension and obesity. Recent Progr Horm Res 2004;59: 169–205.

24. Mancia G, Bousquet P, Elghozi JL, et al. The sympathetic nervous system and the metabolic syndrome. J Hypertens 2007;25:909–20.

25. Landsberg L, Troisi R, Parker D, et al. Obesity, blood pressure, and the sympathetic nervous system. Ann Epidemiol 1991;1:295–303.

26. Massiera F, Bloch-Faure M, Ceiler D, et al. Adipose angiotensinogen is involved in adipose tissue growth and blood pressure regulation. FASEB J 2001;15:2727–9.

27. Frederich RC Jr, Kahn BB, Peach MJ, et al. Tissue-specific nutritional regulation of angiotensinogen in adipose tissue. Am J Hypertens 1992;19:339–44.

28. Serazin V, Dos Santos E, Morot M, et al. Human adipose angiotensinogen gene expression and secretion are stimulated by cyclic AMP via increased DNA cyclic AMP responsive element binding activity. Endocrine 2004;25:97–104.

29. Tuck ML, Sowers J, Dornfield L, et al. The effect of weight reduction on blood pressure plasma renin activity and plasma aldosterone level in obese patients. N Engl J Med 1981;304:930–3.

30. Engeli S, Bohnke J, Gorzelniak K, et al. Weight loss and the renin–angiotensin–aldosterone system. Hypertension 2005;45:356–62.

31. Harp JB, Henry SA, Di Girolamo M. Dietary weight loss decreases serum angiotensin-converting enzyme activity in obese adults. Obes Res 2002; 10:985–90.

32. Engeli S, Boschmann M, Frings P, et al. Influence of salt intake on renin–angiotensin and natriuretic peptide system genes in human adipose tissue. Hypertension 2006;48:1103–8.

33. Jones BH, Standridge MK, Taylor JW, et al. Angiotensinogen gene expression in adipose tissue: analysis of obese models and hormonal and nutritional control. Am J Physiol 1997;273:R236–42.

34. Narkiewicz K, Kato M, Phillips BG, et al. Leptin interacts with heart rate but not sympathetic nerve traffic in healthy male subjects. J Hypertens 2001;19:1089–94.

35. Rumantir MS, Vaz M, Jennings GL, et al. Neural mechanisms in human obesity-related hypertension. J Hypertens 1999;17:1125–33.

36. Krug AW, Vleugels K, Schinner S, et al. Human adipocytes induce an ERK1/2 MAP kinases-mediated upregulation of steroidogenic acute regulatory protein (StAR) and an angiotensin II-sensitization in human adrenocortical cells. Int J Obes (Lond) 2007; 31:1605–16.

37. Lamounier-Zepter V, Ehrhart-Bornstein M, Bornstein SR. Mineralocorticoid-stimulating activity of adipose tissue. Best Pract Res Clin Endocrinol Metab 2005;19:567–75.

38. Huby AC, Antonova G, Groenendyk J, et al. Adipocyte-derived hormone leptin is a direct regulator of aldosterone secretion, which promotes endothelial dysfunction and cardiac fibrosis. Circulation 2015; 132(22):2134–45.

39. Liu J, Yang X, Yu S, et al. The leptin resistance. In: Wu Q, Zheng R, editors. Neural regulation of metabolism. Advances in experimental medicine and biology, vol. 1090. Singapore: Springer; 2018. p. 145–63.

40. Klok MD, Jakobsdottir S, Drent ML. The role of leptin and ghrelin in the regulation of food intake and body weight in humans: a review. Obes Rev 2007;8: 21–34.

41. Schwartz MW, Peskind E, Raskind M, et al. Cerebrospinal fluid leptin levels: relationship to plasma levels and to adiposity in humans. Nat Med 1996; 2:589–93.

42. Potter LR, Abbey-Hosch S, Dickey DM. Natriuretic peptides, their receptors, and cyclic guanosine monophosphate-dependent signaling functions. Endocr Rev 2006;27:47–72.

43. Oliver P, Fox J, Kim R, et al. Hypertension, cardiac hypertrophy and sudden death in mice lacking natriuretic peptide receptor. A Proc Natl Acad Sci U S A 1997;94:24730–5.

44. Knowles J, Esposito G, Mao L, et al. Pressure independent enhancement of cardiac hypertrophy in natriuretic peptide receptor A deficient mice. J Clin Invest 2001;107:975–84.

45. Tamura N, Ogawa Y, Chusho H, et al. Cardiac fibrosis in mice lacking brain natriuretic peptide. Proc Natl Acad Sci U S A 2000;97:4239–44.

46. Jordan J, Stinkens R, Jax T, et al. Improved insulin sensitivity with angiotensin receptor neprilysin inhibition in individuals with obesity and hypertension. Clin Pharmacol Ther 2017;101:254–63.

47. Ghanim H, Monte S, Caruana J, et al. Decreases in neprilysin and vasoconstrictors and increases in vasodilators following bariatric surgery. Diabetes Obes Metab 2018;20:2029–33.

48. Grassi G, Cattaneo BM, Seravalle G, et al. Obesity and the sympathetic nervous system. Blood Press Suppl 1996;1:43–6.

49. Kim JA, Montagnani M, Koh KK, et al. Reciprocal relationships between insulin resistance and endothelial dysfunction: molecular and pathophysiological mechanisms. Circulation 2006;113:1888–904.

50. Ziccardi P, Nappo F, Giugliano G, et al. Reduction of inflammatory cytokine concentrations and improvement of endothelial functions in obese women after weight loss over one year. Circulation 2002;105:804–9.

51. Asadikaram G, Ram M, Izadi A, et al. The study of the serum level of IL-4, TGF-β, IFN-γ, and IL-6 in overweight patients with and without diabetes mellitus and hypertension. J Cell Biochem 2019;120(3):4147–57.

52. Sorop O, Olver TD, van de Wouw J, et al. Microcirculation: a key player in obesity-associated cardiovascular disease. Cardiovasc Res 2017;113(9):1035–45.

53. Trayhurn P. Hypoxia and adipose tissue function and dysfunction in obesity. Physiol Rev 2013;93:1–21.

54. Eringa EC, Bakker W, van Hinsbergh VW. Paracrine regulation of vascular tone, inflammation and insulin sensitivity by perivascular adipose tissue. Vascul Pharmacol 2012;56(5–6):204–9.

55. Schinzari F, Tesauro M, Cardillo C. Endothelial and perivascular adipose tissue abnormalities in obesity-related vascular dysfunction: novel targets for treatment. J Cardiovasc Pharmacol 2017;69(6):360–8.

56. Alpert MA. Obesity, cardiomyopathy, pathophysiology and evolution of the clinical syndrome. Am J Med Sci 2001;321:225–36.

57. Cioffi G, Russo TE, Stefenelli C, et al. Severe obstructive sleep apnea elicits concentric left ventricular geometry. J Hypertens 2010;28(5):1074–82.

58. Dewan NA, Nieto FJ, Somers VK. Intermittent hypoxemia and OSA: implications for comorbidities. Chest 2015;147(1):266–74.

59. Lopes-Vicente WRP, Rodrigues S, Cepeda FX, et al. Arterial stiffness and its association with clustering of metabolic syndrome risk factors. Diabetol Metab Syndr 2017;9:87.

60. Saladini F, Palatini P. Arterial distensibility, physical activity, and the metabolic syndrome. Curr Hypertens Rep 2018;20(5):39.

61. Terentes-Printzios D, Vlachopoulos C, Xaplanteris P, et al. Cardiovascular risk factors accelerate progression of vascular aging in the general population: results from the CRAVE Study (Cardiovascular Risk Factors Affecting Vascular Age). Hypertension 2017;70:1057–64.

62. van den Munckhof ICL, Holewijn S, de Graaf J, et al. Sex differences in fat distribution influence the association between BMI and arterial stiffness. J Hypertens 2017;35:1219–25.

63. Slivovskaja I, Ryliskyte L, Serpytis P, et al. Aerobic training effect on arterial stiffness in metabolic syndrome. Am J Med 2018;131:148–55.

64. Joo HJ, Cho SA, Cho JY, et al. Different relationship between physical activity, arterial stiffness, and metabolic status in obese subjects. J Phys Act Health 2017;14:716–25.

65. Ashor AW, Lara J, Siervo M, et al. Effects of exercise modalities on arterial stiffness and wave reflection: a systematic review and meta-analysis of randomized controlled trials. PLoS One 2014;9:e110034.

66. Mora-Rodriguez R, Ramirez-Jimenez M, Fernandez-Elias VE, et al. Effects of aerobic interval training on arterial stiffness and microvascular function in patients with metabolic syndrome. J Clin Hypertens 2018;20:11–8.

67. Bagi Z, Feher A, Cassuto J. Microvascular responsiveness in obesity: implications of therapeutic intervention. Br J Pharmacol 2012;165:544–60.

68. Ahmari SA, Bunch TJ, Modesto K, et al. Impact of individual and cumulative coronary risk factors on coronary flow reserve assessed by dobutamine stress echocardiography. Am J Cardiol 2008;101:1694–9.

69. Zhang C. The role of inflammatory cytokines in endothelial dysfunction. Basic Res Cardiol 2008;103(5):398–406.

70. de Simone G, Izzo R, De Luca N, et al. Left ventricular geometry in obesity: is it what we expect? Nutr Metab Cardiovasc Dis 2013;23(10):905–12.

Prognostic Markers and Management

Sodium-Glucose Cotransporter-2 Inhibitors, Reverse J-Curve Pattern, and Mortality in Heart Failure

Konstantinos Imprialos, MD, Konstantinos Stavropoulos, MD,
Vasilios Papademetriou, MD*

KEYWORDS

- SGLT-2 inhibitors • Cardiovascular events • Heart failure • Reverse J- curve • Mortality

KEY POINTS

- The therapeutic armamentarium for managing diabetes did not offer drugs with the potential to ameliorate morbidity and mortality outcomes in diabetic patients with heart failure.
- The novel sodium-glucose co-transporters 2 inhibitors are a promising class of drugs, shown to offer multidimensional ameliorating effects on a variety of traditional cardiovascular and heart failure risk factors.
- Most trial data suggest beneficial effects of SGLT-2 inhibitors on cardiovascular events in high-risk diabetic patients and in patients with HF.
- The reverse J-curve pattern between blood pressure levels and mortality has emerged as an important topic in the field of heart failure.
- There is no significant evidence to propose any potential effect of sodium-glucose co-transporters 2 inhibitors on the J-shape-suggested mortality in patients with heart failure.

INTRODUCTION

Type 2 diabetes mellitus is a traditional risk factor for the development of heart failure (HF).[1] The prevalence of both conditions is increasing, worldwide, partially owing to population aging.[2] The epidemic of HF and diabetes mellitus increases the need for efficient treatments to reduce morbidity and mortality in these patients. Although significant progress has been made in reducing cardiovascular (CV) outcomes in patient with type 2 diabetes mellitus, drugs offering reduction in the risk for HF and corresponding outcomes were missing.[3,4] Among novel antidiabetic drug classes, sodium-glucose co-transporters (SGLT)-2 inhibitors have provided incredible CV-ameliorating results. More important, they were shown to decrease HF and CV events in patients with HF.[5,6]

SODIUM-GLUCOSE CO-TRANSPORTER 2 INHIBITORS

During the past decade, the identification and targeting of potential novel mechanisms for the management of hyperglycemia has been at the epicenter of diabetes research. Kidneys seem to play a major role in glucose homeostasis and have been thoroughly examined during recent years. Several pathways involved in glucose homeostasis have been recognized, among which the SGLT-related mechanisms have been

VAMC and Georgetown University, 50 Irving Street, Washington, DC 20422, USA
* Corresponding author.
E-mail address: vpapademetriou@va.gov

Heart Failure Clin 15 (2019) 519–530
https://doi.org/10.1016/j.hfc.2019.06.004
1551-7136/19/© 2019 Elsevier Inc. All rights reserved.

examined as a potential target for the management of diabetes.[7] The SGLT family is located on the apical surface of the proximal convoluted tubule. The transporters are responsible for the active transportation of glucose from the luminal to the intracellular space with the use of a sodium gradient. Two members of the SGLT family, SGLT-1 and SGLT-2, are located in the renal tubules. SGLT-1 is located on the S2 and S3 segment of the proximal convoluted tubules and are responsible for the reabsorption of 10% of the filtered glucose, whereas SGLT-2 is located on the S1 segment and is responsible for the reabsorption of 90% of filtered glucose.[8,9]

The kidney plays an important role in the regulation of blood glucose. Approximately 170 to 180 g of glucose are filtered by the kidney daily, and almost all of glucose is reabsorbed in the renal tubules. However, higher blood glucose levels (approximately 200–250 mg/dL and higher) results in increased glucose filtration rate by the kidney. Saturation of the SLGT is observed when filtration rate is greater than 350 mg of glucose per minute; subsequently, glucose excess is excreted in the urine.[7,8]

In the setting of diabetes, the kidneys seem to present a maladaptive response in terms of glucose homeostasis. In particular, both glucose transporter 2 and SGLT-2 are found overexpressed in tubular cell from urine samples of patients with diabetes mellitus.[10] As a result of the higher SLGT-2 number, glucose reabsorption seems to be increased by approximately 20%.[11] Favoring these findings, glucose urine excretion was found to be lower than anticipated by the corresponding blood glucose levels in patients with type 1 diabetes mellitus.[12] This phenomenon seems to be an attempt to conserve this important metabolic substance, worsening however the diabetes-associated hyperglycemia.

The vital role of SGLT in the management of blood glucose levels has led research efforts to the development of a novel class of drugs that inhibit the SGLT, thus resulting in decreased reabsorption and increased excretion of glucose in the urine. Phlorizin was the first inhibitor of the SGLT family that was developed and tested for the management of hyperglycemia. Use of the drug was found to significantly decrease the reabsorption of glucose by inhibiting both the SGLT-1 and SGLT-2. However, SGLT-1 are also highly expressed in the gastrointestinal system, and thus, phlorizin use resulted in the inhibition of glucose absorption in the small intestine as well. Subsequently, the use of phlorizin resulted in increased adverse events from the gastrointestinal system and the development of the drug was terminated.[13–16] Several newer SGLT-2 inhibitors have been developed since, and currently are available in the United States, Europe, and other parts of the world, including dapagliflozin, canagliflozin, and emoagliflozin. Three other members of this drug class (ipragliflozin, tofogliflozin, and luseogliflozin) have been only approved in Japan.[17]

SODIUM-GLUCOSE CO-TRANSPORTERS 2 INHIBITORS AND EFFECT ON CARDIOVASCULAR RISK FACTORS

Several studies have investigated the impact of SGLT-2 inhibitors on a variety of traditional CV risk factors. Apart from the benefits of SGLT-2 inhibition in glycemic control, it was found that this novel class of drugs offers significant ameliorating effects in an abundance of CV risk factors, such as increased blood pressure, body weight, dyslipidemias, and nonalcoholic fatty liver disease.[4,5]

The paramount importance of glycemic control has been demonstrated in the UKPDS study, where significant reduction in the risks for myocardial infarction (MI), stroke, and all-cause death was shown with the reduction of glycated hemoglobin.[18] The glucose-lowering profile of SGLT-2 inhibitors has been the primary outcome in the majority of the studies with this class of drugs. In general, SGLT-2 inhibitors seem to offer a mild but significant reduction of HbA1c by approximately 0.5% to 1.0%.[18–62] When compared with placebo, SGLT-2 inhibitors were shown to reduce hemoglobin A1c by 0.5% (absolute values). Compared with other antidiabetic drugs, SGLT-2 inhibitors use found that this class of drugs is not inferior to other hypoglycemic drugs, offering similar reduction in hemoglobin A1c.[63] Metaanalytic data of canagliflozin, dapagliflozin, and empagliflozin use showed reduction of approximately 0.70%, 0.66%, and 0.40% to 2.00% with their use, respectively.[63] Of note, other members of this drug class (ipragliflozin, luseogliflozin, tofogliflozin) were shown to offer similar benefits in glycemic control.[54–62]

Elevated blood pressure (BP) is a major risk factor for the development of HF with reduced ejection fraction (HFrEF) or HF with preserved ejection fraction (HFpEF).[64,65] In addition, the management of hypertension (both systolic and diastolic) was found to decrease the risk for incident HF by 50%.[66–70] The SPRINT trial has found significant benefits with the intensive BP treatment and the recent American Heart Association/American College of Cardiology revised guidelines for the management of HF suggest a target BP of less than 130/80 mm Hg in patients with either HFrEF or HFpEF.[71]

Among the various beneficial properties of SGLT-2 inhibitors, this new class of drugs has been associated with mild decreases in BP levels. SGLT-2 uses a sodium gradient for the active reabsorption of filtered glucose, and thus, inhibition of the co-transporter results in increased urine sodium (and water) excretion. This mild diuretic effect is further enhanced owing to the increased glucose excretion in the urine, resulting in clinically meaningful diuresis and changes in patient's hemodynamics.[72] This finding has been demonstrated in studies where increased urine output was observed in patients on SGLT-2 inhibitors compared with placebo or diuretics.[73,74] The effect of SGLT-2 inhibition on BP levels has been examined in the majority of the SGLT-2 inhibitors study. In general a mild decrease in both the systolic BP (SBP) and the diastolic BP (DBP) of 3 to 5 mm Hg and 1 to 2 mm Hg, respectively, is observed. Importantly, this change seems to be a class effect with no clinically meaningful differences among different members of the SGLT-2 inhibitors family.[75–77] The BP-lowering effects of SGLT-2 inhibitors have also been demonstrated by studies assessing BP levels with the use of 24-hour ambulatory BP measurement.[74,78–83] Pooled data from these studies found a reduction in 24-hour SBP and 24-hour DBP by 3.76 and 1.83 mm Hg with either dapagliflozin, canagliflozin, empagliflozin, or ertugliflozin versus placebo, respectively.[84]

Important ameliorating effects of this class of drugs were also observed in the setting of body weight. The SGLT-2 inhibitor-induced glycosuria results in a caloric deficit that enhances the catabolism of visceral and subcutaneous fat. However, the subsequent weight loss is restricted by an increased caloric intake that is observed in patients on SGLT-2 inhibitors, secondary to an increase in appetite.[85–88] In general, a mild decrease of 2 to 3 kg is demonstrated in patients on SGLT-2 inhibitors compared with placebo or other antidiabetic drugs. Compared with hypoglycemic agents that cause an increase in body weight (insulin and insulin secretagogues), the difference is even greater, and favoring the use of SGLT-2 inhibitors, suggesting that addition of an SGLT-2 inhibitor might counterbalance the detrimental effects of these drugs on body weight and fat metabolism.[89]

SGLT-2 inhibitors have also been associated with mild improvement of the lipidemic profile of diabetic patients. Specifically, a mild decrease in triglycerides and a mild increase in high-density lipoprotein cholesterol levels have been observed with their use. In contrast, low-density lipoprotein cholesterol levels seem to slightly increase with SGLT-2 inhibition.[90–92] SGLT-2 inhibitors were also found to ameliorate arterial stiffness indices, which were shown to be independently associated with increased CV risk.[93] In addition, the attenuation of hepatic fibrosis, alanine aminotransferase levels, and markers of liver fibrosis and lipid concentration in the liver was also observed with their use in the setting of nonalcoholic fatty liver disease and steatohepatitis, conditions that are also independently associated with an increased risk for CV events.[94–96] Last, SGLT-2 inhibitors seem to cause a mild decrease in uric acid levels through the more distally located glucose transporter 9 isoform 2.[97]

EFFECT OF SODIUM-GLUCOSE CO-TRANSPORTERS 2 INHIBITORS ON HEART FAILURE OUTCOMES

The multidimensional beneficial profile of the SGLT-2 inhibitors raised expectations for a potential decrease in the risks for CV morbidity and mortality. As of this writing 3 major CV trials have assessed the impact of SGLT-2 on CV outcomes, as well as in HF end points.

As of this writing, 3 major CV trials have assessed the impact of sGLT-2 inhibitors in HF outcomes. The first trial was the EMPAREG-OUTCOMES study that assessed the CV safety of empagliflozin in patients with type 2 diabetes with established CV disease. Patients randomly received either 10 or 25 mg of empagliflozin or placebo and were followed for approximately 3 years. The primary end point of the study was the combination of CV mortality, nonfatal MI, and nonfatal stroke. Empagliflozin was related to a decrease in the risk of the primary outcome, CV death, and all-cause death by 14%, 38%, and 32%, respectively. Importantly, empagliflozin decreased hospitalizations for HF by 35%, whereas HF hospitalization and CV death were also decreased by 26% compared with placebo.[98] A post hoc analysis of the EMPAREG-OUTCOMES trial examined the impact of the drug specifically on HF outcomes. The decrease in HF hospitalization (35%) was found to be the same across doses, sensitivity analyses, and subgroups defined by baseline characteristics. Furthermore, the risk for HF hospitalization or CV death, hospitalization for HF, CV death, and all-cause mortality hospitalization or CV death were significantly lower with empagliflozin compared with placebo in both groups of patients with and without HF at baseline. Importantly, CV mortality in patients hospitalized for HF was lower in the empagliflozin group compared with placebo (13.5% vs 24.2%, respectively). Last, loop diuretics were less frequently introduced in patients on empagliflozin compared with placebo, potentially secondary to the diuretic properties of the SGLT-2 inhibitor.[99]

The second trial examining the CV profile of an SGLT-2 inhibitor was the Canagliflozin Cardiovascular Assessment Study (CANVAS) study. The study assessed the effect of canagliflozin on CV outcomes in high-risk patients with diabetes. The study consisted of 2 arms. In the first arm, 4330 patients received either 100 or 300 mg of canagliflozin or placebo. In the second arm, 5812 patients received 100 mg with a potential up-titration to 300 mg during the study or placebo. The primary outcome was the combination of CV death, nonfatal MI, and nonfatal stroke, and was decrease by 14% compared with placebo. The risks for CV death, nonfatal MI, and nonfatal stroke were all significantly lower in the empagliflozin group by 13%, 15% and 10% compared with placebo, respectively. In terms of HF outcomes, the results were similar to those of empagliflozin. Canagliflozin resulted in a 33% decrease in HF hospitalizations, and the risk for CV death or HF hospitalization was decrease by 22%.[100] A post hoc analysis examined the impact of canagliflozin on HF outcomes based on the ejection fraction of the hospitalized patients. Fatal or hospitalized HF was decreased by 30% with canagliflozin use. Furthermore, canagliflozin significantly decreased the risk for fatal of hospitalized HFrEF by 31%, and for HFpEF by 17% compared with placebo. For cases where the EF of the patients was unknown (HF with unknown EF) canagliflozin use was associated with significant reduction in the risk for fatal or hospitalized HF with unknown EF by 46%. Importantly, adjustment for other competing death risks showed similar decreases with active treatment compared with placebo.[101]

The recent Dapagliflozin Effect on Cardiovascular Events–Thrombolysis in Myocardial Infarction 58 (DECLARE–TIMI 58) trial is the third large CV randomized study of the SGLT-2 inhibitors class. The trial randomized more than 17,000 patients with type 2 diabetes to either 10 mg of dapagliflozin or placebo for approximately 4 years. The primary safety outcome was the combination of CV death, MI, or stroke, and the 2 primary efficacy outcomes were the above and a composite of CV death or hospitalization for HF. A trend for a decrease in the primary safety end point, along with the risks for stroke, MI, all-cause death, and CV death was noted with dapagliflozin compared with placebo; however, this factor did not reach statistical significance. In contrast, the risk for CV death or hospitalization for HF was significantly decreased with dapagliflozin by 17%, mainly driven by the impact of the drug on the risk for hospitalization for HF (a risk reduction of 27%). Importantly, dapagliflozin decreased the risk for HF or CV death in both groups of patients with and without HF at baseline.

Of note, the incidence of HF hospitalization or CV death was significantly lower in patients with overt CV disease, whereas it did not reach statistical significance in patients with multiple risk factors.[102] A recent report of the effect of dapagliflozin on HF outcomes found that SGLT-2 inhibition was associated with a reduction in the risk for CV death or hospitalization for HF in patients with HFrEF compared with placebo users, with a remarkable risk reduction of 38%. However, patients without HFrEF did not benefit from dapagliflozin administration. Furthermore, the effect of dapagliflozin was similar across patients with HF without known reduced EF and those without a history of HF. In contrast, dapagliflozin decreased the risk for hospitalization for HF regardless of EF status, with risk reductions of 36% and 24% for HFrEF and not HFrEF patients, respectively. Last, CV death and all-cause mortality were all significantly lower with dapagliflozin by 45% and 41%, respectively, whereas a nonsignificant decrease in patients with HF with unknown reduced EF was noted with dapagliflozin for both outcomes.[103]

Important data from the real-life setting have emerged from the Comparative Effectiveness of Cardiovascular Outcomes in New Users of SGLT-2 Inhibitors (CVD-REAL) trial. This retrospective international study assessed the impact of SGLT-2 inhibitors on CV morbidity and mortality compared with other antidiabetic drugs. In the more than 190,164 person-years of follow-up, there were 961 hospitalizations for HF events, resulting in a 39% risk reduction with SGLT-2 inhibitors compared with other antidiabetic drugs. In addition, in more than 143,342 person-years of follow-up, there were 1983 events of hospitalization for HF or all-cause death, translating to a significant risk reduction of 46% with SGLT-2 inhibitors use compared with other antidiabetic drugs.[104] After this study, the CVD-REAL 2 trial found that in more than 441,357 person-years, SGLT-2 inhibitors use was related with a decreased risk for hospitalization for HF by 36%. Importantly, hospitalization for FH was significantly lower in all countries included in the study. Last, in more than 441,357 person-years of follow-up, the risk for hospitalization for HF or death was significantly lower with SGLT-2 inhibition by 40% compared with other hypoglycemic agents.[105]

POTENTIAL MECHANISMS EXPLAINING HEART FAILURE BENEFITS WITH SODIUM-GLUCOSE CO-TRANSPORTERS 2 INHIBITORS

To this point, all SGLT-2 inhibitors large randomized CV trials have shown significant ameliorating effects in CV mortality and HF hospitalization, mainly in patients with HF at baseline, whereas SGLT-2 inhibitors seem to offer benefits and in patients without HF at baseline.

Several mechanisms might be implicated in the remarkable effects of SGLT-2 inhibition in HF outcomes. Among these, osmotic diuresis and increased sodium excretion are of paramount importance in the setting of HF to decrease the preload to the heart. Arterial stiffening and the mild decrease in BP with their use may also be implicated. However, the remarkable outcomes in the setting of HF found in all the SGLT-2 inhibitors trials might not be fully explained by these mechanisms.[106]

The use of glucose by the myocardium in the patient with diabetes is found to be decreased, whereas, free fatty acids and their catabolism is increased. The switch toward increased fatty acid metabolism seems to be attributed to the decrease in insulin sensitivity, along with the high bioavailability of free fatty acids in the setting of diabetes. The imbalanced cardiac metabolism along with the type of available metabolic supply in the circulation results in impaired cardiac energetics and dysfunction. Therefore, the alteration of the balance between free fatty acids and glucose in the blood might offer significant improvements in cardiac energetics and function.[107] Ketones seem to be a more powerful fuel for the diabetic heart compared with glucose. It has been observed that patients receiving SGLT-2 inhibitors have even up to 3-fold higher levels of circulation ketones, compared with nonusers. Importantly, beta-hydroxybutyrate is used by the cardiac tissue to produce free fatty acids that offer greater oxygen consumption and oxidation of the mitochondria, enhancing this energy production. In addition, the diuretic potency of SGLT-2 inhibitors results in hemoconcentration and increased oxygen supply to the heart. The combination of these 2 mechanisms might result in an improved and easily used energy supply to the diabetic heart.[108,109] Theoretically, these important metabolic properties of SGLT-2 inhibitors may contribute in their class effect on HF outcomes.

BLOOD PRESSURE DECREASE IN HEART FAILURE AND MORTALITY: IS THERE A J-CURVE RELATIONSHIP?

Almost after antihypertensive drug use was shown to offer CV benefits,[110,111] the J-curve phenomenon emerged as a hot topic in the field of hypertension.[112,113] The J-curve phenomenon was first described by Cruickshank,[113] who found a J-shaped association between the incidence of myocardial infraction and DBP, with the lower

risk for events with DBP between 85 to 90 mm Hg. The Hypertension Optimal Treatment (HOT) trial compared different levels of DBP (<90, <85, and <80 mm Hg) and no difference was observed in CV outcomes between these groups. However, the difference in achieved BP between the groups was small. A post hoc analysis of the HOT trial suggested a nadir BP level of 138.5/82.6 mm Hg.[114] The existence of the J-curve hypothesis with reduction in SBP has been brought to light from various intensive BP-lowering trials. The Action to Control Cardiovascular Risk in Diabetes did not found a significant reduction in major CV events with a target BP of less than 120 mm Hg versus 140 mm Hg.[115] The Ongoing Telmisartan Alone and in Combination With Ramipril Global End Point Trial (ONTARGET) study found a trend for an increase in all-cause death with a target SBP of less than 130 mm Hg,[116] whereas in the INternational VErapamil SR-Trandolapril (INVEST) trial, patients with diabetes had increased risk of all-cause mortality if they achieved an SBP of less than 115 versus an SBP of less than 130 mm Hg.[117] A more recent post hoc analysis by Böhm and colleagues[118] of the ONTARGET and Telmisartan Randomised Assessment Study in ACE Intolerant Participants With Cardiovascular Disease (TRANSCEND) trials in patients aged 55 years or older without symptomatic HF at entry and with a history of chronic coronary artery disease, peripheral artery disease, transient ischemic attack, stroke, or diabetes mellitus found that achieved SBP values of less than 120 mm Hg were not associated with an increased risk of MI or stroke. However, they were related to a greater risk for all-cause and CV death and HF. In contrast, the SPRINT study reported a significant decrease in CV morbidity and mortality with an achieved BP of approximately 121 mm Hg. It has to be noted that most data come from observational studies, and few data exist from randomized trials.[119]

The lack of a J-curve effect on stroke and MI outcomes along with the potential existence of such an effect on all-cause mortality raises the question of whether reverse causality contributes to these findings. One should take into account that low BP levels are significantly associated with increased mortality in patients with HF and renal disease. Therefore, associations should be interpreted cautiously, especially when recording BP before death.

In the setting of HF, however, the J-curve topic has been less examined. It has been shown that low BP levels are associated with increased mortality in patients with HF. Among 5747 patients with New York Heart Association functional class

II or III HF and EF of 0.45 or less, the all-cause mortality rate during the entire study period for patients with a baseline SBP of less than 100 mm Hg was 50%, which is significantly higher than that of patients with SBP of 130 to 139 mm Hg (mortality rate of 32%, a 65% risk increase).[120] In another study assessing baseline BP levels and mortality outcomes, it was found that in more than 7200 patients with mild to moderate chronic systolic and diastolic HF, SPB levels of less than 120 mm Hg were related to a greater CV and HF mortality, by 15% and 30%, respectively, after 5 years compared with patients with an SBP of greater than 120 mm Hg. Of note, all-cause death did not differ significantly between the 2 groups.[121] Metaanalytic data from 10 studies and 8088 patients with chronic HF found a decrease in mortality of 13% with an increase in SBP by 10 mm Hg. Importantly, in the lowest tertile (patients with an SBP of 109 mm Hg), a 10-mm Hg increase in BP resulted in an 18% decrease in the risk for total mortality.[122] Few data exist about the relation of achieved BP and CV or mortality outcomes in HF. Among 7453 patients with chronic HF, the highest mortality was observed in patients with SBP levels of less than 90 mm Hg compared with patients with an SPB of greater than 130 mm Hg. Patients with BP levels between 90 and 129 mm Hg had an in-between risk.[123]

Based on these findings, lower BP levels in various subgroups of patients with HF seem to be associated with worse outcomes. However, none of these studies were able to identify the nadir BP point on which HF patients have less risk for morbidity and mortality. In contrast with other populations where the nadir point seems to range between 100 and 120 mm Hg of SBP, the limited findings in patients with HF suggest that the nadir point is at higher BP levels. In this setting, a recent study suggested a reverse J-curve phenomenon in patients with HF. A study followed more than 5600 patients hospitalized for acute HF for approximately 2 years. The relation of on-treatment BP levels with mortality was assessed at the end of the study. The relationship between BP and all-cause mortality followed a reversed J-shaped curve pattern, with increased risks at lower and higher BPs. More specifically, the event rate increased significantly below and above the reference BP range (130–140/70–80 mm Hg), except for an SBP above the reference BP range, where an insignificant trend for increase in mortality was found above 150 mm Hg. Importantly, a nadir point of 132.4 for SBP and 74.2 mm Hg for DBP was observed, when the event rate was the lowest. The reverse J-curve relationship was observed in both HFrEF and HFpEF for all-cause

mortality, with the lower risk at136.0/76.6 mm Hg and 127.9/72.7 mm Hg, respectively. Mortality risks increased significantly at lower and higher BPs for both SBP and DBP in patients with HFpEF. In contrast, mortality rates were significantly higher only at a lower BP, whereas a trend for an increase was found at higher SBP levels in patients with HFrEF.[124]

It remains a matter of great debate whether there is a causal relationship between the low BP and increased risk for events. Low BP levels result in tissue hypoperfusion, deterioration of cardiac function, and increased events. However, someone should bear in mind that other factors might be in play. Low BP is commonly encountered as a sign of other underlying condition (such as cancer or renal disease),[125–127] and thus reverse causality could result in increased mortality rates. In addition, a low SBP is also found in patients with more severe forms of cardiac dysfunction, suggesting a higher risk for events.[128,129] Low DBP could be an indication of progressed vascular disease and arterial stiffness, conditions that result in a higher risk for CV morbidity and mortality. In this setting, low DBP might result in limited perfusion of the already sclerotic coronary arteries, increasing the risk for coronary events.[130–132] Collectively, current data support the existence of a J-curve phenomenon in HF. The nadir point of the curve seems to be higher than the one in the hypertensive population, in which (if it truly exists) it could be found at BP levels between 100 and 120 mm Hg. Other causes for this observation might be in play and until properly designed studies could address the existence J-curve relation, all data should be interpreted cautiously.

SUMMARY

SGLT-2 inhibition seems to decrease morbidity and mortality in patients with HF. Several mechanisms have been proposed to explain this remarkable effect. The higher bioavailability of ketones seems the most prevalent to explain these effects. The amelioration of other CV risk factors could also contribute to the beneficial impact of SGLT-2 inhibitors of CV and HF events. Of note, the mild reduction in BP might also contribute in these benefits. Because baseline BP levels in patients with HF were approximately 134 to 135 mm Hg in the EMPA-REG outcome study, and given the SGLT-2 inhibitors–induced decrease in BP of 3 to 5/1 to 2 mm Hg, achieved BP at the end of the study was close to the nadir point where maximal mortality improvements have been observed in the abovementioned study by Lee and colleagues.[124] However, subanalyses of outcomes according to baseline and at end-of-study BP levels from all SGLT-2 inhibitors CV trials are required to unveil any potential effect of this class of drugs on the reverse J-curve phenomenon.

REFERENCES

1. Kannel WB, Hjortland M, Castelli WP. Role of diabetes in congestive heart failure: the Framingham study. Am J Cardiol 1974;34:29–34.

2. Thrainsdottir IS, Aspelund T, Thorgeirsson G, et al. The association between glucose abnormalities and heart failure in the population-based Reykjavik study. Diabetes Care 2005;28:612–6.

3. Rawshani A, Rawshani A, Gudbjornsdottir S. Mortality and cardiovascular disease in type 1 and type 2 diabetes. N Engl J Med 2017;377:300–1.

4. Cavender MA, Steg PG, Smith SC Jr, et al. Impact of diabetes mellitus on hospitalization for heart failure, cardiovascular events, and death: outcomes at 4 years from the reduction of atherothrombosis for continued health (REACH) registry. Circulation 2015;132:923–31.

5. Imprialos KP, Stavropoulos K, Doumas M, et al. The effect of SGLT2 inhibitors on cardiovascular events and renal function. Expert Rev Clin Pharmacol 2017;10(11):1251–61.

6. Imprialos K, Faselis C, Boutari C, et al. SGLT-2 inhibitors and cardiovascular risk in diabetes mellitus: a comprehensive and critical review of the literature. Curr Pharm Des 2017;23(10):1510–21.

7. DeFronzo RA, Davidson JA, Del Prato S. The role of the kidneys in glucose homeostasis: a new path towards normalizing glycaemia. Diabetes Obes Metab 2011;14:5–14.

8. Vallon V, Platt KA, Cunard R, et al. SGLT2 mediates glucose reabsorption in the early proximal tubule. J Am Soc Nephrol 2011;22(1):104–12.

9. Kanai Y, Lee WS, You G, et al. The human kidney low affinity Na+/glucose cotransporter SGLT2. Delineation of the major renal reabsorptive mechanism for D-glucose. J Clin Invest 1994;93:397–404.

10. Rahmoune H, Thompson P, Ward J, et al. Glucose transporters in human renal proximal tubular cells isolated from the urine of patients with non-insulin-dependent diabetes. Diabetes 2005;54:3427–34.

11. Vlotides G, Mertens PR. Sodium-glucose cotransport inhibitors: mechanisms, metabolic effects and implications for the treatment of diabetic patients with chronic kidney disease. Nephrol Dial Transplant 2015;30(8):1272–6.

12. Mogensen CE. Maximum tubular reabsorption capacity for glucose and renal hemodynamics during rapid hypertonic glucose infusion in normal and diabetic subjects. Scand J Clin Lab Invest 1971;28:101–9.

13. Alvarado F, Crane RK. Phlorizin as a competitive inhibitor of the active transport of sugars by hamster small intestine, in vitro. Biochim Biophys Acta 1962;56:170–2.

14. Rossetti L, Smith D, Shulman GI, et al. Correction of hyperglycemia with phlorizin normalizes tissue sensitivity to insulin in diabetic rats. J Clin Invest 1987;79:1510–5.

15. Ehrenkranz JR, Lewis NG, Kahn CR, et al. Phlorizin: a review. Diabetes Metab Res Rev 2005;21:31–8.

16. Rossetti L, Shulman GI, Zawalich W, et al. Effect of chronic hyperglycemia on in vivo insulin secretion in partially pancreatectomized rats. J Clin Invest 1987;80:1037–44.

17. Abdul-Ghani MA, Norton L, DeFronzo RA. Efficacy and safety of SGLT2 inhibitors in the treatment of type 2 diabetes mellitus. Curr Diab Rep 2012;12:230–8.

18. Henry RR, Rosenstock J, Edelman S, et al. Exploring the potential of the SGLT2 inhibitor dapagliflozin in type 1 diabetes: a randomized, double-blind placebo-controlled pilot study. Diabetes Care 2015;38(3):412–9.

19. Ferrannini E, Ramos SJ, Salsali A, et al. Dapagliflozin monotherapy in type 2 diabetic patients with inadequate glycemic control by diet and exercise: a randomized, double-blind, placebo-controlled, phase 3 trial. Diabetes Care 2010;33(10):2217–24.

20. Wilding JP, Woo V, Soler NG, et al. Long-term efficacy of dapagliflozin in patients with type 2 diabetes mellitus receiving high doses of insulin: a randomized trial. Ann Intern Med 2012;156(6):405–15.

21. Kohan DE, Fioretto P, Tang W, et al. Long-term study of patients with type 2 diabetes and moderate renal impairment shows that dapagliflozin reduces weight and blood pressure but does not improve glycemic control. Kidney Int 2014;85(4):962–71.

22. Jabbour SA, Hardy E, Sugg J, et al. Dapagliflozin is effective as add-on therapy to sitagliptin with or without metformin: a 24-week, multicenter, randomized, double-blind, placebo-controlled study. Diabetes Care 2014;37(3):740–50.

23. Kaku K, Maegawa H, Tanizawa Y, et al. Dapagliflozin as monotherapy or combination therapy in Japanese patients with type 2 diabetes: an open-label study. Diabetes Ther 2014;5(2):415–33.

24. Leiter LA, Cefalu WT, De Bruin TW, et al. Dapagliflozin added to usual care in individuals with type 2 diabetes mellitus with preexisting cardiovascular disease: a 24-week, multicenter, randomized, double-blind, placebo-controlled study with a 28-week extension. J Am Geriatr Soc 2014;62(7):1252–62.

25. Nauck MA, Del Prato S, Durán-García S, et al. Durability of glycaemic efficacy over 2 years with

dapagliflozin versus glipizide as add-on therapies in patients whose type 2 diabetes mellitus is inadequately controlled with metformin. Diabetes Obes Metab 2014;16(11):1111–2.

26. Strojek K, Yoon KH, Hruba V, et al. Dapagliflozin added to glimepiride in patients with type 2 diabetes mellitus sustains glycemic control and weight loss over 48 weeks: a randomized, double-blind, parallel-group, placebo-controlled trial. Diabetes Ther 2014;5(1):267–83.

27. Del Prato S, Nauck M, Durán-Garcia S, et al. Long-term glycaemic response and tolerability of dapagliflozin versus a sulphonylurea as add -on therapy to metformin in patients with type 2 diabetes: 4-year data. Diabetes Obes Metab 2015;17(6):581–90.

28. Bode B, Stenlöf K, Sullivan D, et al. Efficacy and safety of canagliflozin treatment in older subjects with type 2 diabetes mellitus: a randomized trial. Hosp Pract (1995) 2013;41(2):72–84.

29. Cefalu WT, Stenlöf K, Leiter LA, et al. Effects of canagliflozin on body weight and relationship to HbA1c and blood pressure changes in patients with type 2 diabetes. Diabetologia 2015;58(6):1183–7.

30. Lavalle-González FJ, Januszewicz A, Davidson J, et al. Efficacy and safety of canagliflozin compared with placebo and sitagliptin in patients with type 2 diabetes on background metformin monotherapy: a randomised trial. Diabetologia 2013;56(12):2582–92.

31. Schernthaner G, Gross JL, Rosenstock J, et al. Canagliflozin compared with sitagliptin for patients with type 2 diabetes who do not have adequate glycemic control with metformin plus sulfonylurea: a 52-week randomized trial. Diabetes Care 2013;36(9):2508–15.

32. Stenlöf K, Cefalu WT, Kim KA, et al. Efficacy and safety of canagliflozin monotherapy in subjects with type 2 diabetes mellitus inadequately controlled with diet and exercise. Diabetes Obes Metab 2013;15(4):372–82.

33. Wilding JP, Charpentier G, Hollander P, et al. Efficacy and safety of canagliflozin in patients with type 2 diabetes mellitus inadequately controlled with metformin and sulphonylurea: a randomised trial. Int J Clin Pract 2013;67(12):1267–82.

34. Forst T, Guthrie R, Goldenberg R, et al. Efficacy and safety of canagliflozin over 52 weeks in patients with type 2 diabetes on background metformin and pioglitazone. Diabetes Obes Metab 2014;16(5):467–77.

35. Inagaki N, Kondo K, Yoshinari T, et al. Efficacy and safety of canagliflozin monotherapy in Japanese patients with type 2 diabetes inadequately controlled with diet and exercise: a 24-week, randomized, double-blind, placebo-controlled, Phase III study. Expert Opin Pharmacother 2014;15(11):1501–15.

36. Sha S, Devineni D, Ghosh A, et al. Pharmacodynamic effects of canagliflozin, a sodium glucose co-transporter 2 inhibitor, from a randomized study in patients with type 2 diabetes. PLoS One 2014;9(9):e110069.

37. Sha S, Polidori D, Heise T, et al. Effect of the sodium glucose co-transporter 2 inhibitor canagliflozin on plasma volume in patients with type 2diabetes mellitus. Diabetes Obes Metab 2014;16(11):1087–95.

38. Stenlöf K, Cefalu WT, Kim KA, et al. Long-term efficacy and safety of canagliflozin monotherapy in patients with type 2 diabetes inadequately controlled with diet and exercise: findings from the 52-week CANTATA-M study. Curr Med Res Opin 2014;30(2):163–75.

39. Ji L, Han P, Liu Y, et al. Canagliflozin in Asian patients with type 2 diabetes on metformin alone or metformin in combination with sulphonylurea. Diabetes Obes Metab 2015;17(1):23–31.

40. Leiter LA, Yoon KH, Arias P, et al. Canagliflozin provides durable glycemic improvements and body weight reduction over 104 weeks versus glimepiride in patients with type 2 diabetes on metformin: a randomized, double-blind, phase 3 study. Diabetes Care 2015;38(3):355–64.

41. Neal B, Perkovic V, De Zeeuw D, et al. Efficacy and safety of canagliflozin, an inhibitor of sodium-glucose cotransporter 2, when used in conjunction with insulin therapy in patients with type 2 diabetes. Diabetes Care 2015;38(3):403–11.

42. Weir MR, Januszewicz A, Gilbert RE, et al. Effect of canagliflozin on blood pressure and adverse events related to osmotic diuresis and reduced intravascular volume in patients with type 2 diabetes mellitus. J Clin Hypertens (Greenwich) 2014;16(12):875–82.

43. Yale JF, Bakris G, Cariou B, et al. Efficacy and safety of canagliflozin over 52 weeks in patients with type 2 diabetes mellitus and chronic kidney disease. Diabetes Obes Metab 2014;16(10):1016–27.

44. Häring HU, Merker L, Seewaldt-Becker E, et al. Empagliflozin as add-on to metformin plus sulfonylurea in patients with type 2 diabetes: a 24-week, randomized, double-blind, placebo-controlled trial. Diabetes Care 2013;36(11):3396–404.

45. Kovacs CS, Seshiah V, Swallow R, et al. Empagliflozin improves glycaemic and weight control as add-on therapy to pioglitazone or pioglitazone plus metformin in patients with type 2 diabetes: a 24-week, randomized, placebo-controlled trial. Diabetes Obes Metab 2014;16(2):147–58.

46. Roden M, Weng J, Eilbracht J, et al. Empagliflozin monotherapy with sitagliptin as an active

comparator in patients with type 2 diabetes: a randomised, double-blind, placebo-controlled, phase 3 trial. Lancet Diabetes Endocrinol 2013; 1(3):208–19.

47. Rosenstock J, Seman LJ, Jelaska A, et al. Efficacy and safety of empagliflozin, a sodium glucose co-transporter 2 (SGLT2) inhibitor, as add-on to metformin in type 2 diabetes with mild hyperglycaemia. Diabetes Obes Metab 2013; 15(12):1154–60.

48. Barnett AH, Mithal A, Manassie J, et al. Efficacy and safety of empagliflozin added to existing anti-diabetes treatment in patients with type 2 diabetes and chronic kidney disease: a randomised, double-blind, placebo-controlled trial. Lancet Diabetes Endocrinol 2014;2(5):369–84.

49. Häring HU, Merker L, Seewaldt-Becker E, et al. Empagliflozin as add-on to metformin in patients with type 2 diabetes: a 24-week, randomized, double-blind, placebo-controlled trial. Diabetes Care 2014;37(6):1650–9.

50. Kadowaki T, Haneda M, Inagaki N, et al. Empagliflozin monotherapy in Japanese patients with type 2 diabetes mellitus: a randomized, 12-week, double-blind, placebo-controlled, phase II trial. Adv Ther 2014;31(6):621–38.

51. Ridderstråle M, Andersen KR, Zeller C, et al. Comparison of empagliflozin and glimepiride as add-on to metformin in patients with type 2 diabetes: a 104-week randomised, active-controlled, double-blind, phase 3 trial. Lancet Diabetes Endocrinol 2014;2(9):691–700.

52. DeFronzo RA, Lewin A, Patel S, et al. Combination of empagliflozin and linagliptin as second-line therapy in subjects with type 2 diabetes inadequately controlled on metformin. Diabetes Care 2015; 38(3):384–93.

53. Nishimura R, Tanaka Y, Koiwai K, et al. Effect of empagliflozin monotherapy on postprandial glucose and 24-hour glucose variability in Japanese patients with type 2 diabetes mellitus: a randomized, double-blind, placebo-controlled, 4-week study. Cardiovasc Diabetol 2015;14(1):11.

54. Kashiwagi A, Kazuta K, Goto K, et al. Ipragliflozin in combination with metformin for the treatment of Japanese patients with type 2 diabetes: ILLUMINATE, a randomized, double-blind, placebo-controlled study. Diabetes Obes Metab 2015; 17(3):304–8.

55. Kashiwagi A, Takahashi H, Ishikawa H, et al. A randomized, double-blind, placebo-controlled study on long-term efficacy and safety of ipragliflozin treatment in patients with type 2 diabetes mellitus and renal impairment: results of the long-term ASP1941 safety evaluation in patients with type 2 diabetes with renal impairment (LANTERN) study. Diabetes Obes Metab 2015;17(2):152–60.

56. Wilding JP, Ferrannini E, Fonseca VA, et al. Efficacy and safety of ipragliflozin in patients with type 2 diabetes inadequately controlled on metformin: a dose-finding study. Diabetes Obes Metab 2013; 15(5):403–9.

57. Inagaki N, Seino Y, Sasaki T, et al. Luseogliflozin, a selective SGLT2 inhibitor, added on to glimepiride for 52 weeks improves glycaemic control with no major hypoglycaemia in Japanese type 2 diabetes patients. Diabetologia 2013;56(suppl 1):S82.

58. Haneda M, Seino Y, Fukatsu A, et al. Luseogliflozin, a SGLT2 inhibitor, as add-on therapy to 5 types of oral antidiabetic drugs improves glycaemic control and reduces body weight in Japanese patients with type 2 diabetes mellitus. Diabetologia 2013; 56(suppl 1):S384.

59. Seino Y, Sasaki T, Fukatsu A, et al. Efficacy and safety of luseogliflozin monotherapy in Japanese patients with type 2 diabetes mellitus: a 12-week, randomized, placebo-controlled, phase II study. Curr Med Res Opin 2014;30(7):1219–30.

60. Seino Y, Sasaki T, Fukatsu A, et al. Efficacy and safety of luseogliflozin as monotherapy in Japanese patients with type 2 diabetes mellitus: a randomized, double-blind, placebo-controlled, phase 3 study. Curr Med Res Opin 2014;30(7):1245–55.

61. Kaku K, Watada H, Iwamoto Y, et al. Efficacy and safety of monotherapy with the novel sodium/glucose cotransporter-2 inhibitor tofogliflozin in Japanese patients with type 2 diabetes mellitus: a combined Phase 2 and 3 randomized, placebo-controlled, double-blind, parallel-group comparative study. Cardiovasc Diabetol 2014;13:65.

62. Ikeda S, Takano Y, Cynshi O, et al. A novel and selective SGLT2 inhibitor, tofogliflozin improves glycaemic control and lowers body weight in patients with type 2 diabetes mellitus. Diabetologia 2012;55(suppl 1):S1–538.

63. Liu XY, Zhang N, Chen R, et al. Efficacy and safety of sodium-glucose cotransporter 2 inhibitors in type 2 diabetes: a meta-analysis of randomized controlled trials for 1 to 2 years. J Diabetes Complications 2015;29:1295–303.

64. Levy D, Larson MG, Vasan RS, et al. The progression from hypertension to congestive heart failure. JAMA 1996;275:1557–62.

65. Wilhelmsen L, Rosengren A, Eriksson H, et al. Heart failure in the general population of men: morbidity, risk factors and prognosis. J Intern Med 2001;249:253–61.

66. Kostis JB, Davis BR, Cutler J, et al. Prevention of heart failure by antihypertensive drug treatment in older persons with isolated systolic hypertension: SHEP Cooperative Research Group. JAMA 1997;278:212–6.

67. Beckett NS, Peters R, Fletcher AE, et al. Treatment of hypertension in patients 80 years of age or older. N Engl J Med 2008;358:1887–98.

68. Sciarretta S, Palano F, Tocci G, et al. Antihypertensive treatment and development of heart failure in hypertension: a Bayesian network metaanalysis of studies in patients with hypertension and high cardiovascular risk. Arch Intern Med 2011;171:384–94.

69. Staessen JA, Wang JG, Thijs L. Cardiovascular prevention and blood pressure reduction: a quantitative overview updated until 1 March 2003. J Hypertens 2003;21:1055–76.

70. Verdecchia P, Sleight P, Mancia G, et al. Effects of telmisartan, ramipril, and their combination on left ventricular hypertrophy in individuals at high vascular risk in the ongoing telmisartan alone and in combination with ramipril global end point trial and the telmisartan randomized assessment study in ACE intolerant subjects with cardiovascular disease. Circulation 2009;120:1380–9.

71. Yancy CW, Jessup M, Bozkurt B, et al. 2017 ACC/AHA/HFSA focused update of the 2013 ACCF/AHA guideline for the management of heart failure: a report of the American College of Cardiology/American Heart Association Task Force on clinical practice guidelines and the Heart Failure Society of America. Circulation 2017;136(6):e137–61.

72. Muskiet MH, van Bommel EJ, van Raalte DH. Antihypertensive effects of SGLT2 inhibitors in type 2 diabetes. Lancet Diabetes Endocrinol 2016;4:188–9.

73. List JF, Woo V, Morales E, et al. Sodium-glucose cotransport inhibition with dapagliflozin in type 2 diabetes. Diabetes Care 2009;32(4):650–7.

74. Lambers-Heerspink HJ, De Zeeuw D, Wie L, et al. Dapagliflozin a glucose-regulating drug with diuretic properties in subjects with type 2 diabetes. Diabetes Obes Metab 2013;15:853–62.

75. Imprialos KP, Sarafidis PA, Karagiannis AI. Sodium-glucose cotransporter-2 inhibitors and blood pressure decrease: a valuable effect of a novel antidiabetic class? J Hypertens 2015;33:2185–97.

76. Mazidi M, Rezaie, Gao HK, et al. Effect of sodium-glucose cotransport-2 inhibitors on blood pressure in people with type 2 diabetes mellitus: a systematic review and meta-analysis of 43 randomized control trials with 22 528 Patients. J Am Heart Assoc 2017;6(6). https://doi.org/10.1161/JAHA.116.004007.

77. Baker WL, Smyth LR, Riche DM, et al. Effects of sodium-glucose co-transporter 2 inhibitors on blood pressure: a systematic review and meta-analysis. J Am Soc Hypertens 2014;8(4):262–75.e9.

78. Townsend RR, Machin I, Ren J, et al. Reductions in mean 24-hour ambulatory blood pressure after 6-week Treatment with canagliflozin in patients with type 2 diabetes mellitus and hypertension. J Clin Hypertens (Greenwich) 2016;18:43–52.

79. Stavropoulos K, Imprialos KP, Boutari C, et al. Canagliflozin and hypertension: is it the optimal choice for all hypertensive patients? J Clin Hypertens (Greenwich) 2016;18(10):1073.

80. Weber MA, Mansfield TA, Alessi F, et al. Effects of dapagliflozin on blood pressure in hypertensive diabetic patients on renin angiotensin system blockade. Blood Press 2016;25:93–103.

81. Weber MA, Mansfield TA, Cain VA, et al. Blood pressure and glycaemic effects of dapagliflozin versus placebo in patients with type 2 diabetes on combination antihypertensive therapy: a randomised, double-blind, placebo-controlled, phase 3 study. Lancet Diabetes Endocrinol 2016;4:211–20.

82. Tikkanen I, Narko K, Zeller C, et al. Empagliflozin reduces blood pressure in patients with type 2 diabetes and hypertension. Diabetes Care 2015;38:420–8.

83. Amin NB, Wang X, Mitchell JR, et al. Blood pressure lowering effect of the sodium glucose cotransporter-2 inhibitor, ertugliflozin, assessed via ambulatory blood pressure monitoring in patients with type 2 diabetes and hypertension. Diabetes Obes Metab 2015;17:805–8.

84. Baker WL, Buckley LF, Kelly MS, et al. Effects of sodium-glucose cotransporter 2 inhibitors on 24-hour ambulatory blood pressure: a systematic review and meta-analysis. J Am Heart Assoc 2017;6(5). https://doi.org/10.1161/JAHA.117.005686.

85. Ribola FA, Cançado FB, Schoueri JH, et al. Effects of SGLT2 inhibitors on weight loss in patients with type 2 diabetes mellitus. Eur Rev Med Pharmacol Sci 2017;21(1):199–211.

86. Barnett AH. Impact of sodium glucose cotransporter 2 inhibitors on weight in patients with type 2 diabetes mellitus. Postgrad Med 2013;125(5):92–100.

87. Ferrannini G, Hach T, Crowe S, et al. Energy balance following sodium-glucose co-transporter-2 (SGLT2) inhibition. Diabetologia 2014;38(9):1730–5.

88. Tsimihodimos V, Filippatos TD, Elisaf MS. Effects of sodium-glucose co-transporter 2 inhibitors on metabolism: unanswered questions and controversies. Expert Opin Drug Metab Toxicol 2017;13(4):399–408.

89. Zaccardi F, Webb DR, Htike ZZ, et al. Efficacy and safety of sodium-glucose co-transporter-2 inhibitors in type 2 diabetes mellitus: systematic review and network meta-analysis. Diabetes Obes Metab 2016;18(8):783–94.

90. Hardy E, Ptanszynska A, de Bruin TWA, et al. Changes in lipid profiles of patients with type 2 diabetes mellitus on dapagliflozin therapy. Diabetologia 2013;(Suppl 947):61.

91. Sinclair A, Bode B, Harris S, et al. Efficacy and safety of canagliflozin compared with placebo in older patients with type 2 diabetes mellitus: a pooled analysis of clinical studies. BMC Endocr Disord 2014;14:37.

92. Hach T, Gerich J, Salsali A, et al. Empagliflozin improves glycaemic parameters and cardiovascular risk factors in patients with type 2 diabetes: pooled data from four pivotal phase III trials. Diabetes 2013;62(Suppl. 1):LB19.

93. Cherney DZ, Perkins BA, Soleymanlou N, et al. The effect of empagliflozin on arterial stiffness and heart rate variability in subjects with uncomplicated type 1 diabetes mellitus. Cardiovasc Diabetol 2014;13:28.

94. Qiang S, Nakatsu Y, Seno Y, et al. Treatment with the SGLT2 inhibitor luseogliflozin improves nonalcoholic steatohepatitis in a rodent model with diabetes mellitus. Diabetol Metab Syndr 2015;7:104.

95. Nishimura N, Kitade M, Noguchi R, et al. Ipragliflozin, a sodium-glucose cotransporter 2 inhibitor, ameliorates the development of liver fibrosis in diabetic Otsuka Long-Evans Tokushima fatty rats. J Gastroenterol 2016;51(12):1141–9.

96. Honda Y, Imajo K, Kato T, et al. The selective SGLT2 inhibitor ipragliflozin has a therapeutic effect on nonalcoholic steatohepatitis in mice. PLoS One 2016;11:e0146337.

97. Katsiki N, Athyros VG, Mikhailidis DP. Cardiovascular effects of sodium-glucose cotransporter 2 inhibitors: multiple actions. Curr Med Res Opin 2016;14:1–2.

98. Zinman B, Wanner C, Lachin JM, et al. Empagliflozin, cardiovascular outcomes, and mortality in type 2 diabetes. N Engl J Med 2015;373:2117–28.

99. Fitchett D, Butler J, van de Borne P, et al. Effects of empagliflozin on risk for cardiovascular death and heart failure hospitalization across the spectrum of heart failure risk in the EMPA-REG OUTCOME® trial. Eur Heart J 2018;39(5):363–70.

100. Neal B, Perkovic V, Mahaffey KW, et al. Canagliflozin and cardiovascular and renal events in type 2 diabetes. N Engl J Med 2017;377(7):644–57.

101. Figtree GA, Rådholm K, Barrett TD, et al. Effects of canagliflozin on heart failure outcomes associated with preserved and reduced ejection fraction in type 2 diabetes: results from the CANVAS program. Circulation 2019. https://doi.org/10.1161/CIRCULATIONAHA.119.040057.

102. Wiviott SD, Raz I, Bonaca MP, et al. Dapagliflozin and cardiovascular outcomes in type 2 diabetes. N Engl J Med 2019;380(4):347–57.

103. Kato ET, Silverman MG, Mosenzon O, et al. Effect of dapagliflozin on heart failure and mortality in type 2 diabetes mellitus. Circulation 2019. https://doi.org/10.1161/CIRCULATIONAHA.119.040130.

104. Kosiborod M, Cavender MA, Fu AZ, et al. Lower risk of heart failure and death in patients initiated on sodium-glucose cotransporter-2 inhibitors versus other glucose-lowering drugs: the CVD-REAL Study (Comparative Effectiveness of Cardiovascular Outcomes in New Users of Sodium-Glucose Cotransporter-2 Inhibitors). Circulation 2017;136(3):249–59.

105. Kosiborod M, Lam CSP, Kohsaka S, et al. Cardiovascular events associated with SGLT-2 inhibitors versus other glucose-lowering drugs: the CVD-REAL 2 study. J Am Coll Cardiol 2018;71(23):2628–39.

106. Athyros VG, Imprialos K, Doumas M, et al. Beneficial effects of sodium glucose co-transporter 2 inhibitors (SGLT2i) on heart failure and cardiovascular death in patients with type 2 diabetes might be due to their off-target effects on cardiac metabolism. Clin Lipidol 2016;11(1):2–5.

107. Mudaliar S, Alloju S, Henry RR. Can a shift in fuel energetics explain the beneficial cardiorenal outcomes in the EMPAREG OUTCOME study? A unifying hypothesis. Diabetes Care 2016;39:1115–22.

108. Ferrannini E, Mark M, Mayoux E. CV protection in the EMPA-REG OUTCOME trial: a "Thrifty Substrate" hypothesis. Diabetes Care 2016;39:1108–14.

109. Barsotti A, Giannoni A, Di Napoli P, et al. Energy metabolism in the normal and in the diabetic heart. Curr Pharm Des 2009;15:836–40.

110. Veterans Administration Cooperative Study Group on Antihypertensive Agents. Effects of treatment on morbidity in hypertension. Results in patients with diastolic blood pressures averaging 115 through 129 mm Hg. JAMA 1967;202:1028–34.

111. Veterans Administration Cooperative Study Group on Antihypertensive Agents. Effects of treatment on morbidity in hypertension. II. Results in patients with diastolic blood pressure averaging 90 through 114 mm Hg. JAMA 1970;213:1143–52.

112. Stewart IMG. Relation of reduction in pressure to first myocardial infarction in patients receiving treatment for severe hypertension. Lancet 1979;313:861–5.

113. Cruickshank JM. Coronary flow reserve and the J curve relation between diastolic blood pressure and myocardial infarction. BMJ 1988;297:1227–30.

114. Hansson L, Zanchetti A, Carruthers SG, et al. Effects of intensive blood-pressure lowering and low-dose aspirin in patients with hypertension: principal results of the Hypertension Optimal Treatment (HOT) randomised trial. HOT Study Group. Lancet 1998;351(9118):1755–62.

115. Group AS, Cushman WC, Evans GW, et al. Effects of intensive blood-pressure control in type 2 diabetes mellitus. N Engl J Med 2010;362(17):1575–85.

116. Mancia G, Schumacher H, Redon J, et al. Blood pressure targets recommended by guidelines and incidence of cardiovascular and renal events in the ongoing telmisartan alone and in combination with ramipril global endpoint trial (ONTARGET). Circulation 2011;124(16):1727–36.

117. Cooper-DeHoff RM, Gong Y, Handberg EM, et al. Tight blood pressure control and cardiovascular outcomes among hypertensive patients with diabetes and coronary artery disease. JAMA 2010; 304(1):61–8.

118. Böhm M, Schumacher H, Teo KK, et al. Achieved blood pressure and cardiovascular outcomes in high-risk patients: results from ONTARGET and TRANSCEND trials. Lancet 2017;389:2226–37.

119. Wright JT Jr, Williamson JD, Whelton PK, et al, SPRINT Research Group. A randomized trial of intensive versus standard blood-pressure control. N Engl J Med 2015;373(22):2103–16.

120. Lee TT, Chen J, Cohen DJ, et al. The association between blood pressure and mortality in patients with heart failure. Am Heart J 2006;151(1):76–83.

121. Banach M, Bhatia V, Feller MA, et al. Relation of baseline systolic blood pressure and long-term outcomes in ambulatory patients with chronic mild to moderate heart failure. Am J Cardiol 2011; 107(8):1208–14.

122. Raphael CE, Whinnett ZI, Davies JE, et al. Quantifying the paradoxical effect of higher systolic blood pressure on mortality in chronic heart failure. Heart 2009;95:56–62.

123. Schmid FA, Schlager O, Keller P, et al. Prognostic value of long-term blood pressure changes in patients with chronic heart failure. Eur J Heart Fail 2017;19:837–42.

124. Lee SE, Lee HY, Cho HJ, et al. Reverse J-curve relationship between on-treatment blood pressure and mortality in patients with heart failure. JACC Heart Fail 2017;5(11):810–9.

125. Hakala SM, Tilvis RS. Determinants and significance of declining blood pressure in old age. A prospective birth cohort study. Eur Heart J 1998; 19:1872–8.

126. Langer RD, Criqui MH, Barrett-Connor EL, et al. Blood pressure change and survival after age 75. Hypertension 1993;22:551–9.

127. Boutitie F, Gueyffier F, Pocock S, et al. J-shaped relationship between blood pressure and mortality in hypertensive patients: new insights from a meta-analysis of individual-patient data. Ann Intern Med 2002;136:438–48.

128. Tuomilehto J, Ryynanen OP, Koistinen A, et al. Low diastolic blood pressure and mortality in a population based cohort of 16913 hypertensive patients in North Karelia, Finland. J Hypertens 1998;16: 1235–42.

129. Oakley C. Diagnosis and natural history of congested (dilated) cardiomyopathies. Postgrad Med J 1978;54:440–50.

130. Boutouyrie P, Tropeano AI, Asmar R, et al. Aortic stiffness is an independent predictor of primary coronary events in hypertensive patients: a longitudinal study. Hypertension 2002;39:10–5.

131. Franklin SS, Lopez VA, Wong ND, et al. Single versus combined blood pressure components and risk for cardiovascular disease: the Framingham Heart Study. Circulation 2009;119:243–50.

132. Vaccarino V, Holford TR, Krumholz HM. Pulse pressure and risk for myocardial infarction and heart failure in the elderly. J Am Coll Cardiol 2000;36: 130–8.

Hypertension and Heart Failure

Jeremy Slivnick, MD[a], Brent C. Lampert, DO[b],*

KEYWORDS

- Hypertension • Heart failure • LVH • HFpEF • HFrEF • Heart failure drug therapy

KEY POINTS

- Hypertension leads to heart failure through pathologic left ventricular hypertrophy (LVH) and diastolic dysfunction. A subset of these patients ultimately develops systolic heart failure owing to ischemia, genetic polymorphisms, or other insults to the cardiac myocytes.
- LVH represents the inciting event in the development of heart failure owing to hypertension.
- Early screening and intervention are keys to preventing hypertensive heart failure. Even after the onset of LVH, prompt initiation of therapy may still lead to reversal of remodeling.
- Once heart failure develops, the outlook declines significantly. Treatment should be in accordance with current guidelines for heart failure.

INTRODUCTION

Hypertension is the leading risk factor for numerous cardiovascular diseases, including stroke, coronary artery disease, atrial fibrillation, and peripheral vascular disease. In particular, hypertension contributes significantly to the incidence of heart failure, a condition responsible for 1 in 9 annual deaths in the United States and approximately $30.7 billion in annual health care costs.[1,2] Hypertension is highly prevalent in the heart failure population. In the Framingham study, 91% of patients with new heart failure had underlying hypertension.[3] History of hypertension has also been noted in up to 70% of patients in the PARADIGM-HF trial.[4] Hypertension appears to have a dose-dependent impact on heart failure incidence.[5] In all, hypertension is the single greatest risk factor for heart failure at a population level, owing to its high prevalence.[3] Hypertension is also a leading cause of myocardial infarction, the second greatest risk factor. Hypertensive heart disease is therefore a major concern to anyone caring for heart failure patients.

PATHOPHYSIOLOGY

In the most widely accepted model of hypertensive heart failure, chronic pressure overload leads to the development of left ventricular hypertrophy (LVH). Progressive hypertrophy and fibrotic changes in the heart lead to progressive diastolic dysfunction ultimately leading to elevated left-sided filling pressures and diastolic heart failure. Eventually, a subset of patients progresses to systolic dysfunction in the presence of chronic volume and pressure overload.[6]

Multiple mechanisms appear to contribute to this disease progression. Chronic pressure overload appears to lead to alterations in gene expression resulting in both myocyte hypertrophy and alterations in the extracellular matrix. At the myocyte level, increased microtubule density initially leads to improved contractility and left ventricular mass.[7] In the later stages, derangements within the cardiac myocyte lead to impaired relaxation and increased stiffness. Abnormal calcium handling, microtubule disarray, and hyperphosphorylation of

Disclosure Statement: The authors have nothing to disclose.
Funding sources: No research funding was used in this research.
Relevant disclosures: None.
[a] Ohio State University Wexner Medical Center, 473 West 12th Avenue, Suite 200, Columbus, OH 43210, USA;
[b] Heart Transplantation and Mechanical Circulatory Support, Ohio State University Wexner Medical Center, 473 West 12th Avenue, Suite 200, Columbus, OH 43210, USA
* Corresponding author.
E-mail address: Brent.Lampert@osumc.edu

heartfailure.theclinics.com

titin protein have been implicated in this pathologic process.[8,9] Increased collagen turnover owing to enzymes called membranometalloproteases is also linked to increased fibrotic remodeling and ultimately the development of both diastolic and systolic dysfunction in hypertensive patients.[10,11] The microvasculature may also play a role; both microvascular resistance and reactivity are impaired in hypertension and may contribute to the development of both systolic and diastolic heart failure.[12,13]

Increased neurohormonal stress also appears to play a powerful role in remodeling, and ultimately, heart failure (**Fig. 1**).[14] Elevated levels of renin and aldosterone have been implicated in the development of LVH and fibrotic remodeling.[15,16] Polymorphisms in these pathways may be partially responsible for the variability in remodeling seen in different patient populations.

STAGES OF HYPERTENSIVE HEART FAILURE

Based on the pathophysiologic mechanisms described above, Messerli and colleagues[6,17] proposed the following stages in the evolution of hypertensive heart disease (**Fig. 2**):

- Degree I: Hypertension without LVH
- Degree II: Asymptomatic hypertension with LVH
- Degree III: Symptomatic heart failure with preserved ejection fraction (HFpEF)

- Degree IV: Symptomatic heart failure with reduced ejection fraction

These stages draw similarities from the American College of Cardiology/American Heart Association (ACC/AHA) stages in which those with stage A possess risk factors without overt disease; stage B patients have underlying structural heart disease, and stage C/D patients are those with overt, clinical heart failure.

LEFT VENTRICULAR HYPERTROPHY

Chronic pressure overload resulting in LVH appears to be the inciting event in the cascade ultimately leading to hypertensive heart failure. Concentric hypertrophy represents, at least initially, an attempt by the left ventricle to maintain wall stress in response to elevated systemic pressures in accordance with Laplace's law (**Fig. 3**).

Classically, LVH was diagnosed by electrocardiography (ECG); however, although specific, ECG criteria appear to lack sensitivity for this finding.[18] When more sensitive modalities such as cardiac MRI are used, the prevalence of LVH in the population ranges from 9% to 13%.[19]

The link between hypertension and the incidence of LVH is well established and has been demonstrated using multiple imaging modalities, including ECG, echocardiography, and cardiac MRI.[20,21] Hypertension appears to result in LVH in a dose-dependent fashion with even prehypertensive

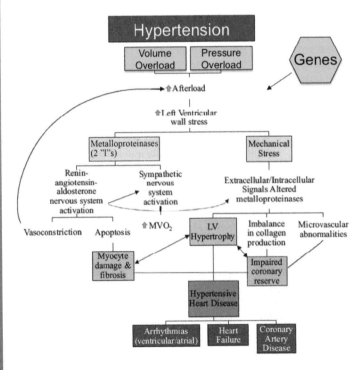

Fig. 1. Cellular pathways contributing to LVH in hypertensive heart disease. Both physical and neurohormonal stresses contribute to alterations in gene expression resulting in myocyte hypertrophy and pathologic remodeling. LV, left ventricular; MVO$_2$, Myocardial oxygen consumption. (*From* Shenasa M, Shenasa H. Hypertension, left ventricular hypertrophy, and sudden cardiac death. Int J Cardiol 2017;237:61; with permission.)

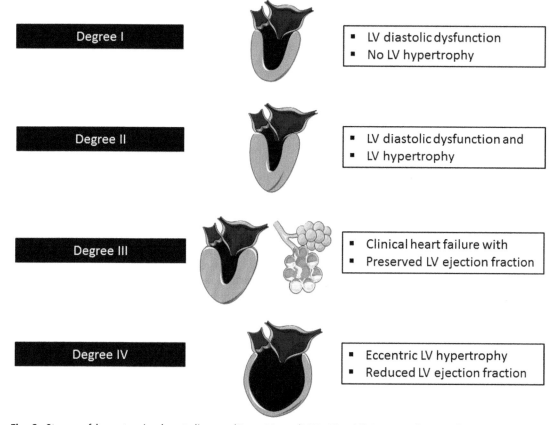

Fig. 2. Stages of hypertensive heart disease. (*From* Messerli FH, Rimoldi SF, Bangalore S. The Transition From Hypertension to Heart Failure: Contemporary Update. JACC Heart Fail 2017;5(8):546; with permission.)

patients at risk for remodeling.[21–23] This correlation appears to be much stronger when ambulatory or workplace blood pressure monitoring is used as compared with physician's office measurements.[24]

It should be noted that other factors besides blood pressure also modulate the development of LVH. Not all patients with hypertension develop LVH and not all LVH occur secondary to hypertension. In a review of major trials by Devereux and colleagues,[24] the prevalence of LVH among hypertensive patients was only 23% to 48%. In addition, LVH was seen in 0% to 10% of normal subjects. In regression models, hypertension only explained 50% to 68% of the variance in left ventricular mass.[21,25] Race appears to play a significant role. On average, blacks have significantly higher left ventricular mass and are over twice as likely to develop LVH as their white counterparts.[18,19] These racial differences suggest the possible role of genetics in the remodeling process. This is supported by sibling studies from the Framingham cohort, which demonstrated a significant heritable component of hypertrophy in response to hypertension.[26] Last, classical cardiovascular risk factors, such as diabetes, active smoking, and obesity, also significantly contribute to LVH irrespective of blood pressure.[21,27,28] Thus, this process appears to be multifactorial in nature.

FROM REMODELING TO HEART FAILURE

Although initially adaptive, LVH in response to hypertension ultimately becomes pathologic. There are clear differences in the pattern of hypertrophy in patients with LVH owing to hypertension when compared with those with physiologic hypertrophy, such as in athletes. In a study by Galderisi and colleagues,[29] patients with hypertensive hypertrophy

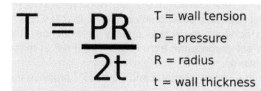

$$T = \frac{PR}{2t}$$

T = wall tension
P = pressure
R = radius
t = wall thickness

Fig. 3. Law of Laplace.

had significantly lower global longitudinal strain and greater degrees of diastolic dysfunction than age-matched competitive athletes despite lower mean left ventricular mass. As discussed above, impairments in active myocyte relaxation and extracellular fibrosis appear to contribute to the process. In addition, left ventricular mass inversely correlates with cardiac index in hypertensive patients, which also argues against a physiologic benefit to this pattern of hypertrophy.[24]

Regardless of how it occurs, once LVH develops, the risk of developing heart failure increases dramatically.[21,30] This remains true for both HFpEF and heart failure with reduced ejection fraction (HFrEF), even when controlling for known heart failure risk factors, such as age, gender, blood pressure, myocardial infarction, and diabetes.[30] This relationship appears to be dose dependent. In a study by de Simone and colleagues,[30] each 1% increase in left ventricular mass above the normal range on echocardiogram was associated with a 1% increased incidence of heart failure after controlling for risk factors, such as prior myocardial infarction. Several studies have shown that elevations in biomarkers, such as N-terminal-prohormone brain natriuretic peptide (NT-proBNP) and troponin, may identify patients with LVH at higher risk of heart failure and death.[31,32]

DIASTOLIC DYSFUNCTION

Following left ventricular remodeling, ongoing pressure overload leads to diastolic dysfunction, a finding that heralds the transition to symptomatic heart failure. At this stage, abnormalities in myocyte relaxation and progressive extracellular fibrosis lead to impaired ventricular filling. This ultimately leads to elevation in left atrial pressure and dyspnea. As discussed above, this process is mediated by both pressure overload and neurohormonal influences.

Diastolic dysfunction is common in hypertensive patients with LVH and appears to precede changes in systolic function.[33–35] Increased left ventricular mass is not just associated with echocardiographic changes but clinical heart failure as well. It is therefore not surprising that hypertension is highly prevalent in patients with HFpEF in major clinical trials.[36,37] In subanalysis of HFpEF patients from the CHARM and I-PRESERVE trials, the presence of LVH was also associated with increased risk of major adverse events in this population.[38]

Once clinical HFpEF has manifested, there is minimal hope for reversing the disease process. Despite advances in treatment of HFrEF, therapeutic options for HFpEF remain limited. At present, no medical intervention has been shown to alter mortality in HFpEF and very few medications appear to alter the disease process at all. This highlights the importance of the early detection and treatment of hypertension and LVH before onset of HFpEF.

HEART FAILURE WITH REDUCED EJECTION FRACTION

Eventually, a subset of patients with longstanding hypertension progresses to develop systolic dysfunction and clinical HFrEF. Unlike those who develop HFpEF, these patients appear to develop disproportionate myocyte loss rather than hypertrophy. Myocyte death leads to increased wall stress and the shift toward a dilated cardiomyopathy phenotype.[13] Interestingly, eccentric hypertrophy appears to be as common as concentric hypertrophy in patients with hypertension.[39] The pattern of hypertrophy may be influenced, in part, by variable levels of pressure and volume overload. Indeed, patients with eccentric hypertrophy have lower systolic blood pressure and systemic vascular resistance than their concentric counterparts.[38] Those with eccentric hypertrophy are also more likely to develop HFrEF than those with concentric hypertrophy.[40] Conversely, in the same study, the pattern of hypertrophy did not appear to impact the risk of developing HFpEF.

The combination of LVH with elevated biomarkers, such as NT-proBNP and troponin, may identify a subgroup of patients at particularly high risk of developing symptomatic HFrEF as compared with HFpEF.[32] This finding also supports the contribution of low-grade myocardial injury in the development of systolic dysfunction. Moreover, these biomarkers may identify higher-risk patients in whom intensified treatment may prevent progression.

Unlike in HFpEF, defining how hypertension causes systolic heart failure is more complex. It is clear that hypertension is a strong risk factor for the development of systolic dysfunction.[41] In addition, there is evidence that systolic strain is abnormal in hypertensive patients; these abnormalities in strain appear to be proportional to increases in wall stress, suggesting a relationship between afterload and systolic performance.[24,42,43] However, in epidemiologic studies, hypertension does not appear to be a common sole cause of HFrEF.[44] In addition, there is a paucity of evidence of a direct progression from HFpEF to HFrEF in these patients.

In a review, Borlaug and Redfield[45] propose the idea of a "second hit" leading to accelerated myocyte dysfunction in the background of hypertensive remodeling. Hypertensive heart disease that progresses for a long time before a second hit may closely resemble HFpEF. Such a second hit may occur from myocardial infarction, medications (eg, anthracyclines), toxins (eg, alcohol or cocaine), or genetic polymorphisms. The longer that concentric hypertrophy develops before the onset of HFrEF, the more a patient's phenotype is likely to overlap HFpEF. Ischemia is by far the most common insult. In the Framingham cohort, 42% of hypertensive heart failure patients had preceding myocardial infarction.[3] In addition, LVH and hypertension are potent risk factors for coronary artery disease, creating a synergistic risk profile.[46,47] In a review article, Levy and colleagues[48] propose myocardial infarction as an obligate step in the incidence of systolic heart failure in their population. This likely applies to many but not all patients. In large observational studies, nearly half of patients with hypertensive heart disease appear to progress to systolic dysfunction in the absence of coronary

artery disease.[3,49] Other mechanisms, such as toxins, genetic factors, or environmental exposures, may be responsible for accelerated myocyte loss leading to HFrEF.

Decreased renin-angiotensin-aldosterone activity and accelerated collagen breakdown have also been linked to dilated hypertrophy in hypertensive patients.[50,51] Overall, the authors agree with the concept that HFpEF represents the natural trajectory of uncontrolled hypertensive heart disease, with a second insult likely being required in order to develop HFrEF (Fig. 4).

Similar to HFpEF, once HFrEF develops in patients with hypertensive heart disease, the prognosis becomes markedly worse. Despite significant advances in therapy for systolic heart failure, the estimated 4-year survival for a patient with symptomatic New York Heart Association (NYHA) class II–III heart failure is only 60%; survival is markedly worse for those with NYHA class IV symptoms.[52,53]

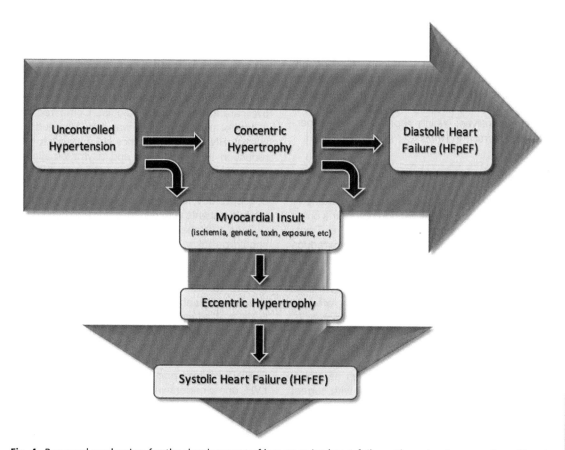

Fig. 4. Proposed mechanism for the development of hypertensive heart failure. The natural progression of heart failure owing to hypertension is concentric hypertrophy leading to diastolic heart failure. A subset of patients will develop systolic heart failure, generally through a second insult leading to myocyte loss. (Modified from Borlaug BA, Redfield MM. Diastolic and systolic heart failure are distinct phenotypes within the heart failure spectrum. Circulation 2011;123(18).)

ADVANCED HEART FAILURE WITH REDUCED EJECTION FRACTION

In patients with end-stage systolic heart failure owing to hypertension, blood pressure may paradoxically be low. In their review article, Messerli and colleagues[6] coin the term "decapitated hypertension" to refer to the lower mean blood pressures frequently seen in hypertensive heart failure patients with reduced EF. This finding of low blood pressure may confound the diagnosis of hypertensive heart disease in patients with HFrEF. Elevation in blood pressure after initiation of goal-directed medical therapy may be a clue to underlying hypertensive heart disease.

Some have postulated a possible protective role of high blood pressure in patients with reduced ejection fraction. This finding is supported by the observation that lower pretreatment blood pressure is associated with an increased risk for mortality.[54–56] Improvements in blood pressure may also herald clinical improvement in response to common heart failure therapies.[57,58] However, it is unclear if this relationship is correlative or causative in nature, because lower pretreatment blood pressures may identify sicker patients with a greater degree of left ventricular dysfunction. This theoretic protective effect should by no means be used as evidence to support withholding guideline-directed medical therapy with antihypertensives, which represent the cornerstone of therapy in HFrEF.

TREATMENT

The most effective method of treating hypertensive heart failure is primary prevention before the onset of pathologic remodeling and heart failure. Treatment of blood pressure has been shown to reduce LVH and reduce the risk of developing heart failure.[59] This benefit also appears to be dose dependent.[60] Multiple agents have shown benefit in large randomized trials. Thiazide diuretics, angiotensin-converting-enzyme inhibitors (ACEi), angiotensin-receptor blockers (ARB), and dihydropyridine calcium channel blockers (CCB) appear to be the most effective agents at reducing heart failure risk as compared with other agents, such as alpha- and beta-blockers.[61–63] This is in line with current hypertension guidelines that list these as first-line agents.[64] In a large meta-analysis, thiazide diuretics appeared to confer the lowest risk of heart failure of the 3 agents.[65] In addition, in a Cochrane Review, ACEi/ARBs outperformed CCBs with respect to heart failure endpoints.[66] Thus, thiazides are likely the ideal agent for heart failure prevention followed by ACEi/ARBs. For primary prevention,

blood pressure targets should be in accordance with the ACC/AHA Eighth Joint National Committee (JNC-8) guidelines.[65]

In patients at elevated cardiovascular risk, strong consideration should be given for more stringent blood pressure control. The landmark SPRINT trial demonstrated a reduction in major adverse cardiac events with intensive blood pressure control (systolic blood pressure <120 mm Hg) in hypertensive patients at increased cardiovascular risk.[67] This benefit was accompanied by greater reductions in LVH and new heart failure incidence.[68] In addition, a greater number of intensively treated patients had resolution of LVH, which fits with the observed dose-dependent relationship between blood pressure and LVH discussed above. Based on these findings, the JNC-8 guidelines were updated to support a blood pressure target of 130/90 mm Hg in patients at high cardiovascular risk (atherosclerotic cardiovascular disease >10%), a recommendation that these authors strongly support.[65]

Biomarkers may also be useful in identifying an at-risk patient population that may benefit from more aggressive therapy. In the STOP-HF trial, patients with multiple risk factors for heart failure were screened for risk using B-type natriuretic peptide (BNP).[69] Those with elevated biomarkers underwent echocardiography and were referred for collaborative care involving a cardiologist. Compared with a control population that was not screened, the use of BNP screening showed a trend toward reduction in heart failure and asymptomatic left ventricular systolic dysfunction. Although it did not reach significance, this is an interesting proof-of-concept study; further research is warranted, particularly in patients with hypertension and LVH.

Once LVH has developed, aggressive efforts should be taken to control blood pressure in the hopes of halting or reversing the remodeling process. Antihypertensive therapy has been shown to lead to reduction in left ventricular mass by echocardiography, with corresponding reduction in risks of adverse events.[70–73] ACEi, ARBs, and CCBs appear to be most effective at reducing LVH.[74] Once developed, the hypertrophy process may take years to improve.[75] Given the above SPRINT findings and the known associated with LVH, one wonders whether hypertensive patients with LVH would also benefit from more intensive blood pressure control in the absence of other indications. Further studies are needed to address this important question.

Once heart failure has developed, treatment should be in accordance with available heart failure guidelines.[76] In patients with HFpEF, spironolactone and ACEi/ARBs can be considered for the management of hypertension based on some suggesting benefit at decreasing heart failure hospitalizations. Based on results from the SPRINT trial, recent heart failure guidelines advocate for stringent blood pressure control with a blood pressure target of less than 130/80 mm Hg.

For patients in all stages of systolic heart failure, ACEi/ARBs and beta-blockers represent the cornerstone of antihypertensive therapy based on high-quality, randomized controlled data. The combination of these agents carries a class I indication in patients with systolic dysfunction regardless of NYHA class.[77] The evidence for ACEi/ARB originated from several trials, most notably the SOLVD, CONSENSUS, Val-HEFT, and CHARM trials.[77–80] In these trials, ACEi/ARB were initiated at lower doses and titrated to reach the maximum tolerated dose based on symptoms and renal function. Evidence for beta-blockers arose from the COPERNICUS and MERIT-HF trials.[81,82] As with ACEi/ARBs, these agents were titrated to maximally tolerated dosages based on symptoms and heart rate. For those with NYHA class II–IV who are maximally titrated on the above medications and have acceptable renal function, the use of aldosterone antagonists is a class I indication.[83] Hydralazine and long-acting nitrates should also be considered in African Americans with NYHA class III–IV heart failure already on an ACEi/ARB, beta-blocker, and a mineralocorticoid antagonist.[84] More recently, with the publication of the PARADIGM-HF trial, angiotensin-neprilysin inhibitors (ARNI) have been shown to reduce mortality in patients with HFrEF and NYHA class II–III symptoms despite above agents.[4] These promising data were reflected in the 2017 updated heart failure guidelines, which assigned a class I recommendation for the use of ARNIs, ACEi, or ARBs in this population.[77] Given the success of ARNI in HFrEF, there are now ongoing trials evaluating the use of these agents in patients with HFpEF. With regards to blood pressure targets, the most recent ACC/AHA heart failure guidelines advocate for treating to achieve a blood pressure less than 130/80 mm Hg.[77] However, as discussed above, in most of the landmark systolic heart failure trials, these medications were titrated to maximum tolerated dosages rather than a blood pressure cutoff.

Recently, the concept of heart failure with midrange EF (HFmrEF) has been increasingly recognized and was described as its own distinct heart failure subset in the most recent European Society of Cardiology Heart Failure Guidelines.[85] This group comprises nearly one-quarter of all heart failure patients and suffers similar morbidity and mortality as patients with HFpEF and HFrEF.[86,87] Despite this, HFmrEF is largely underrepresented in large clinical trials.[88] One factor that complicates this is the group's heterogeneity, because it appears to be composed of patients with stable systolic function, HFrEF patients with recovering EF, and HFpEF patients in decline.[89,90] Much of the available data comes from subgroup analysis of major heart failure trials, which included patients with HFmrEF. Based on subgroup analysis from the CHARM and TOPCAT trials, candesartan and spironolactone appeared to reduce major adverse heart failure events in patients with HFmrEF.[91,92] Similar benefits were also seen with betablockers based on meta-analyses in patients with HFmrEF.[93] Although there have been insufficient data to provide strong guideline recommendations, it is the opinion of these authors that these agents should be preferentially used based on the evidence available. Further research is indicated to determine optimal management strategies in this population.

RISK FACTOR MODIFICATION

In all stages of treatment, it is imperative to prevent coronary artery disease. Coronary artery disease is highly prevalent among hypertensive patients, particularly those with LVH.[47,48] In addition, as discussed above, myocardial infarction is likely the most common accelerant to systolic heart failure in patients with hypertensive heart disease. This should be accomplished by appropriate initiation of antiplatelet, lipid-lowering, and antihypertensive medications in patients who have or are at risk for developing coronary artery disease. Efforts to address diabetes, obesity, sleep apnea, and salt intake may also help to prevent pathologic remodeling and reduce the future risk of heart failure.[94–97]

SUMMARY

Hypertensive heart disease describes a spectrum of illness spanning from uncontrolled hypertension to the ultimate development of heart failure. The inciting event in hypertensive heart disease is the development of LVH, a process that may be reversible if recognized early and treated aggressively. LVH appears to be a pathologic process ultimately leading to fibrosis, impaired left ventricular compliance, and ultimately, diastolic heart failure. A subset of patients ultimately develops systolic heart failure, generally because of a subsequent insult leading to accelerated myocyte loss. Once developed, heart failure owing to hypertension is often irreversible and results in significant morbidity and mortality. Once heart failure is diagnosed, patients should be treated in accordance with available heart failure guidelines.

REFERENCES

1. Writing Group Members, Mozaffarian D, Benjamin EJ, Go AS, et al. Heart disease and stroke statistics—2016 update: a report from the American Heart Association. Circulation 2016;133(4):e38–360.
2. Whelton PK, Carey RM, Aronow WS, et al. ACC/AHA/AAPA/ABC/ACPM/AGS/APhA/ASH/ASPC/NMA/PCNA Guideline for the prevention, detection, evaluation, and management of high blood pressure in adults: a report of the American College of Cardiology/American Heart Association Task Force on Clinical Practice Guidelines. Hypertension 2018;71:e13–115.
3. Levy D, Larson MG, Vasan RS, et al. The progression from hypertension to congestive heart failure. JAMA 1996;275(20):1557–62.
4. McMurray JJV, Packer M, Desai AS, et al. Angiotensin-neprilysin inhibition versus enalapril in heart failure. N Engl J Med 2014;371(11):993–1004.
5. Haider AW, Larson MG, Franklin SS, et al, Framingham Heart Study. Systolic blood pressure, diastolic blood pressure, and pulse pressure as predictors of risk for congestive heart failure in the Framingham Heart Study. Ann Intern Med 2003;138(1):10–6.
6. Messerli FH, Rimoldi SF, Bangalore S. The transition from hypertension to heart failure: contemporary update. JACC Heart Fail 2017;5(8):543–51.
7. Tagawa H, Rozich JD, Tsutsui H, et al. Basis for increased microtubules in pressure-hypertrophied cardiocytes. Circulation 1996;93(6):1230–43.
8. Shah SJ, Aistrup GL, Gupta DK, et al. Ultrastructural and cellular basis for the development of abnormal myocardial mechanics during the transition from hypertension to heart failure. Am J Physiol Heart Circ Physiol 2014;306(1):H88–100.
9. Borbély A, Falcao-Pires I, van Heerebeek L, et al. Hypophosphorylation of the Stiff N2B titin isoform raises cardiomyocyte resting tension in failing human myocardium. Circ Res 2009;104(6):780–6.
10. Ahmed SH, Clark LL, Pennington WR, et al. Matrix metalloproteinases/tissue inhibitors of metalloproteinases: relationship between changes in proteolytic determinants of matrix composition and structural, functional, and clinical manifestations of hypertensive heart disease. Circulation 2006;113(17):2089–96.
11. López B, González A, Querejeta R, et al. Alterations in the pattern of collagen deposition may contribute to the deterioration of systolic function in hypertensive patients with heart failure. J Am Coll Cardiol 2006;48(1):89–96.
12. Levy BI, Ambrosio G, Pries AR, et al. Microcirculation in hypertension: a new target for treatment? Circulation 2001;104(6):735–40.
13. Paulus WJ, Tschöpe C. A novel paradigm for heart failure with preserved ejection fraction: comorbidities drive myocardial dysfunction and remodeling through coronary microvascular endothelial inflammation. J Am Coll Cardiol 2013;62(4):263–71.
14. Shenasa M, Shenasa H. Hypertension, left ventricular hypertrophy, and sudden cardiac death. Int J Cardiol 2017;237:60–3.
15. Iwai N, Ohmichi N, Nakamura Y, et al. DD genotype of the angiotensin-converting enzyme gene is a risk factor for left ventricular hypertrophy. Circulation 1994;90(6):2622–8.
16. Qin W, Rudolph AE, Bond BR, et al. Transgenic model of aldosterone-driven cardiac hypertrophy and heart failure. Circ Res 2003;93(1):69–76.
17. Iriarte M, Murga N, Sagastagoitia D, et al. Classification of hypertensive cardiomyopathy. Eur Heart J 1993;14(Suppl J):95–101.
18. Jain A, Tandri H, Dalal D, et al. Diagnostic and prognostic utility of electrocardiography for left ventricular hypertrophy defined by magnetic resonance imaging in relationship to ethnicity: the Multi-Ethnic Study of Atherosclerosis (MESA). Am Heart J 2010;159(4):652–8.
19. Drazner MH, Dries DL, Peshock RM, et al. Left ventricular hypertrophy is more prevalent in blacks than whites in the general population: the Dallas Heart Study. Hypertension 2005;46(1):124–9.
20. Kannel WB, Gordon T, Offutt D. Left ventricular hypertrophy by electrocardiogram. prevalence, incidence, and mortality in the Framingham study. Ann Intern Med 1969;71(1):89–105.
21. Heckbert SR, Post W, Pearson GDN, et al. Traditional cardiovascular risk factors in relation to left ventricular mass, volume, and systolic function by cardiac magnetic resonance imaging: the Multi-ethnic Study of Atherosclerosis. J Am Coll Cardiol 2006;48(11):2285–92.
22. Parati G, Pomidossi G, Albini F, et al. Relationship of 24-hour blood pressure mean and variability to severity of target-organ damage in hypertension. J Hypertens 1987;5(1):93–8.
23. Santos ABS, Gupta DK, Bello NA, et al. Prehypertension is associated with abnormalities of cardiac structure and function in the atherosclerosis risk in communities study. Am J Hypertens 2016;29(5):568–74.
24. Devereux RB, Pickering TG, Alderman MH, et al. Left ventricular hypertrophy in hypertension. Prevalence and relationship to pathophysiologic variables. Hypertension 1987;9(2 Pt 2):II53–60.
25. Devereux RB, Roman MJ, de Simone G, et al. Relations of left ventricular mass to demographic and hemodynamic variables in American Indians: the Strong Heart Study. Circulation 1997;96(5):1416–23.
26. Post WS, Larson MG, Myers RH, et al. Heritability of left ventricular mass: the Framingham Heart Study. Hypertension 1997;30(5):1025–8.

27. Gardin JM, Arnold A, Gottdiener JS, et al. Left ventricular mass in the elderly. The Cardiovascular Health Study. Hypertension 1997;29(5):1095–103.
28. Savage DD, Levy D, Dannenberg AL, et al. Association of echocardiographic left ventricular mass with body size, blood pressure and physical activity (the Framingham Study). Am J Cardiol 1990;65(5):371–6.
29. Galderisi M, Lomoriello VS, Santoro A, et al. Differences of myocardial systolic deformation and correlates of diastolic function in competitive rowers and young hypertensives: a speckle-tracking echocardiography study. J Am Soc Echocardiogr 2010;23(11):1190–8.
30. de Simone G, Gottdiener JS, Chinali M, et al. Left ventricular mass predicts heart failure not related to previous myocardial infarction: the Cardiovascular Health Study. Eur Heart J 2008;29(6):741–7.
31. Neeland IJ, Drazner MH, Berry JD, et al. Biomarkers of chronic cardiac injury and hemodynamic stress identify a malignant phenotype of left ventricular hypertrophy in the general population. J Am Coll Cardiol 2013;61(2):187–95.
32. Seliger SL, de Lemos J, Neeland IJ, et al. Older adults, "malignant" left ventricular hypertrophy, and associated cardiac-specific biomarker phenotypes to identify the differential risk of new-onset reduced versus preserved ejection fraction heart failure: CHS (Cardiovascular Health Study). JACC Heart Fail 2015;3(6):445–55.
33. Krepp JM, Lin F, Min JK, et al. Relationship of electrocardiographic left ventricular hypertrophy to the presence of diastolic dysfunction. Ann Noninvasive Electrocardiol 2014;19(6):552–60.
34. Inouye I, Massie B, Loge D, et al. Abnormal left ventricular filling: an early finding in mild to moderate systemic hypertension. Am J Cardiol 1984;53(1):120–6.
35. Bonaduce D, Breglio R, Conforti G, et al. Myocardial hypertrophy and left ventricular diastolic function in hypertensive patients: an echo Doppler evaluation. Eur Heart J 1989;10(7):611–21.
36. Shah AM, Claggett B, Sweitzer NK, et al. Cardiac structure and function and prognosis in heart failure with preserved ejection fraction: findings from the echocardiographic study of the Treatment of Preserved Cardiac Function Heart Failure with an Aldosterone Antagonist (TOPCAT) Trial. Circ Heart Fail 2014;7(5):740–51.
37. Zile MR, Gottdiener JS, Hetzel SJ, et al. Prevalence and significance of alterations in cardiac structure and function in patients with heart failure and a preserved ejection fraction. Circulation 2011;124(23):2491–501.
38. Hawkins NM, Wang D, McMurray JJV, et al. Prevalence and prognostic implications of electrocardiographic left ventricular hypertrophy in heart failure: evidence from the CHARM programme. Heart 2007;93(1):59–64.
39. Ganau A, Devereux RB, Roman MJ, et al. Patterns of left ventricular hypertrophy and geometric remodeling in essential hypertension. J Am Coll Cardiol 1992;19(7):1550–8.
40. Velagaleti RS, Gona P, Pencina MJ, et al. Left ventricular hypertrophy patterns and incidence of heart failure with preserved versus reduced ejection fraction. Am J Cardiol 2014;113(1):117–22.
41. Drazner MH, Rame JE, Marino EK, et al. Increased left ventricular mass is a risk factor for the development of a depressed left ventricular ejection fraction within five years: the Cardiovascular Health Study. J Am Coll Cardiol 2004;43(12):2207–15.
42. Shimizu G, Hirota Y, Kita Y, et al. Left ventricular midwall mechanics in systemic arterial hypertension. Myocardial function is depressed in pressure-overload hypertrophy. Circulation 1991;83(5):1676–84.
43. de Simone G, Devereux RB, Roman MJ, et al. Assessment of left ventricular function by the midwall fractional shortening/end-systolic stress relation in human hypertension. J Am Coll Cardiol 1994;23(6):1444–51.
44. Felker GM, Thompson RE, Hare JM, et al. Underlying causes and long-term survival in patients with initially unexplained cardiomyopathy. N Engl J Med 2000;342(15):1077–84.
45. Borlaug BA, Redfield MM. Diastolic and systolic heart failure are distinct phenotypes within the heart failure spectrum. Circulation 2011;123(18):2006–13 [discussion: 2014].
46. Yeh RW, Sidney S, Chandra M, et al. Population trends in the incidence and outcomes of acute myocardial infarction. N Engl J Med 2010;362(23):2155–65.
47. Yusuf S, Hawken S, Ounpuu S, et al. Effect of potentially modifiable risk factors associated with myocardial infarction in 52 countries (the INTERHEART study): case-control study. Lancet 2004;364(9438):937–52.
48. Vasan RS, Levy D. The role of hypertension in the pathogenesis of heart failure. A clinical mechanistic overview. Arch Intern Med 1996;156(16):1789–96.
49. Rame JE, Ramilo M, Spencer N, et al. Development of a depressed left ventricular ejection fraction in patients with left ventricular hypertrophy and a normal ejection fraction. Am J Cardiol 2004;93(2):234–7.
50. du Cailar G, Pasquié JL, Ribstein J, et al. Left ventricular adaptation to hypertension and plasma renin activity. J Hum Hypertens 2000;14(3):181–8.
51. Nakahara T, Takata Y, Hirayama Y, et al. Left ventricular hypertrophy and geometry in untreated essential hypertension is associated with blood levels of aldosterone and procollagen type III amino-terminal peptide. Circ J 2007;71(5):716–21.

52. SOLVD Investigators, Yusuf S, Pitt B, Davis CE, et al. Effect of enalapril on mortality and the development of heart failure in asymptomatic patients with reduced left ventricular ejection fractions. N Engl J Med 1992; 327(10):685–91.

53. Frazier CG, Alexander KP, Newby LK, et al. Associations of gender and etiology with outcomes in heart failure with systolic dysfunction: a pooled analysis of 5 randomized control trials. J Am Coll Cardiol 2007; 49(13):1450–8.

54. Fonarow GC, Adams KF, Abraham WT, et al, ADHERE Scientific Advisory Committee, Study Group, and Investigators. Risk stratification for in-hospital mortality in acutely decompensated heart failure: classification and regression tree analysis. JAMA 2005;293(5):572–80.

55. Gheorghiade M, Abraham WT, Albert NM, et al. Systolic blood pressure at admission, clinical characteristics, and outcomes in patients hospitalized with acute heart failure. JAMA 2006;296(18): 2217–26.

56. Lee TT, Chen J, Cohen DJ, et al. The association between blood pressure and mortality in patients with heart failure. Am Heart J 2006;151(1):76–83.

57. McAlister FA, Wiebe N, Ezekowitz JA, et al. Meta-analysis: beta-blocker dose, heart rate reduction, and death in patients with heart failure. Ann Intern Med 2009;150(11):784–94.

58. Ather S, Bangalore S, Vemuri S, et al. Trials on the effect of cardiac resynchronization on arterial blood pressure in patients with heart failure. Am J Cardiol 2011;107(4):561–8.

59. Moser M, Hebert PR. Prevention of disease progression, left ventricular hypertrophy and congestive heart failure in hypertension treatment trials. J Am Coll Cardiol 1996;27(5):1214–8.

60. Ettehad D, Emdin CA, Kiran A, et al. Blood pressure lowering for prevention of cardiovascular disease and death: a systematic review and meta-analysis. Lancet 2016;387(10022):957–67.

61. ALLHAT Officers and Coordinators for the ALLHAT Collaborative Research Group, The Antihypertensive and Lipid-Lowering Treatment to Prevent Heart Attack Trial. Major outcomes in high-risk hypertensive patients randomized to angiotensin-converting enzyme inhibitor or calcium channel blocker vs diuretic: The Antihypertensive and Lipid-Lowering Treatment to Prevent Heart Attack Trial (ALLHAT). JAMA 2002;288(23):2981–97.

62. Prevention of stroke by antihypertensive drug treatment in older persons with isolated systolic hypertension. Final results of the Systolic Hypertension in the Elderly Program (SHEP). SHEP Cooperative Research Group. JAMA 1991;265(24):3255–64.

63. Beckett NS, Peters R, Fletcher AE, et al. Treatment of hypertension in patients 80 years of age or older. N Engl J Med 2008;358(18):1887–98.

64. Whelton PK, Carey RM, Aronow WS, et al. 2017 ACC/AHA/AAPA/ABC/ACPM/AGS/APhA/ASH/ASPC/NMA/PCNA guideline for the prevention, detection, evaluation, and management of high blood pressure in adults: executive summary: a report of the American College of Cardiology/American Heart Association Task Force on Clinical Practice Guidelines. Circulation 2018;138(17):e426–83.

65. Sciarretta S, Palano F, Tocci G, et al. Antihypertensive treatment and development of heart failure in hypertension: a Bayesian network meta-analysis of studies in patients with hypertension and high cardiovascular risk. Arch Intern Med 2011;171(5):384–94.

66. Chen N, Zhou M, Yang M, et al. Calcium channel blockers versus other classes of drugs for hypertension. Cochrane Database Syst Rev 2010;(8): CD003654.

67. SPRINT Research Group, Wright JT, Williamson JD, Whelton PK, et al. A randomized trial of intensive versus standard blood-pressure control. N Engl J Med 2015;373(22):2103–16.

68. Soliman EZ, Ambrosius WT, Cushman WC, et al. Effect of intensive blood pressure lowering on left ventricular hypertrophy in patients with hypertension: SPRINT (systolic blood pressure intervention trial). Circulation 2017;136(5):440–50.

69. Ledwidge M, Gallagher J, Conlon C, et al. Natriuretic peptide-based screening and collaborative care for heart failure: the STOP-HF randomized trial. JAMA 2013;310(1):66–74.

70. Devereux RB, Dahlöf B, Gerdts E, et al. Regression of hypertensive left ventricular hypertrophy by Losartan compared with atenolol: the Losartan Intervention for Endpoint Reduction in Hypertension (LIFE) trial. Circulation 2004;110(11): 1456–62.

71. Levy D, Salomon M, D'Agostino RB, et al. Prognostic implications of baseline electrocardiographic features and their serial changes in subjects with left ventricular hypertrophy. Circulation 1994;90(4): 1786–93.

72. Pierdomenico SD, Lapenna D, Cuccurullo F. Regression of echocardiographic left ventricular hypertrophy after 2 years of therapy reduces cardiovascular risk in patients with essential hypertension. Am J Hypertens 2008;21(4):464–70.

73. Mathew J, Sleight P, Lonn E, et al. Reduction of cardiovascular risk by regression of electrocardiographic markers of left ventricular hypertrophy by the angiotensin-converting enzyme inhibitor ramipril. Circulation 2001;104(14):1615–21.

74. Klingbeil AU, Schneider M, Martus P, et al. A meta-analysis of the effects of treatment on left ventricular mass in essential hypertension. Am J Med 2003; 115(1):41–6.

75. Franz IW, Ketelhut R, Behr U, et al. Time course of reduction in left ventricular mass during long-term

antihypertensive therapy. J Hum Hypertens 1994; 8(3):191–8.

76. Yancy CW, Jessup M, Bozkurt B, et al. 2017 ACC/AHA/HFSA focused update of the 2013 ACCF/AHA guideline for the management of heart failure: a report of the American College of Cardiology/American Heart Association Task Force on Clinical Practice Guidelines and the Heart Failure Society of America. J Card Fail 2017;23(8):628–51.

77. SOLVD Investigators, Yusuf S, Pitt B, Davis CE, et al. Effect of enalapril on survival in patients with reduced left ventricular ejection fractions and congestive heart failure. N Engl J Med 1991;325(5):293–302.

78. Cohn JN, Tognoni G, Valsartan Heart Failure Trial Investigators. A randomized trial of the angiotensin-receptor blocker valsartan in chronic heart failure. N Engl J Med 2001;345(23):1667–75.

79. McMurray JJV, Ostergren J, Swedberg K, et al. Effects of candesartan in patients with chronic heart failure and reduced left-ventricular systolic function taking angiotensin-converting-enzyme inhibitors: the CHARM-Added trial. Lancet 2003;362(9386):767–71.

80. CONSENSUS Trial Study Group. Effects of enalapril on mortality in severe congestive heart failure. Results of the Cooperative North Scandinavian Enalapril Survival Study (CONSENSUS). N Engl J Med 1987;316(23):1429–35.

81. Effect of metoprolol CR/XL in chronic heart failure: Metoprolol CR/XL Randomised Intervention Trial in Congestive Heart Failure (MERIT-HF). Lancet 1999;353(9169):2001–7.

82. Packer M, Fowler MB, Roecker EB, et al. Effect of carvedilol on the morbidity of patients with severe chronic heart failure: results of the carvedilol prospective randomized cumulative survival (COPERNICUS) study. Circulation 2002;106(17):2194–9.

83. Pitt B, Zannad F, Remme WJ, et al. The effect of spironolactone on morbidity and mortality in patients with severe heart failure. Randomized Aldactone Evaluation Study Investigators. N Engl J Med 1999;341(10):709–17.

84. Cohn JN, Archibald DG, Ziesche S, et al. Effect of vasodilator therapy on mortality in chronic congestive heart failure. Results of a Veterans Administration Cooperative Study. N Engl J Med 1986;314(24):1547–52.

85. Ponikowski P, Voors AA, Anker SD, et al. 2016 ESC guidelines for the diagnosis and treatment of acute and chronic heart failure: the task force for the diagnosis and treatment of acute and chronic heart failure of the European Society of Cardiology (ESC). Developed with the special contribution of the Heart Failure Association (HFA) of the ESC. Eur J Heart Fail 2016;18(8):891–975.

86. Cheng RK, Cox M, Neely ML, et al. Outcomes in patients with heart failure with preserved, borderline, and reduced ejection fraction in the Medicare population. Am Heart J 2014;168(5):721–30.

87. Tsuji K, Sakata Y, Nochioka K, et al. Characterization of heart failure patients with mid-range left ventricular ejection fraction-a report from the CHART-2 Study. Eur J Heart Fail 2017;19(10):1258–69.

88. Lopatin Y. Heart failure with mid-range ejection fraction and how to treat it. Card Fail Rev 2018;4(1):9–13.

89. Rastogi A, Novak E, Platts AE, et al. Epidemiology, pathophysiology and clinical outcomes for heart failure patients with a mid-range ejection fraction. Eur J Heart Fail 2017;19(12):1597–605.

90. Hsu JJ, Ziaeian B, Fonarow GC. Heart failure with mid-range (borderline) ejection fraction: clinical implications and future directions. JACC Heart Fail 2017;5(11):763–71.

91. Lund LH, Claggett B, Liu J, et al. Heart failure with mid-range ejection fraction in CHARM: characteristics, outcomes and effect of candesartan across the entire ejection fraction spectrum. Eur J Heart Fail 2018;20(8):1230–9.

92. Solomon SD, Claggett B, Lewis EF, et al. Influence of ejection fraction on outcomes and efficacy of spironolactone in patients with heart failure with preserved ejection fraction. Eur Heart J 2016;37(5):455–62.

93. Cleland JGF, Bunting KV, Flather MD, et al. Beta-blockers for heart failure with reduced, mid-range, and preserved ejection fraction: an individual patient-level analysis of double-blind randomized trials. Eur Heart J 2018;39(1):26–35.

94. MacMahon SW, Wilcken DE, Macdonald GJ. The effect of weight reduction on left ventricular mass. A randomized controlled trial in young, overweight hypertensive patients. N Engl J Med 1986;314(6):334–9.

95. Ferrara LA, de Simone G, Pasanisi F, et al. Left ventricular mass reduction during salt depletion in arterial hypertension. Hypertension 1984;6(5):755–9.

96. Holt A, Bjerre J, Zareini B, et al. Sleep apnea, the risk of developing heart failure, and potential benefits of continuous positive airway pressure (CPAP) therapy. J Am Heart Assoc 2018;7(13) [pii:e008684].

97. Zinman B, Wanner C, Lachin JM, et al. Empagliflozin, cardiovascular outcomes, and mortality in type 2 diabetes. N Engl J Med 2015;373(22):2117–28.

Hypertension and Arrhythmias

Muhammad R. Afzal, MD, Salvatore Savona, MD, Omar Mohamed, MD,
Aayah Mohamed-Osman, MD, Steven J. Kalbfleisch, MD, FHRS*

KEYWORDS

- Hypertension • Atrial fibrillation • Ventricular tachycardia • Sudden cardiac death

KEY POINTS

- Hypertension is the most common risk factor for cardiovascular diseases and is associated with development and progression of various atrial and ventricular arrhythmias.
- Left ventricular hypertrophy resulting from chronic hypertension leads to progressive ventricular dysfunction and left atrial enlargement, which predispose for development of atrial and ventricular arrhythmias.
- Prompt intervention, including preemptive screening for hypertension in high-risk patients, aggressive lifestyle modifications, and pharmacotherapy, can halt the progression of hypertensive heart disease and thus development of atrial and ventricular arrhythmias.

INTRODUCTION

Hypertension remains a significant risk for the development of adverse cardiovascular events and continues to increase in prevalence.[1] The increase in the prevalence of hypertension is attributed to multiple risk factors including dietary indiscretions, obesity, obstructive sleep apnea and aging populations.[2] Hypertension manifests in the form of various cardiovascular diseases including heart failure (HF), coronary artery disease, and various arrhythmias including atrial fibrillation (AF), ventricular arrhythmias, and sudden cardiac death.[1,3]

Hypertension is the most common risk factor for the development of AF.[4–9] Development of AF in patients with hypertension has several implications, the most important of which is the increased risk of thromboembolism and stroke. Depending on the degree of left ventricular hypertrophy (LVH), AF can be a precipitant of HF, particularly HF with preserved ejection fraction (HFpEF).[10] The combination of pharmacotherapy for hypertension and AF can increase the risk of orthostatic hypotension, especially in the elderly.[11] The development of hypertension increases the risk of sudden cardiac death and ventricular arrhythmias, as well as adversely affecting the conduction system.[7,12–14]

The complex interplay between hypertension and cardiac arrhythmias in the face of increasing prevalence of both disorders warrants a detailed understanding of the pathogenesis to appropriately curtail the implications of hypertensive heart disease and cardiac arrhythmias. This review summarizes the existing literature on the association of hypertension and cardiac arrhythmias with an emphasis on the pathophysiology and management.

EPIDEMIOLOGY

Hypertension is the most common risk factor for cardiovascular diseases with an estimated prevalence of 29% in 2011 to 2014.[2] The prevalence of hypertension increased with age, from 7.3%

Conflict of Interest: None.
Division of Cardiovascular Medicine, The Ohio State University Wexner Medical Center, 473 West 12th Avenue, Suite 200, Columbus, OH 43210, USA
* Corresponding author.
E-mail address: steven.kalbfleisch@osumc.edu

among adults aged 18% to 39% to 32.2% among those aged 40% to 59%, and 64.9% among those aged 60 and over. A similar pattern was found among both men (8.4% for those aged 18%–39%, 34.6% for 40%–59%, and 63.1% for ≥60) and women (6.1% for those aged 18%–39%, 29.9% for 40%–59%, and 66.5% for ≥60). The increased prevalence in hypertension is depicted in **Fig. 1**. The prevalence is projected to increase to 41.4% in 2030.

Hypertension is associated with cardiac arrhythmias and particularly AF, which is considered the most common sustained arrhythmia in adults. The estimated prevalence of AF in the United States is approximately 5.2 million, and is expected to increase to 12.1 million by 2030.[15] Hypertension is associated with a 1.8-fold increased risk of developing new-onset AF and a 1.5-fold increased risk of progression to permanent AF.[4] The lifetime risk for the development of AF in this population is as high as 25% at 40 years of age.[5] Almost 60% of patients with AF have hypertension.[7] Owing to the aging population, a 2 to 3 times increase in the total number of patients with AF is expected over the next 20 to 30 years.[16–18]

Hypertension is also associated with ventricular arrhythmias and sudden cardiac death. The incidence of sudden cardiac death is 350,000 events per year in United States.[13] The presence of LVH and AF increase the risk of sudden cardiac death by 3- to 4-fold as shown in a secondary analysis of the LIFE study.[19] Similarly, a history of hypertension was an independent predictor of in-hospital ventricular fibrillation.[20]

PATHOGENESIS OF ARRHYTHMIAS IN HYPERTENSION

The association between hypertension and arrhythmias is complex. In hypertensive patients with no other cardiac risk factors, the incidence and prevalence of cardiac arrhythmias is directly related to the status of hypertensive heart disease.[21] With the progression of hypertensive heart disease as manifested by cardiac remodeling, the incidence of AF, ventricular arrhythmias, and sudden death increases. The following factors are attributed to the development of cardiac arrhythmias in patients with hypertension: LVH, increased left atrial size, activation of the sympathetic nervous system (SNS) and renin–angiotensin–aldosterone system (RAAS), electrical abnormalities, and microvascular ischemia. **Fig. 2** depicts the various aspects of arrhythmogenesis in patients with hypertension, and **Box 1** outlines risk factors modification in patients diagnosed with hypertension.

Left Ventricular Hypertrophy

Chronic hypertension is strongly related to the development of LVH that promotes the development of cardiac arrhythmias. Chronic increases in afterload and intracardiac pressure promote hypertrophy of cardiac myocytes and stimulates cardiac fibroblasts. Hypertrophy of the cardiac myocytes and collagen deposition from cardiac fibroblasts result in increased mass of the myocardium.[22] Diastolic dysfunction is the initial functional maladaptation from LVH, with progressive remodeling resulting in decreased systolic function.[10]

Increased Left Atrial Size

Left atrial size is a valuable parameter to assess the chronicity of AF.[23] Chronic elevation in the left ventricular end-diastolic pressure leads to increased left atrial pressure. Chronic elevation of the left atrial pressure results in chamber enlargement.[24] Atrial stretch leads to electrical dissociation among muscle bundles and facilitates the initiation and maintenance of AF as it allows multiple small reentrant wavelet to sustain AF. Thus, AF is maintained and induced by tissue

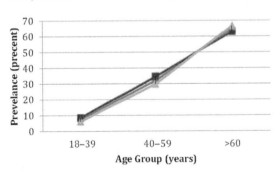

Fig. 1. The increase in prevalence of hypertension as a function of age is depicted from 2011 to 2014. The increase is consistent regardless of gender.

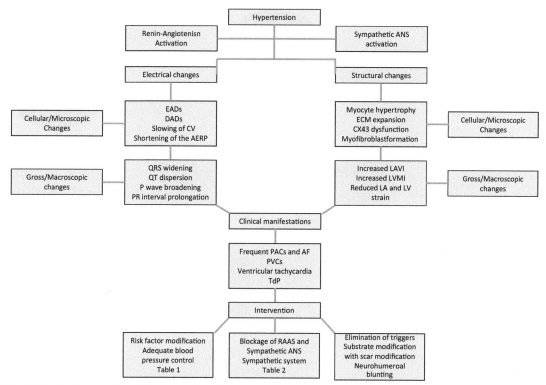

Fig. 2. Mechanisms and manifestations of arrhythmogenesis in patients with hypertension. Hypertension influences arrhythmia genesis through macro and microscopic modifications to the cardiac environment, resulting in electrical and structural changes. The clinical manifestations of these changes are arrhythmias and electrophysiologic alterations such as PACs, PVCs, AF, bundle branch block, QT prolongation, etc. Blood pressure control targeting the renin-angiotensin system and SNS may abate these processes. AERP, atrial effective refractory period; ANS, autonomic nervous system; CV, conduction velocity; CX43, Connexin 43; DAD, delayed afterpolarization; EAD, early afterpolarization; ECM, extracellular matrix; LAVI, left atrial volume index; LVMI, left ventricular mass index; PACs, premature atrial contractions; PVCs, premature ventricular contractions; TdP, torsades de pointes.

remodeling owing to the changes in essential characteristics of the atria.[25,26]

Activation of Sympathetic Nervous System and Renin–Angiotensin–Aldosterone System

Activation of the SNS and the RAAS plays a key role in the development, maintenance, and

---

Box 1
Risk factor modification in hypertension

Blood pressure control per current guidelines

Cessation from tobacco containing products

Minimizing alcohol intake (men ≤2 and women ≤1 drink per day)

Regular physical activity

Assessment and treatment of sleep apnea

Screening for diabetes and hyperlipidemia

Weight reduction and dietary modification

---

progression of both hypertension and various cardiac arrhythmias.[27] **Fig. 3** depicts the renin–angiotensin system with associated therapeutic targets.

Activation of the SNS results in peripheral vasoconstriction, which leads to increased systemic blood pressure. A heightened SNS reduces the refractory period of myocytes and promotes both atrial and ventricular arrhythmias. Angiotensin II, a mediator of RAAS, is implicated for progression of atrial and ventricular fibrosis. Pharmacologic interventions targeting the SNS and the RAAS have been shown to be beneficial for both hypertension and cardiac arrhythmias.[28,29]

Electrical Abnormalities Promoting Arrhythmogenesis in Patients with Hypertension

Electrical changes occur early in hypertensive heart disease. Two distinct abnormalities include the prolongation of atrial conduction velocity and a decrease

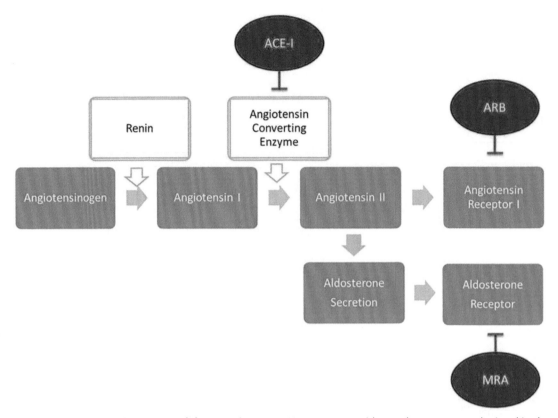

Fig. 3. Renin–angiotensin system and therapeutic targets. Hormones, peptides, and receptors are depicted in the blue boxes. Enzymes are depicted in the green boxes. Therapeutic agents are depicted in the red circles. ACE-I, angiotensin-converting enzyme inhibitor; ARB, angiotensin receptor blocker; MRA, mineralocorticoid antagonist.

in atrial refractoriness. Additionally, triggered activity through both early and delayed after depolarizations are thought to play a role in the initiation of AF related to hypertensive heart disease.[27,30] LVH also results in QRS and QT prolongation as a result of prolonged action potential duration and QT dispersion, which can increase the propensity for early after depolarization, the mechanism for polymorphic ventricular tachycardia/torsades de pointes.[19,20,31]

Microvascular Ischemia Leading to Ventricular Arrhythmia

LVH is also associated with subendocardial ischemia as a result of changes to the microvasculature.[32] Local areas of ischemia produce myocardial scar, as well as fibrosis, which are well-documented substrates for ventricular arrhythmias and sudden cardiac death.[33] Additionally, hypertension is a strong risk factor for the development of macrovascular ischemia through obstructive coronary disease. Infarction scar provides a substrate for macro reentrant arrhythmias such as ventricular tachycardia. LVH also decreases coronary flow reserve owing to

increased left ventricular mass. As coronary flow reserve decreases, there is an increased risk of further ischemia and thus ventricular arrhythmias.[34]

MANAGEMENT OF ARRHYTHMIAS IN PATIENTS WITH HYPERTENSION
Atrial Fibrillation

Appropriate control of blood pressure is associated with a decreased incidence of AF in several studies. This decrease has been partly attributed to the antiarrhythmic properties of antihypertensive medications. The RAAS is the therapeutic target for the prevention of AF. Higher levels of angiotensin II and angiotensin-converting enzymes are observed in patients with AF. In addition to improved blood pressure control, angiotensin-converting enzyme inhibitors and angiotensin receptor blockers theoretically provide antifibrotic and antiapoptotic actions.[35,36] The antiarrhythmic effects of angiotensin receptor blockers was observed in LIFE study, in which new-onset AF occurred in only 150 losartan-treated patients compared with 221 atenolol-treated patients.

These findings suggest a RAAS-specific effect. Stronger evidence for prevention of AF by RAAS blockage with angiotensin-converting enzyme inhibitors or angiotensin receptor blockers was shown in hypertensive patients with LVH and systolic HF.[37] **Table 1** outlines therapies that have been shown to decrease the incidence of new-onset AF.

Optimal blood pressure control to prevent LVH and left atrial enlargement with antihypertensive drugs seems to be important to prevent progression of AF. Although beta-blockers are frequently used for acute and chronic rate control in AF, they are not considered first-line therapies for hypertension. In a study of patients with hypertension, 85 patients with or without LVH had more atrial premature beats than an age-matched control group.[18] Beta-blockers and calcium antagonists resulted in a decreased frequency of premature atrial contractions. In a review of 12,000 patients with HF, the incidence of new-onset AF was significantly lower in patients who received beta-blockers, with a risk reduction of 27%. However, the findings of the LIFE study suggest RAAS blockade is superior to beta-blockade in treating patients with hypertension.[9] Therapies with associated trial results for the prevention of new onset AF can be found in **Table 1**.

Premature Ventricular Beats

Ventricular arrhythmias are common among hypertensive patients, and this association may have important clinical implications. Data from the Atherosclerosis Risk in Communities (ARIC) study of more than 15, 000 African American and white men and women showed that frequent or complex ventricular ectopic beats are associated with high blood pressure.[38] Epidemiologic data have shown that hypertension induced LVH is associated with sustained ventricular arrhythmias.[39] High blood pressure is not arrhythmogenic per se; however, acute or chronic ventricular overload can lead to electrophysiologic properties that may be even more important under pathologic conditions, such as ischemic scars.[40]

The management of PVCs in patients with and without hypertension is similar. A 12-lead electrocardiogram and a 24-hour Holter recording may help to potentially localize the site of origin and to quantify premature ventricular beats.[41] Transthoracic echocardiography may be useful to assess for other signs of hypertensive or structural heart disease, as well as to assess left ventricular systolic function. With regard to treatments for sustained ventricular arrhythmias and prevention of sudden cardiac death, hypertension does not modify the indications for implantable cardioverter-defibrillators or ablation, as recommended by current guidelines.[42,43]

Ventricular Tachycardia, Ventricular Fibrillation, and Sudden Cardiac Death

Hypertension is a risk factor for sudden cardiac death, particularly in the context of increased LV mass.[37] LVH is associated with long-term risk of sudden cardiac death independent of blood pressure, and the risk of sudden cardiac death increases progressively with LV mass. The proposed mechanisms to explain the relationship between the presence of LVH and sudden cardiac death include prolongation of repolarization, mismatch between oxygen supply and demand, reduced coronary flow reserve and subsequent myocardial ischemia.[44]

There is evidence that optimal control of blood pressure and regression of LVH can result in a decreased incidence of sudden cardiac death.[1,45] It is also important to consider the potential influence of antihypertensive drugs on the risk of sudden cardiac death. The use of thiazide diuretics

Table 1
Anti-hypertensive medications and prevention of new-onset AF

Treatment	Trial/Study	Results
Losartan	Losartan Intervention For EndPoint reduction in hypertension (LIFE)	A 33% decrease in new-onset AF compared with treatment with atenolol (3.5% vs 5.3%)
Valsartan	Valsartan Antihypertensive Long-term Use Evaluation Trial (VALUE)	A 16% decrease in new-onset AF compared with amlodipine
Beta-blockers (bisoprolol, metoprolol, bucindolol, Carvedilol, nebivolol)	Prevention of atrial fibrillation onset by beta-blocker treatment in heart failure: a meta-analysis	A 27% decrease in new-onset AF in beta-blocker treated patients with congestive heart failure compared with placebo

has been associated with a dose-dependent increase in sudden cardiac death, probably by increasing the risk of hypokalemia, QT prolongation, QT dispersion, and the propensity for arrhythmogenic early and delayed after-depolarizations.[44] Antihypertensive therapy with angiotensin receptor blockers and angiotensin-converting enzyme inhibitors was associated with a decreased risk of sudden cardiac death.[29,46] This finding provides some supportive evidence for blocking the RAAS in hypertensive patients at high risk of sudden cardiac death.

IMPLICATIONS OF SUBOPTIMAL TREATMENT OF ARRHYTHMIAS AND HYPERTENSION
Heart Failure

Almost 50% of patients with HF have HFpEF.[10] Most common precipitants for HFpEF include uncontrolled hypertension and AF, the 2 conditions that require aggressive management during an episode of decompensated HF. The incidence of HFpEF increases with advancing age, hypertension, diabetes, obesity, and chronic renal dysfunction. All these risk factors are also implicated for the onset and progression of AF. Rhythm control or aggressive rate control for AF is needed for the appropriate management of HFpEF. Similarly, aggressive blood pressure control is crucial during an acute exacerbation of HFpEF.[43,47]

Orthostatic Hypotension

Treatment of hypertension in elderly patients with AF has implications. The incidence of orthostatic hypotension in elderly patients receiving antihypertensive medications is high and an anticipated increased risk of falling may inappropriately prevent the use of anticoagulation for stroke prevention.[48] Similarly, the concomitant use of certain antidepressants, antipsychotics, or drugs for Parkinson disease with antihypertensive medications (eg, diuretics, alpha-blockers, beta-blockers, calcium channel blockers, RAAS blockers, and nitrates) may increase the risk of orthostatic hypotension. When possible, patients should be monitored for ambulatory standing blood pressure to appropriately screen for fall risk.[49]

Thromboembolism and Increased Bleeding Risk

Optimal blood pressure control is crucial for both stroke and bleeding risk reduction in patients with AF taking oral anticoagulation.[50] Given its high prevalence among patients with AF, hypertension may often be the single risk factor requiring a decision on oral anticoagulation use, and data from contemporary real-world AF registries shows that physicians often underestimate the significance of hypertension as a stroke risk factor, despite clearly positive net clinical benefit (the balance of stroke reduction against serious bleeding) of oral anticoagulation in patients with 1 or more stroke risk factors in contemporary large AF cohorts.[51]

ECONOMIC IMPACT OF HYPERTENSION AND ARRHYTHMIAS

The high prevalence of both hypertension and AF and the increasing costs for their treatment constitute an important financial burden; therefore, many economic analyses have been done with the aim to assess the cost effectiveness of treating these diseases. In these analyses the focus is mainly on the risk of stroke and the savings that can be obtained by preventing stroke occurrence and the consequent health care resources for hospitalization, rehabilitation, and assistance resulting from disability, which are associated with high direct and indirect costs.[43,52]

The stroke associated with AF lead to significant debility and the cost of taking care of such patients is greater than the costs for stroke unrelated to AF. Several studies performed after novel oral anticoagulants became available have shown that these medications are cost effective despite a higher initial cost owing to the significant decrease in intracranial bleeding and stroke prevention.[53]

Finally, from an economic perspective, it is noteworthy to stress that, because AF is frequently asymptomatic, opportunistic screening for asymptomatic AF is indicated to institute antithromboembolic prophylaxis in patients at risk, and proved to be cost effective.[54,55]

SUMMARY

Experimental and epidemiologic studies have established a close link between hypertension, LVH, and various cardiac arrhythmias. Chronic hypertension results in the alteration of cardiac hemodynamic, structural, and electrophysiological properties and leads to the development of AF, ventricular arrhythmias, and sudden cardiac death. Optimal management of hypertension with different agents to lower blood pressure and, more important, to regress LVH can prevent AF and sudden cardiac death. Treatment with angiotensin-converting enzyme inhibitors and angiotensin receptor blockers has been shown to decrease ventricular ectopy and sudden cardiac death. Beta-blocker therapy also should be considered in patients who require additional antihypertensive therapy. Mineralocorticoid receptor antagonists remain a promising therapeutic approach to reduce myocardial fibrosis, though further studies are needed to validate its use in prevention of ventricular arrhythmia and sudden cardiac death in hypertensive heart disease.

REFERENCES

1. Mancia G, Fagard R, Narkiewicz K, et al. 2013 ESH/ESC guidelines for the management of arterial hypertension: the Task Force for the Management of Arterial Hypertension of the European Society of Hypertension (ESH) and of the European Society of Cardiology (ESC). Eur Heart J 2013;34:2159–219.
2. Zhang Y, Moran AE. Trends in the prevalence, awareness, treatment, and control of hypertension among young adults in the United States, 1999 to 2014. Hypertension 2017;70:736–42.
3. Egan BM, Zhao Y, Axon RN. US trends in prevalence, awareness, treatment, and control of hypertension, 1988-2008. Jama 2010;303:2043–50.
4. Dzeshka MS, Shahid F, Shantsila A, et al. Hypertension and Atrial fibrillation: an intimate association of epidemiology, pathophysiology, and outcomes. Am J Hypertens 2017;30:733–55.
5. Ghiadoni L, Taddei S, Virdis A. Hypertension and atrial fibrillation: any change with the new anticoagulants. Curr Pharm Des 2014;20:6096–105.
6. Kannel WB, Wolf PA, Benjamin EJ, et al. Prevalence, incidence, prognosis, and predisposing conditions for atrial fibrillation: population-based estimates. Am J Cardiol 1998;82:2n–9n.
7. Lau YF, Yiu KH, Siu CW, et al. Hypertension and atrial fibrillation: epidemiology, pathophysiology and therapeutic implications. J Hum Hypertens 2012;26:563–9.
8. Manolis AJ, Rosei EA, Coca A, et al. Hypertension and atrial fibrillation: diagnostic approach, prevention and treatment. Position paper of the Working Group 'Hypertension Arrhythmias and Thrombosis' of the European Society of Hypertension. J Hypertens 2012;30:239–52.
9. Ogunsua AA, Shaikh AY, Ahmed M, et al. Atrial fibrillation and hypertension: mechanistic, epidemiologic, and treatment parallels. Methodist DeBakey Cardiovasc J 2015;11:228–34.
10. Redfield MM. Heart failure with preserved ejection fraction. N Engl J Med 2016;375:1868–77.
11. Figueroa JJ, Basford JR, Low PA. Preventing and treating orthostatic hypotension: as easy as A, B, C. Cleve Clin J Med 2010;77:298–306.
12. Ijiri H, Kohno I, Yin D, et al. Cardiac arrhythmias and left ventricular hypertrophy in dipper and nondipper patients with essential hypertension. Jpn Circ J 2000; 64:499–504.
13. Messerli FH. Hypertension and sudden cardiac death. Am J Hypertens 1999;12:181s–8s.
14. Pringle SD, Dunn FG, Macfarlane PW, et al. Significance of ventricular arrhythmias in systemic hypertension with left ventricular hypertrophy. Am J Cardiol 1992;69:913–7.
15. Ball J, Carrington MJ, McMurray JJ, et al. Atrial fibrillation: profile and burden of an evolving epidemic in the 21st century. Int J Cardiol 2013;167:1807–24.
16. Seccia TM, Caroccia B, Muiesan ML, et al. Atrial fibrillation and arterial hypertension: a common duet with dangerous consequences where the renin angiotensin-aldosterone system plays an important role. Int J Cardiol 2016;206:71–6.
17. Verdecchia P, Reboldi G, Gattobigio R, et al. Atrial fibrillation in hypertension: predictors and outcome. Hypertension 2003;41:218–23.
18. Zhao LQ, Liu SW. Atrial fibrillation in essential hypertension: an issue of concern. J Cardiovasc Med (Hagerstown) 2014;15:100–6.
19. Morin DP, Oikarinen L, Viitasalo M, et al. QRS duration predicts sudden cardiac death in hypertensive patients undergoing intensive medical therapy: the LIFE study. Eur Heart J 2009;30:2908–14.
20. Al-Khatib SM, Granger CB, Huang Y, et al. Sustained ventricular arrhythmias among patients with acute coronary syndromes with no ST-segment elevation: incidence, predictors, and outcomes. Circulation 2002;106:309–12.
21. Nattel S. New ideas about atrial fibrillation 50 years on. Nature 2002;415:219–26.
22. Kahan T, Bergfeldt L. Left ventricular hypertrophy in hypertension: its arrhythmogenic potential. Heart 2005;91:250–6.
23. de Vos CB, Pisters R, Nieuwlaat R, et al. Progression from paroxysmal to persistent atrial fibrillation clinical correlates and prognosis. J Am Coll Cardiol 2010;55:725–31.
24. Henry WL, Morganroth J, Pearlman AS, et al. Relation between echocardiographically determined left atrial size and atrial fibrillation. Circulation 1976;53:273–9.
25. Tribulova N, Okruhlicova L, Novakova S, et al. Hypertension-related intermyocyte junction remodelling is associated with a higher incidence of low-K(+)-induced lethal arrhythmias in isolated rat heart. Exp Physiol 2002;87:195–205.
26. Zou R, Kneller J, Leon LJ, et al. Substrate size as a determinant of fibrillatory activity maintenance in a mathematical model of canine atrium. Am J Physiol Heart Circ Physiol 2005;289:H1002–12.
27. Patterson E, Po SS, Scherlag BJ, et al. Triggered firing in pulmonary veins initiated by in vitro autonomic nerve stimulation. Heart Rhythm 2005;2:624–31.
28. Xiao P, Gao C, Fan J, et al. Blockade of angiotensin II improves hyperthyroid induced abnormal atrial electrophysiological properties. Regul Pept 2011; 169:31–8.
29. Yusuf S, Sleight P, Pogue J, et al. Effects of an angiotensin-converting-enzyme inhibitor, ramipril,

on cardiovascular events in high-risk patients. N Engl J Med 2000;342:145–53.

30. Voigt N, Heijman J, Wang Q, et al. Cellular and molecular mechanisms of atrial arrhythmogenesis in patients with paroxysmal atrial fibrillation. Circulation 2014;129:145–56.

31. Kannel WB, Schatzkin A. Sudden death: lessons from subsets in population studies. J Am Coll Cardiol 1985;5:141b–9b.

32. Goette A, Bukowska A, Dobrev D, et al. Acute atrial tachyarrhythmia induces angiotensin II type 1 receptor-mediated oxidative stress and microvascular flow abnormalities in the ventricles. Eur Heart J 2009;30:1411–20.

33. Goette A, Bukowska A, Lillig CH, et al. Oxidative stress and microcirculatory flow abnormalities in the ventricles during atrial fibrillation. Front Physiol 2012;3:236.

34. Emiroglu MY, Bulut M, Sahin M, et al. Assessment of atrial conduction time in patients with essential hypertension. J Electrocardiol 2011;44:251–6.

35. Mayet J, Chapman N, Shahi M, et al. The effects on cardiac arrhythmias of antihypertensive therapy causing regression of left ventricular hypertrophy. Am J Hypertens 1997;10:611–8.

36. Hirsh BJ, Copeland-Halperin RS, Halperin JL. Fibrotic atrial cardiomyopathy, atrial fibrillation, and thromboembolism: mechanistic links and clinical inferences. J Am Coll Cardiol 2015;65:2239–51.

37. Wachtell K, Hornestam B, Lehto M, et al. Cardiovascular morbidity and mortality in hypertensive patients with a history of atrial fibrillation: the Losartan Intervention For End Point Reduction in Hypertension (LIFE) study. J Am Coll Cardiol 2005;45:705–11.

38. Simpson RJ Jr, Cascio WE, Crow RS, et al. Association of ventricular premature complexes with electrocardiographic-estimated left ventricular mass in a population of African-American and white men and women (The Atherosclerosis Risk in Communities. Am J Cardiol 2001;87:49–53.

39. Chatterjee S, Bavishi C, Sardar P, et al. Meta-analysis of left ventricular hypertrophy and sustained arrhythmias. Am J Cardiol 2014;114:1049–52.

40. Calkins H, Maughan WL, Weisman HF, et al. Effect of acute volume load on refractoriness and arrhythmia development in isolated, chronically infarcted canine hearts. Circulation 1989;79:687–97.

41. Baman TS, Lange DC, Ilg KJ, et al. Relationship between burden of premature ventricular complexes and left ventricular function. Heart Rhythm 2010;7:865–9.

42. Priori SG, Blomstrom-Lundqvist C, Mazzanti A, et al. 2015 ESC guidelines for the management of patients with ventricular arrhythmias and the prevention of sudden cardiac death: the Task Force for the Management of Patients with Ventricular Arrhythmias and the Prevention of Sudden Cardiac Death of the European Society of Cardiology (ESC) Endorsed by:

Association for European Paediatric and Congenital Cardiology (AEPC). Europace 2015;17:1601–87.

43. Lip GYH, Coca A, Kahan T, et al. Hypertension and cardiac arrhythmias: a consensus document from the European Heart Rhythm Association (EHRA) and ESC Council on Hypertension, endorsed by the Heart Rhythm Society (HRS), Asia-Pacific Heart Rhythm Society (APHRS) and Sociedad Latinoamericana de Estimulacion Cardiaca y Electrofisiologia (SOLEACE). Europace 2017;19:891–911.

44. Osadchii OE. Mechanisms of hypokalemia-induced ventricular arrhythmogenicity. Fundam Clin Pharmacol 2010;24:547–59.

45. Novo S, Abrignani MG, Novo G, et al. Effects of drug therapy on cardiac arrhythmias and ischemia in hypertensives with LVH. Am J Hypertens 2001;14:637–43.

46. Lindholm LH, Dahlof B, Edelman JM, et al. Effect of losartan on sudden cardiac death in people with diabetes: data from the LIFE study. Lancet 2003;362:619–20.

47. Lam CS, Donal E, Kraigher-Krainer E, et al. Epidemiology and clinical course of heart failure with preserved ejection fraction. Eur J Heart Fail 2011;13:18–28.

48. Shen S, He T, Chu J, et al. Uncontrolled hypertension and orthostatic hypotension in relation to standing balance in elderly hypertensive patients. Clin Interv Aging 2015;10:897–906.

49. Jones PK, Shaw BH, Raj SR. Orthostatic hypotension: managing a difficult problem. Expert Rev Cardiovasc Ther 2015;13:1263–76.

50. Independent predictors of stroke in patients with atrial fibrillation: a systematic review. Neurology 2007;69:546–54.

51. Angaran P, Dorian P, Tan MK, et al. The risk stratification and stroke prevention therapy care gap in Canadian atrial fibrillation patients. Can J Cardiol 2016;32:336–43.

52. Hannon N, Callaly E, Moore A, et al. Improved late survival and disability after stroke with therapeutic anticoagulation for atrial fibrillation: a population study. Stroke 2011;42:2503–8.

53. Bruggenjurgen B, Rossnagel K, Roll S, et al. The impact of atrial fibrillation on the cost of stroke: the Berlin Acute Stroke Study. Value Health 2007;10:137–43.

54. Nasir JM, Pomeroy W, Marler A, et al. Predicting determinants of atrial fibrillation or flutter for therapy elucidation in patients at risk for thromboembolic events (PREDATE AF) study. Heart Rhythm 2017;14:955–61.

55. Kusumoto FM, Hao SC, Slotwiner DJ, et al. Arrhythmia care in a value-based environment: past, present, and future: developed and endorsed by the Heart Rhythm Society (HRS). Heart Rhythm 2018;15:e5–15.

Hypertension Treatment in Diabetes
Focus on Heart Failure Prevention

Hannah F. Bensimhon, MD*, Matthew A. Cavender, MD, MPH

KEYWORDS

• Diabetes • Hypertension • Heart failure

KEY POINTS

• Diabetes is strongly associated with the development of cardiovascular disease and poor cardiovascular outcomes.
• Management of hypertension has been shown to reduce cardiovascular outcomes among patients with diabetes.
• The American Diabetes Association has a target blood pressure goal of less than 140/90 for patients with diabetes.
• Angiotensin-converting enzyme inhibitors (ACEIs) or an aldosterone receptor blocker (ARBs) should be considered as first-line therapy, followed by calcium channel blockers and diuretics.
• Sodium glucose transporter 2 (SGLT-2) inhibitors are a promising novel therapeutic that impacts blood pressure and cardiovascular risk in patients with diabetes.

Diabetes is strongly associated with the development of cardiovascular (CV) disease and adverse CV events. Although the management of diabetes has improved in the last several decades, the increasing prevalence of diabetes has led to a subsequent rise of CV disease. Although 382 million people were estimated to be living with diabetes in 2013 across the world, this number is projected to rise and reach 592 million by the year 2035.[1] Most adverse outcomes among patients with diabetes result from vascular disease, including macrovascular complications (including coronary artery disease, peripheral artery disease, and stroke) and microvascular complications (including retinopathy, neuropathy, and nephropathy). The impact of diabetes on the development of macrovascular complications and heart disease has major economic and public health implications.[2]

DIABETES AND HEART FAILURE

There is a clear and well-established link between diabetes and the incidence of coronary artery disease. Given the high rates of coronary artery disease among patients with diabetes, it is not surprising that patients with diabetes are also at a high risk of developing ischemic cardiomyopathy and heart failure. Although it was previously believed that the link between heart failure and diabetes was predominantly mediated through a higher burden of ischemic heart disease and resulting ischemic cardiomyopathy, heart failure occurs at higher rates in patients with diabetes

Disclosure Statement: Research support (nonsalary) from AstraZeneca, Bristol Myers Squibb, Chiesi, GlaxoSmithKline, Novartis, Takeda, and The Medicines Company. Research support (salary) from Novo-Nordisk. Consulting fees from AstraZeneca, Boehringer-Ingelheim, Chiesi, Edwards Lifesciences, Janssen, Merck, and Sanofi-Aventis.
Division of Cardiology, Department of Medicine, University of North Carolina, Burnett-Womack Building, 160 Dental Circle, CB# 7075, Chapel Hill, NC 27599, USA
* Corresponding author.
E-mail address: Hannah.Bensimhon@unchealth.unc.edu

Heart Failure Clin 15 (2019) 551–563
https://doi.org/10.1016/j.hfc.2019.06.008
1551-7136/19/© 2019 Elsevier Inc. All rights reserved.

even in the absence of overt atherosclerosis and risk factors for coronary artery disease, such as hypertension and obesity.[3]

The Framingham Heart Study, published in 1974, was one of the first studies to demonstrate that patients with diabetes were at increased risk of heart failure.[4] Data from a pooled cohort (from the Cardiovascular Disease Lifetime Risk Pooling Project) showed that among five modifiable risk factors for heart failure (current smoking, diabetes, elevated low-density lipoprotein, hypertension, and obesity), diabetes was associated most strongly with heart failure–free survival.[5] From these data, subjects without diabetes at age 45 years compared with those with diabetes were more than 60% less likely to develop heart failure.[5] Heart failure also represents a risk factor for diabetes. In a survey of 3580 patients admitted with heart failure in a large, multicenter European study, 40% had diabetes.[6] This high prevalence was replicated in the EVEREST analysis[7] and in a CHARM study group analysis where more than 25% of patients with heart failure had diabetes.[8]

Although most heart failure in patients with diabetes results from progression of coronary vascular disease to ischemic cardiomyopathy, the long-standing metabolic perturbations of diabetes also seem to be directly toxic to the myocardium.[3,9] Diabetic cardiomyopathy (defined as systolic or diastolic dysfunction in the absence of coronary artery disease, hypertension, valvular disease, and congenital abnormalities) was found in 15% of patients with diabetes.[10] Another community-based cohort study that followed patients for nearly 30 years revealed several biomarkers (serving as surrogates for insulin resistance) that were associated with heart failure, independent of ischemic CV disease and other established risk factors for heart failure.[11]

In addition to increasing the risk of heart disease, the presence of diabetes worsens the outcomes of patients with CV disease, including heart failure. Patients with heart failure with preserved ejection fraction and diabetes have been shown to have more numerous comorbidities; increased left ventricular hypertrophy; and increased circulating markers of vasoconstriction, oxidative stress, inflammation, and fibrosis.[12] Among these patients, there are also increased signs and symptoms of fluid retention at baseline and these patients were at increased risk for hospitalization for heart failure and death from heart failure during the study period.[13] In one population of patients admitted with new or worsening heart failure, diabetes increased the mortality risk, an effect that was similar in patients with depressed and normal left ventricular systolic function.[14]

Four-year data from the REACH Registry (an international registry of more than 45,000 patients) demonstrated that the presence of diabetes was associated with a 33% increase in the odds of hospitalization for heart failure. The presence of diabetes and heart failure at baseline was independently associated with increase in CV death.[15]

HYPERTENSION AND CARDIOVASCULAR EVENTS

Hypertension is also a well-established risk factor for CV disease regardless of the presence of diabetes. In a meta-analysis of studies that included data from more than 1 million patients, reduction in blood pressure resulted in a significant reduction in the risk of vascular death with no lower limit of benefit seen.[16] Furthermore, in a cohort of 1.25 million subjects followed over time, increasing systolic blood pressure was associated with a higher risk of all types of CV disease including an approximately 30% increase in the risk of subsequent heart failure.[17]

The effects of hypertension on the vasculature, as measured by increasing aortic stiffness on aortic pulse wave velocity, are seen even in the young. In the heart, long-standing pressure overload results in compensatory hypertrophy in the myocardium. As the left ventricle hypertrophies and left ventricular mass increases, perturbations in myocardial relaxation are seen resulting in diastolic dysfunction.[18] These changes in myocardial relaxation make patients more susceptible to pulmonary edema and other clinical symptoms of heart failure, particularly during episodes of acute elevation in blood pressure, volume retention, or coronary ischemia. If the heart remains exposed to elevated pressure and elevated volume, heart failure with reduced ejection fraction can develop (**Fig. 1**).[19]

DIABETES, HYPERTENSION, AND HEART FAILURE

Given the overlapping risk factors for diabetes and hypertension, the two diseases frequently coexist. In one meta-analysis, the prevalence of hypertension was found to range from 60% to 75% among patients with diabetes.[20] There are also data to suggest that precedent hypertension is associated with a 35% increased risk of diabetes.[21] The risk of macrovascular complications in patients with hypertension and diabetes is greater than in patients with just one of these conditions.[22]

There is also a clear link between diabetes, renal dysfunction, and CV events. Microalbuminuria or proteinuria can develop in patients with diabetes

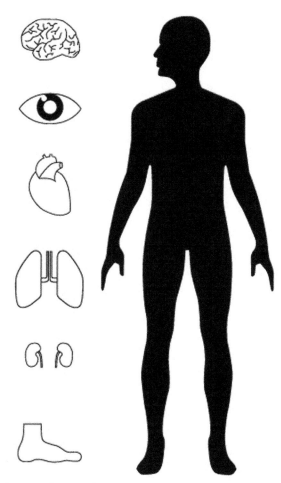

- **Vascular Dementia**
- **CVA**
- **Intracranial Hemorrhage**

- **Retinopathy**
- **Choroidopathy**
- **Optic Neuropathy**

- **Cardiomyopathy**
- **LVH**
- **CAD**
- **Diastolic Dysfunction**

- **Obstructive Sleep Apnea**

- **Glomerulosclerosis**
- **Renal Artery Aneurysm**
- **Renal Failure**

- **Osteoporosis**

Fig. 1. End organ damage in chronic hypertension. CAD, Coronary artery disease; CVA, Cerebrovascular vascular accident; LVH, left ventricular hypertrophy.

as a manifestation of long-standing hyperglycemia resulting in microvascular damage to the renal glomerulus. The presence of albuminuria has also been shown to increase the risk of hypertension in patients with diabetes.[23] When taken together, those patients with diabetes and albuminuria are at the highest subsequent risk of CV disease.[24,25] Increased serum glucose and insulin may also result in increased renal sodium and water retention, further contributing to hypertension and risk of heart failure. The renin-angiotensin-aldosterone system (RAAS), which is an important mediator of high blood pressure, left ventricular mass, and volume status, has been shown to be inhibited by diabetes through a process mediated by incretin hormones further strengthening the degree of interconnectivity of the CV, renal, and endocrine systems.[26]

Thus, managing hypertension in patients with diabetes remains one of the key strategies for reducing heart failure in this population because

of evidence for pronounced reduction in CV outcomes.[27–29] Several large trials have attempted to identify appropriate blood pressure targets among this population, and there has also been considerable efforts to identify the best therapeutic approach in the management of hypertension among patients with diabetes (**Table 1**).

BLOOD PRESSURE LOWERING AND CLINICAL OUTCOMES IN DIABETES

The United Kingdom Prospective Diabetes Study (UKPDS-38) was one of the earliest studies that attempted to define appropriate blood pressure targets for patients with diabetes. In this study, more than 1000 patients with type 2 diabetes and hypertension were randomized to strict versus lenient blood pressure control and followed over time. Those randomized to a more aggressive blood pressure target achieved an average blood pressure of 144/82 mm Hg compared with the

Table 1
Key trials: blood pressure management in patients with diabetes

Trial Name	Year Published	Study Design	Drugs Tested	Key Cardiovascular Outcome	Results
SHEP[43]	1996	Drug vs placebo	Chlorthalidone	Combined major cardiovascular event[a]	Chlorthalidone: RR, 0.66; HR, 0.46–0.94; P<.05[a]
HOT[31]	1998	Intense vs less intense control	1°: Felodipine	Major cardiovascular event[b]	Diastolic BP <90 vs <80: RR, 2.06; P = .005
UKPDS[68]	1998	Intense vs less intense control	1°: Captopril and atenolol	Combined macrovascular disease[c]	Intense control: RR, 0.76; 95% CI, 0.62–0.92; P .00046
ABCD-H[46]	1998	Drug vs drug	Nisoldipine vs enalapril	Fatal and nonfatal MI	Nisoldipine: RR, 7.0; 95% CI, 2.3–21.4; P = .001
CAPPP[47]	1999	Drug vs drug	Captopril vs beta/diuretic	Cardiovascular mortality[d]	Captopril: RR, 0.59; 95% CI, 0.38–0.91; P.018
HOPE[50]	2000	Drug vs placebo	Ramipril vs placebo	Combined end point[e]	Ramipril: RRR, 25%; 95% CI, 12–36; P = .0004
IDN[52]	2001	Drug vs drug vs placebo	Irbesartan vs amlodipine vs placebo	Heart failure	Irbesartan vs placebo: HR, 0.72; 95% CI, 0.52–1.00; P = .048 Irbesartan vs amlodipine: HR, 0.65; 95% CI, 0.48–0.87; P = .004

Trial	Year	Comparison	Drugs	Outcome	Result
ALLHAT[28] (diabetes subgroup)	2002	Drug vs drug	Chlorthalidone, amlodipine, lisinopril	Heart failure	Amlodipine: RR, 1.39; 95% CI, 1.22–1.59 / Lisinopril: RR, 1.15; 95% CI, 1.00–1.32
LIFE[48]	2002	Drug vs drug	Losartan vs atenolol	Combined cardiovascular outcome[f]	Losartan: RR, 0.87; 95% CI, 0.77–0.98; P = .021
ADVANCE[34]	2007	Drug vs placebo	Perindopril and indapamide vs placebo	Vascular complications	Perindopril and indapamide: HR, 0.91; 95% CI, 0.83–1.00; P = .04
DIRECT-protect 2[51]	2008	Drug vs placebo	Candesartan vs placebo	Combined cardiovascular event[g]	Candesartan: HR, 0.67; 95% CI, 0.42–1.07
ACCORD[33]	2010	Intense vs less intense control	N/A	Composite end point[h]	No difference
ACCOMPLISH[55]	2010	Drug vs drug	ACEI + CCB vs ACEI + diuretic	Combined cardiovascular event[i]	ACEI + CCB: HR, 0.79; 95% CI, 0.68–0.92; P = .003

Abbreviations: ACEI, angiotensin-converting enzyme inhibitors; BP, blood pressure; CCB, calcium channel blocker; CI, confidence interval; HR, hazard ratio; MI, myocardial infarction; N/A, Not applicable; RR, relative risk; RRR, relative risk reduction.

[a] Nonfatal or fatal MI, sudden cardiac death, rapid cardiac death, coronary artery bypass graft, angioplasty, nonfatal or fatal stroke, transient ischemic attack, aneurysm, and endarterectomy.
[b] Nonfatal or fatal MI, nonfatal or fatal stroke, and cardiovascular death.
[c] MI, sudden death, stroke, and peripheral vascular disease.
[d] Fatal stroke and MI, sudden death, and other cardiovascular death.
[e] MI, stroke, and cardiovascular death.
[f] Death, MI, and stroke.
[g] Cardiovascular death, nonfatal MI, and stroke.
[h] Deaths caused by cardiovascular disease, nonfatal MI, and nonfatal stroke.
[i] Cardiovascular death, MI, stroke, hospitalization for angina, resuscitated arrest, and coronary revascularization.

other group who had an average blood pressure of 154/87 mm Hg. After a median follow-up of more than 8 years, patients treated with more intensive blood pressure control had a 34% reduction in macrovascular disease events (a composite end point that included sudden death, myocardial infarction [MI], stroke, or peripheral vascular disease).[29] An important finding from this trial was the need for sustained blood pressure control: in longer term follow-up, the difference in blood pressure between the groups was lost, as were clinical improvements, within 2 years of the study termination.[30]

In the Hypertension Optimization Trial (HOT), the effects of treating to diastolic blood pressure goals were tested. In this trial, 18,790 patients, of which 1501 patients had diabetes, were randomized to target diastolic blood pressure goals of 80, 85, and 90. Felodipine was the first-line blood pressure agent used and angiotensin-converting enzyme inhibitors (ACEI), β-blockers, and then diuretics were added in subsequent stepwise fashion. In patients with diabetes, there was a 50% reduction in the risk of CV death, MI, or stroke in those patients randomized to diastolic blood pressure less than or equal to 80 mm Hg when compared with patients randomized to diastolic blood pressure less than or equal to 80 mm Hg (P for trend = .005).[31]

However, the findings were in contrast to the ACCORD trial, a 2 × 2 factorial designed trial that evaluated intensive glucose-lowering therapy and intensive blood pressure control in patients with diabetes. Despite significant differences in blood pressure after almost 5 years of follow-up, in the 4733 patients with type 2 diabetes, targeting a systolic blood pressure less than 120 mm Hg did not reduce rates of CV death, MI, or stroke when compared with a target systolic blood pressure less than 140 mm Hg.[32] With regards to heart failure, there were also no differences in the rates of heart failure (hazard ratio [HR], 0.94; 95% confidence interval [CI], 0.70–1.26; P = .67). Although this trial may have suggested more lenient blood pressure goals, there was a major limitation in sampling in this trial; because this arm was embedded in a larger trial, many of the subjects were "lower risk" than the general population given that higher risk patients had been selected for other study arms (notably the ACCORD lipid arm). This reality was evident in the 50% lower-than-expected mortality rate observed in the control arm.[33]

The blood pressure arm of the ADVANCE trial randomized 11,000 participants with type 2 diabetes to a fixed dose of a thiazide diuretic–ACEI combination pill (indapamide and perindopril) or control. The treatment arm achieved a blood pressure of 136/73 mm Hg compared with the control arm whose average blood pressure was 142/75. This resulted in a 9% relative risk (RR) reduction of major macrovascular or microvascular events (15.5% [thiazide-ACEI combination] vs 16.8% [placebo]; HR, 0.91; 95% CI, 0.83–1.00; P = .04). The RR of death from CV disease was reduced by 18% (3.8% [thiazide-ACEI combination] vs 4.6% [placebo]; HR, 0.82; 95% CI, 0.68–0.98; P = .03) and death was reduced by 14% (7.3% active vs 471 8.5% placebo; HR, 0.86; 95% CI, 0.75–0.98; P = .03).[34] Following these trials, a subsequent meta-analysis of 13 trials and 37,736 patients found that intensive blood pressure control to a systolic blood pressure of less than or equal to 135 mm Hg reduced mortality and stroke. However, there were no significant effects on heart failure (RR, 0.90; 95% CI, 0.75–1.06) with more intensive blood pressure control.[35]

BLOOD PRESSURE TARGETS

Current guidelines offer clinicians guidance on blood pressure control in patients with diabetes. The American Diabetes Association (ADA) consensus report remains committed to a blood pressure goal of less than 140/90 mm Hg for patients with diabetes.[27] Although they acknowledge that some patients with increased risk of CV disease might benefit from a lower blood pressure target, they are compelled by the strongest evidence from the ACCORD trial, which failed to demonstrate this benefit from lower blood pressure targets among patients with diabetes. The 2017 American College of Cardiology (ACC)/American Heart Association (AHA) hypertension guidelines recommend initiating antihypertensives for blood pressure greater than 130/80 in patients with diabetes.[36] The 2018 European Society of Cardiology and the European Society of Hypertension joint task force on blood pressure control recommends targeting blood pressure management in patients with diabetes to a blood pressure of 130/80, and lower if possible, without going below a systolic blood pressure of 120 mm Hg. They do not recommend the initiation of antihypertensives until blood pressure is greater than 140/90 mm Hg.[37]

In patients with heart failure, irrespective of the presence or absence of diabetes, similar blood pressure targets have been proposed. The SPRINT trials specifically evaluated patients without diabetes who were at increased risk of CV events, greater than or equal to 50 years old, and had a systolic blood pressure between 130 and 180 mm Hg. In this trial MI, acute coronary syndrome, stroke, heart failure, or death from CV causes was lower in patients treated to a goal blood pressure of less than 120 mm Hg.[38] In the 2017 ACC/AHA focused update for the treatment of patients with heart failure, a class I (strong) recommendation was made to treat patients at risk for heart failure and those with both heart failure and reduced ejection fraction and heart failure with preserved ejection fraction to a goal blood pressure of less than 130/80 mm Hg.[39]

THERAPEUTIC OPTIONS FOR THE TREATMENT OF HYPERTENSION
Thiazide Therapy

Thiazide diuretics work by inhibiting Na^+/Cl^- cotransporter in the distal convoluted tubules of the kidneys, resulting in a mild volume loss and subsequent decline in blood pressure. The Antihypertensive and Lipid-Lowering Treatment to Prevent Heart Attack Trial (ALLHAT) found chlorthalidone, a long-acting thiazide diuretic, to be as effective as doxazosin, amlodipine, and lisinopril in a broad composite end point of CV events.[40] However, chlorthalidone significantly reduced the risk of heart failure when compared with doxazosin and amlodipine and was similar to therapy with lisinopril.[41] In the subgroup of patients with diabetes, chlorthalidone was found to be particularly effective with regards to reduction in the risk of heart failure (when compared with chlorthalidone, RR with amlodipine 1.39; 95% CI, 1.22–1.59; and RR lisinopril, 1.15; 95% CI, 1.00–1.32).[42] Similar results were found in the subgroup of patients with diabetes in the systolic hypertension in the elderly program, which found lower rates of major CV events in patients with diabetes receiving a diuretic compared with placebo (20% vs 27%; RR, 0.66 [0.46–0.94]; P<.05).[43]

Renin-angiotensin system
There is a clear link between diabetes, renal disease, and CV events. Patients at increased risk of CV events are identified by the presence of albuminuria, the incidence of which is increased in patients with diabetes and hypertension.[44] Diabetic nephropathy and hypertension result in perturbations in the renin-angiotensin system (RAS); however, inhibition of the RAS with ACEIs and angiotensin receptor blockers (ARBs) has been shown to decrease albuminuria, retard the decline in glomerular filtration rate, and reduce CV events in patients with diabetes.[45]

The Appropriate Blood Pressure Control in Diabetes (ABCD) trial evaluated the impact of ACEI therapy in 950 patients with noninsulin-dependent diabetes. This trial revealed a significantly higher incidence of fatal and nonfatal MI in patients with diabetes and hypertension who were randomized to receive nisoldipine compared with those receiving the ACEI enalapril (RR, 7.0; 95% CI, 2.3–21.4; P = .001).[46] In the Captopril Prevention Project (CAPPP), patients were randomized to captopril to standard diuretic and β-blocker based antihypertensive therapy. In the subgroup of patients with diabetes, captopril reduced a composite end point of CV events (MI, stroke, or other CV deaths; RR, 0.59; 95% CI, 0.38–0.91; P .018).[47] The LIFE Trial compared the effect of an ARB and a β-blocker on CV outcomes among patients with hypertension and diabetes who had already developed left ventricular hypertrophy. The patients assigned to the ARB group had statistically significantly lower rates of CV events and death, despite achieving nearly identical blood pressure levels (RR, 0.87; 95% CI, 0.77–0.98; P = .021).[48]

The ADVANCE trial set out to assess the benefit of a fixed-dose ACEI (perindopril) and a diuretic (indapamide) in the absence of a blood pressure target among patients with type 2 diabetes. More than 11,000 patients with type 2 diabetes and an average baseline blood pressure of 145/81 mm Hg were enrolled and exposed to a randomization of perindopril-indapamide or control. Although the difference in blood pressure between the two groups was only 5.6/2.2 mm Hg, there was a reduction in major macrovascular and microvascular events (HR, 0.91; 95% CI, 0.83–1.00; P = .04), and lower rates of CV and all-cause mortality, suggesting a benefit of RAAS-oriented therapy in this population separate from their impact on blood pressure.[34] In this study group, the reduced rates of death and major CV events was preserved (despite loss of the small blood pressure difference) during the post-trial observational period.[49] This finding was reiterated by the HOPE trial, which randomized patients to ramipril versus placebo.[50] In this trial, systolic blood pressure was only mildly elevated and reduction in blood pressure was minimal (2/1 mm Hg). Nonetheless, patients randomized to ramipril had a 25% RR reduction of the combined outcome of MI, stroke, and CV death (95% CI, 12–36; P = .0004)[43] and the trial was terminated early for efficacy.

ARBs have also been shown to be effective. The DIRECT-PROTECT 2 trial randomized patients with type 2 diabetes with or without hypertension to receive candesartan or placebo. Patients were followed for more than 4 years and outcomes included microvascular and macrovascular complications. Overall, candesartan reduced the rates of vascular complications. Candesartan reduced microvascular (microalbuminuria and retinopathy) complications in all patients (HR, 0.85; 95% CI, 0.72–0.99; P = .040), but only reduced macrovascular complications (CV death, nonfatal MI, and stroke) in those patients with baseline hypertension (HR, 0.67; 95% CI, 0.42–1.07).[51] The Irbesartan Diabetic Nephropathy trial, published in 2003, looked directly at the impact of RAAS-oriented drugs on the development of heart failure in this population. The administration of irbesartan reduced the risk of heart failure in patients with diabetes and nephropathy compared with control and amlodipine (HR, 0.72; 95% CI, 0.52–1.00; $P = .048$).[52]

Of note, despite the benefit seen in prior trials with ACEI and ARBs, there does not seem to be a role for these drugs to be used in combination, given the higher risk of adverse events and little additional clinical benefit.[53]

Calcium Channel Blockers

Although RAS inhibitors have been shown to be more effective in reducing CV events, calcium channel blockers (CCBs) are effective therapies in reducing blood pressure and have a role in the treatment of blood pressure in patients with diabetes. In the large diabetic subgroup of the ASCOT (Anglo Scandinavian Cardiac Outcomes Trial), amlodipine was shown to reduce CV events when compared with atenolol (HR, 0.86; 95% CI, 0.76–0.98; $P = .026$). There were consistent effects in patients with and without diabetes.[54] The ACCOMPLISH (Avoiding Cardiovascular Events Through COMbination Therapy in Patients Living With Systolic Hypertension) trial compared the effects of an ACEI combined with a CCB to an ACEI combined with a diuretic. The combination of an ACEI with a CCB was shown to have greater benefit in reducing CV events among patients with diabetes compared with an ACEI combined with a diuretic (HR, 0.79; 95% CI, 0.68–0.92; $P = .003$).[55] This effect was primarily driven through coronary events, and there was a statistically nonsignificant trend toward benefit of the diuretic group for the heart failure hospitalization end point. These effects are in contrast with data suggesting that thiazide diuretics are more effective in reducing subsequent heart failure.[41] When the data regarding CCBs are evaluated in totality, those studies comparing CCBs with placebo found decreased risk of heart failure; this likely represents the effects of blood pressure control on subsequent heart failure (odds ratio [OR], 0.72; 95% CI, 0.59–0.87). In contrast, when compared with other active agents (most commonly diuretics or RAS inhibitors), CCBs were less effective in reducing the risk of heart failure (OR, 1.17; 95% CI, 1.11–1.24; $P = .0001$ for heterogeneity).[56] These findings do not suggest that CCBs increase the risk of heart failure but rather that thiazides and RAS inhibitors should be the preferred therapy in patients with diabetes and hypertension who are at risk for heart failure.[27]

Mineralocorticoid Receptor Antagonists

The mineralocorticoid receptor antagonists (MRAs) spironolactone and eplerenone have been shown to be effective in reduction of blood pressure in patients with hypertension. A meta-analysis of trials with spironolactone found an average reduction in systolic blood pressure of more than 20 mm Hg (95% CI, 16.58–23.06; $P<.00001$).[57] There is good evidence that MRAs can be used to supplement the inhibition of the RAAS by ACEIs and ARBs to further reduce proteinuria in patients with type 2 diabetes and chronic kidney disease.[58,59] Furthermore, they have an established role in the treatment of heart failure.[60] Given their tendency to cause hyperkalemia, they must be used with caution in patients with renal disease. In a retrospective analysis of patients hospitalized with heart failure and diabetes, use of MRAs at discharge was associated with an increased risk of readmission for acute renal failure and hyperkalemia.[61] However, their use did reduce the risk of long-term, all-cause readmissions. The Mineralocorticoid Receptor Antagonist Tolerability Study-Diabetic Nephropathy (ARTS-DN) randomized patients with diabetes and albuminuria, who were already receiving a RAAS blocking agent, to the novel selective nonsteroidal MRA, finerenone, or placebo.[62] Those receiving finerenone showed reduction in urine creatinine to albumin ratio and fewer than 2% required discontinuation because of hyperkalemia. There were no CV outcomes examined in this trial.

Meta-Analyses

Several recent meta-analyses have been undertaken to further clarify the varied data produced from these trials. In one meta-analysis published in 2015 that included 33 randomized trials, a 10 mm Hg reduction in blood pressure from baseline was associated with significantly lower risk of mortality and CV disease. There were no major differences in outcomes when comparing different therapeutic approaches with the exception of a reduction in heart failure among patients treated with chlorthalidone, an effect driven by the data from ALLHAT.[28] A meta-analysis published in 2017 identified 41 randomized control trials that evaluated blood pressure management in patients with diabetes. The target blood pressure of less than 140/90 was again noted to offer the greatest benefit for patients with diabetes. ACEI showed the greatest benefit in this group relative to other classes.[63]

GLUCOSE-LOWERING THERAPIES: NEW FRONTIER OF BLOOD PRESSURE CONTROL

Although diabetes is driven by different mechanisms with various underlying causes, all forms of the disease result in elevated serum glucose levels and long-term risk of ischemic and heart failure events. Although there is a clear association between chronic hyperglycemia (as measured by glycated hemoglobin A_{1c} [HbA_{1c}]) and ischemic events, the relationship is also seen with regards to heart failure but is not as strong.[64] No glucose-lowering agents have shown a relationship between degree of HbA_{1c} reduction and reduction in the incidence of heart failure.[65] Among patients with heart failure enrolled in the Candesartan in Heart failure: Assessment of Reduction in Mortality and Morbidity (CHARM) program, an increase in HbA_{1c} level of 1% was shown to confer a 25% increased risk of CV death, hospitalization for worsening heart failure, and all-cause death.[66] These findings differ slightly from a Veterans Affair registry study that examined data on more than 5000 outpatients with heart failure and diabetes, and found a U-shaped relationship between HbA_{1c} and mortality wherein patients who achieved moderate glucose control (HbA_{1c} >7.1% and <7.8%) had the lowest mortality.[67]

Ultimately, the relationship between glucose control and heart failure outcomes has led to efforts to reduce morbidity and mortality from heart failure through glucose-lowering therapies. Although intensive glucose control has been shown to reduce microvascular complications of diabetes,[68] until recently, aggressive glucose control had failed to show significant reduction in CV mortality among patients with diabetes.[69] Additionally, certain antihyperglycemia medications have been found to worsen outcomes among patients with diabetes and heart failure, and have therefore required caution when used in this population.

SGLT-2 INHIBITORS

More recent data have shown CV benefit of novel antihyperglycemics. One class, the SGLT-2 inhibitors, block the renal sodium glucose cotransporter-2, increasing urinary excretion of glucose, and resulting in subsequent osmotic diuresis. The multicenter Empagliflozin, Cardiovascular Outcomes, and Mortality in Type 2 Diabetes trial (EMPA-REG OUTCOME) was the first trial to show benefits of the SGLT-2 inhibitors in CV outcomes.[70] More than 7000 patients with established atherosclerosis were randomized to daily empagliflozin (10 or 25 mg) or placebo. Empagliflozin reduced the combined end point of CV mortality, nonfatal MI, or nonfatal stroke (10.5% vs 12.1%; $P = .04$; number needed to treat [NNT], 62), and a reduction in all-cause mortality (5.7% vs 8.3%; $P<.001$; NNT, 38) and CV mortality (3.7% vs 5.9%; $P<.001$; NNT, 45). In addition, there were significant reductions in heart failure.

In the CANagliflozin cardioVascular Assessment Study (CANVAS), 10,142 participants with type 2 diabetes and high CV risk (including those with and without established CV disease) were randomly assigned to receive canagliflozin or placebo and were followed for more than 3.5 years. Canagliflozin showed a reduction in the primary composite end point (death from CV causes, nonfatal MI, or nonfatal stroke; HR, 0.86; 95% CI, 0.75–0.97; $P<.001$ for noninferiority; $P = .02$ for superiority). This trial assessed hospitalization for heart failure as a secondary outcome and also found a reduction in this end point among patients treated with canagliflozin (HR, 0.67; 95% CI, 0.52–0.87). Similar data with regards to the effects on blood pressure and heart failure hospitalization have also been shown with dapagliflozin in a trial that predominantly included those patients without established CV disease and in observational studies.[71,72]

Although CV disease (and CV disease risk factors, such as diabetes and hypertension) disproportionally impact African-American patients, this population has been largely underrepresented in trials evaluating SGLT-2 inhibitors.[73] To date, only one randomized trial has been performed specifically in minority populations. In this trial, 150 African- Americans with diabetes and hypertension were randomized to empaglilozin or placebo. Empagliflozin led to reductions in blood pressure (−8.39 mm Hg; 95% CI, −13.74 to −3.04; $P = .0025$), body weight (−1.23 kg; 95% CI, −2.39 to −0.07; $P = .0382$), and HbA_{1c} (−0.78%; 95% CI, −1.18 to −0.38; $P = .0002$).[74] These data were subsequently extrapolated to a large real-world population of African-American patients with diabetes and hypertension from the Diabetes Collaborative Registry (an observational US registry of patients recruited from primary care, cardiology, and endocrinology practices). Among the 74,290 African-American patients with diabetes in this registry, 34.5% had a systolic blood pressure greater than or equal to 140 mm Hg. Of these, only 1.7% had been prescribed an SGLT-2 inhibitor. Assuming an 8 mm Hg reduction in blood pressure with the use of these medications, the mean estimated 5-year risk of CV death was estimated to be reduced from 7.7% to 6.2% if SGLT-2 inhibitors were used in this population.[75]

Review of the data on SGLT-2 inhibitors has shown that the reduction in CV events seen with these drugs is likely attributed to their effect on obesity and blood pressure rather than their impact on blood glucose levels.[73,74] The mechanism by which these drugs decrease blood pressure is not fully understood, but it is probably a multifactorial effect that includes diuresis (osmotic and natriuretic) and decrease in arterial stiffness and sympathetic tone.[75] The decongesting effect of these drugs suggests their impact on CV outcomes may reduce risk of heart failure more than that of atherothrombotic-related outcomes.[76] Several studies are currently underway to specifically assess the impact of SGLT-2 inhibitors on heart failure in patients including in patients without diabetes.[77]

CURRENT GUIDELINE RECOMMENDATIONS

Based on the large body of research evaluating blood pressure management in patients with diabetes, the ADA has released guidelines that advise a blood pressure target of 140/90 for patients with diabetes.[27] These guidelines recommend that the first line of blood pressure treatment include an ACEI or an ARB to reduce RAAS activation, particularly in patients with evidence of microalbuminuria. Following initiation of an ACEI or and ARB, CCBs or diuretics are recommended. Mineralocorticoids are recommended as additional therapy when these other classes fail to control blood pressure effectively. In patients with established heart failure, irrespective of whether they have reduced or preserved ejection fraction, current ACC/AHA guidelines recommend treating patients to a goal blood pressure of less than 130 mm Hg.[39] In the most recently published 2019 ACC/AHA Guidelines, patients with a 10-year ASCVD risk of 10% or greater, and those with diabetes and chronic kidney disease, are recommended to begin blood pressure–lowering medications to achieve a blood pressure target of less than 130/80 mm Hg.[78] The ADA guidelines are similar and support a blood pressure target of 130/80 mm Hg in patients at high risk of CV events, and a blood pressure target of 140/90 mm Hg for those at lower risk of CV events.[27]

SUMMARY

Reducing CV risk in patients with diabetes is of paramount importance given the association between diabetes and CV events, such as MI, stroke, and heart failure. Current guidelines, including those from CV and endocrine societies, are largely similar and support treating most patients to achieve blood pressure target of less than 130 mm Hg. Many patients need multidrug strategies to achieve these goals with thiazide diuretics and RAS inhibitors having the most evidence to support reduction in CV events. Novel medications, such as SGLT-2 inhibitors, have been shown to reduce CV events, such as heart failure, in patients with diabetes and are an attractive option for patients with diabetes.

REFERENCES

1. Guariguata L, Whiting DR, Hambleton I, et al. Global estimates of diabetes prevalence for 2013 and projections for 2035. Diabetes Res Clin Pract 2014; 103(2):137–49.
2. Beckman JA, Creager MA, Libby P. Diabetes and atherosclerosis epidemiology, pathophysiology, and management. J Am Med Assoc 2002;287(19): 2570–81.
3. Marwick TH. Diabetic heart disease. Postgrad Med J 2008;84(990):188–92.
4. Kannel WB, Hjortland M, Castelli WP. Role of diabetes in congestive heart failure: the Framingham study. Am J Cardiol 1974;34(1):29–34.
5. Ahmad FS, Ning H, Rich JD, et al. Hypertension, obesity, diabetes, and heart failure-free survival: the cardiovascular disease lifetime risk pooling project. JACC Heart Fail 2016;4(12):911–9.
6. Nieminen MS, Brutsaert D, Dickstein K, et al. Euro-Heart Failure Survey II (EHFS II): a survey on hospitalized acute heart failure patients: description of population. Eur Heart J 2006;27(22):2725–36.
7. Sarma S, Mentz RJ, Kwasny MJ, et al. Association between diabetes mellitus and post-discharge outcomes in patients hospitalized with heart failure: findings from the EVEREST trial. Eur J Heart Fail 2013;15(2):194–202.
8. Yusuf S, Ostergren JB, Gerstein HC, et al. Effects of candesartan on the development of a new diagnosis of diabetes mellitus in patients with heart failure. Circulation 2005;112(1):48–53.
9. Marwick TH, Ritchie R, Shaw JE, et al. Implications of underlying mechanisms for the recognition and management of diabetic cardiomyopathy. J Am Coll Cardiol 2018;71(3):339–51.
10. Dandamudi S, Slusser J, Mahoney DW, et al. The prevalence of diabetic cardiomyopathy: a population-based study in Olmsted County, Minnesota. J Card Fail 2014;20(5):304–9.
11. Ingelsson E, Ärnlöv J, Sundström J, et al. Novel metabolic risk factors for heart failure. J Am Coll Cardiol 2005;46(11):2054–60.

12. Lindman BR, Dávila-Román VG, Mann DL, et al. Cardiovascular phenotype in HFpEF patients with or without diabetes: a RELAX trial ancillary study. J Am Coll Cardiol 2014;64(6):541–9.

13. Aguilar D, Deswal A, Ramasubbu K, et al. Comparison of patients with heart failure and preserved left ventricular ejection fraction among those with versus without diabetes mellitus. Am J Cardiol 2010;105(3):373–7.

14. Gustafsson I, Brendorp B, Seibaek M, et al. Heart failure influence of diabetes and diabetes-gender interaction on the risk of death in patients hospitalized with congestive heart failure. J Am Coll Cardiol 2004;43:771–8.

15. Cavender MA, Steg PG, Smith SC, et al. Impact of diabetes mellitus on hospitalization for heart failure, cardiovascular events, and death. Circulation 2015;132(10):923–31.

16. Lewington S, Clarke R, Qizilbash N, et al, Prospective Studies Collaboration. Age-specific relevance of usual blood pressure to vascular mortality: a meta-analysis of individual data for one million adults in 61 prospective studies. Lancet 2002; 360(9349):1903–13.

17. Rapsomaniki E, Timmis A, George J, et al. Blood pressure and incidence of twelve cardiovascular diseases: lifetime risks, healthy life-years lost, and age-specific associations in 1·25 million people. Lancet 2014;383(9932):1899–911.

18. Mayet J, Hughes A. Cardiac and vascular pathophysiology in hypertension. Heart 2003;89(9):1104–9.

19. Messerli FH, Rimoldi SF, Bangalore S. The transition from hypertension to heart failure. JACC Heart Fail 2017;5(8):543–51.

20. Colosia AD, Palencia R, Khan S. Prevalence of hypertension and obesity in patients with type 2 diabetes mellitus in observational studies: a systematic literature review. Diabetes Metab Syndr Obes 2013;6:327–38.

21. Li X, Wang J, Shen X, et al. Higher blood pressure predicts diabetes and enhances long-term risk of CVD events in individuals with impaired glucose tolerance- 23-year follow-up of the Daqing Diabetes Prevention Study. J Diabetes 2019. https://doi.org/10.1111/1753-0407.12887.

22. Hypertension in Diabetes Study (HDS): I. Prevalence of hypertension in newly presenting type 2 diabetic patients and the association with risk factors for cardiovascular and diabetic complications. J Hypertens 1993;11(3):309–17. Available at: http://www.ncbi.nlm.nih.gov/pubmed/8387089. Accessed January 1, 2019.

23. Ali A, Taj A, Amin MJ, et al. Correlation between microalbuminuria and hypertension in type 2 diabetic patients. Pak J Med Sci 2014;30(3):511–4.

24. Jarrett RJ, Viberti GC, Argyropoulos A, et al. Microalbuminuria predicts mortality in noninsulin-dependent diabetes. Diabet Med 1984;1(1):17–9.

25. Gerstein HC, Mann JF, Yi Q, et al. Albuminuria and risk of cardiovascular events, death, and heart failure in diabetic and nondiabetic individuals. JAMA 2001; 286(4):421–6. Available at: http://www.ncbi.nlm.nih.gov/pubmed/11466120. Accessed December 2, 2018.

26. Wang B, Ni Y, Zhong J, et al. Effects of incretins on blood pressure: a promising therapy for type 2 diabetes mellitus with hypertension. J Diabetes 2012; 4(1):22–9.

27. de Boer IH, Bangalore S, Benetos A, et al. Diabetes and hypertension: a position statement by the American Diabetes Association. Diabetes Care 2017; 40(9):1273–84.

28. Emdin CA, Rahimi K, Neal B, et al. Blood pressure lowering in type 2 diabetes. JAMA 2015;313(6):603.

29. Turner R, Holman R, Stratton, et al. Tight blood pressure control and risk of macrovascular and microvascular complications in type 2 diabetes: UKPDS 38. UK Prospective Diabetes Study Group. BMJ 1998;317(7160):703–13. Available at: http://www.ncbi.nlm.nih.gov/pubmed/9732337. Accessed December 27, 2018.

30. Holman RR, Paul SK, Bethel MA, et al. Long-term follow-up after tight control of blood pressure in type 2 diabetes. N Engl J Med 2008;359(15):1565–76.

31. Hansson L, Zanchetti A, Carruthers SG, et al. Effects of intensive blood-pressure lowering and low-dose aspirin in patients with hypertension: principal results of the Hypertension Optimal Treatment (HOT) randomized trial. Lancet 1998;351(9118):1755–62.

32. Cushman WC, Evans GW, Byington RP, et al. Effects of intensive blood-pressure control in type 2 diabetes mellitus. N Engl J Med 2010;362(17):1575–85.

33. Margolis KL, O'Connor PJ, Morgan TM, et al. Outcomes of combined cardiovascular risk factor management strategies in type 2 diabetes: the ACCORD randomized trial. Diabetes Care 2014; 37(6):1721–8.

34. Patel A, ADVANCE Collaborative Group, MacMahon S, et al. Effects of a fixed combination of perindopril and indapamide on macrovascular and microvascular outcomes in patients with type 2 diabetes mellitus (the ADVANCE trial): a randomised controlled trial. Lancet 2007;370(9590):829–40.

35. Bangalore S, Kumar S, Lobach I, et al. Blood pressure targets in subjects with type 2 diabetes mellitus/impaired fasting glucose. Circulation 2011; 123(24):2799–810.

36. Whelton PK, Carey RM, Aronow WS, et al. 2017 ACC/AHA/AAPA/ABC/ACPM/AGS/APhA/ASH/ASPC/NMA/PCNA Guideline for the Prevention, Detection, Evaluation, and Management of High Blood Pressure in Adults: a report of the American College of Cardiology/American Heart Association task force on clinical practice guidelines. J Am Coll Cardiol 2018;71: e127–248.

37. Williams B, Mancia G, Spiering W, et al. 2018 ESC/ESH guidelines for the management of arterial hypertension. Eur Heart J 2018;39(33):3021–104.

38. Wright JT, Williamson JD, Whelton PK, et al. A randomized trial of intensive versus standard blood-pressure control. N Engl J Med 2015; 373(22):2103–16.

39. Yancy CW, Jessup M, Bozkurt B, et al. 2017 ACC/AHA/HFSA focused update of the 2013 ACCF/AHA guideline for the management of heart failure: a report of the American College of Cardiology/American Heart Association task force on clinical practice guidelines and the Heart Failure Society of America. Circulation 2017;136(6):e137–61.

40. ALLHAT Officers and Coordinators for the ALLHAT Collaborative Research Group. The Antihypertensive and Lipid-Lowering Treatment to Prevent Heart Attack Trial. Major outcomes in high-risk hypertensive patients randomized to angiotensin-converting enzyme inhibitor or calcium channel blocker vs diuretic: the antihypertensive and lipid-lowering treatment to prevent heart attack trial (ALLHAT). JAMA 2002;288(23):2981–97.

41. Davis BR, Piller LB, Cutler JA, et al. Role of diuretics in the prevention of heart failure. Circulation 2006; 113(18):2201–10.

42. Whelton PK, Barzilay J, Cushman WC, et al. Clinical outcomes in antihypertensive treatment of type 2 diabetes, impaired fasting glucose concentration, and normoglycemia. Arch Intern Med 2005; 165(12):1401.

43. Curb JD, Pressel SL, Cutler JA, et al. Effect of diuretic-based antihypertensive treatment on cardiovascular disease risk in older diabetic patients with isolated systolic hypertension. JAMA 1996; 276(23):1886.

44. Ninomiya T, Perkovic V, de Galan BE, et al. Albuminuria and kidney function independently predict cardiovascular and renal outcomes in diabetes. J Am Soc Nephrol 2009;20(8):1813–21.

45. de Zeeuw D, Remuzzi G, Parving H-H, et al. Albuminuria, a therapeutic target for cardiovascular protection in type 2 diabetic patients with nephropathy. Circulation 2004;110(8):921–7.

46. Estacio RO, Jeffers BW, Hiatt WR, et al. The effect of nisoldipine as compared with enalapril on cardiovascular outcomes in patients with non-insulin-dependent diabetes and hypertension. N Engl J Med 1998;338(10):645–52.

47. Niskanen L, Hedner T, Hansson L, et al. Reduced cardiovascular morbidity and mortality in hypertensive diabetic patients on first-line therapy with an ACE inhibitor compared with a diuretic/β-blocker–based treatment regimen. Diabetes Care 2001; 24(12):2091–6.

48. Lindholm LH, Ibsen H, Dahlöf B, et al. Cardiovascular morbidity and mortality in patients with diabetes in the losartan intervention for endpoint reduction in hypertension study (LIFE): a randomised trial against atenolol. Lancet 2002;359(9311):1004–10.

49. Zoungas S, Chalmers J, Neal B, et al. Follow-up of blood-pressure lowering and glucose control in type 2 diabetes. N Engl J Med 2014;371(15):1392–406.

50. Effects of ramipril on cardiovascular and microvascular outcomes in people with diabetes mellitus: results of the HOPE study and MICRO-HOPE substudy. Heart Outcomes Prevention Evaluation Study Investigators. Lancet 2000;355(9200):253–9.

51. Tillin T, Orchard T, Malm A, et al. The role of antihypertensive therapy in reducing vascular complications of type 2 diabetes. Findings from the Diabetic Retinopathy Candesartan Trials-protect 2 study. J Hypertens 2011;29(7):1457–62.

52. Berl T, Hunsicker LG, Lewis JB, et al. Cardiovascular outcomes in the irbesartan diabetic nephropathy trial of patients with type 2 diabetes and overt nephropathy. Ann Intern Med 2003;138(7):542.

53. Yusuf S, Teo KK, Pogue J, et al. Telmisartan, ramipril, or both in patients at high risk for vascular events. N Engl J Med 2008;358(15):1547–59.

54. Ostergren J, Poulter NR, Sever PS, et al. The Anglo-Scandinavian cardiac outcomes trial: blood pressure-lowering limb: effects in patients with type Ii diabetes. J Hypertens 2008;26(11):2103–11.

55. Weber MA, Bakris GL, Jamerson K, et al. Cardiovascular events during differing hypertension therapies in patients with diabetes. J Am Coll Cardiol 2010; 56(1):77–85.

56. Costanzo P, Perrone-Filardi P, Petretta M, et al. Calcium channel blockers and cardiovascular outcomes: a meta-analysis of 175 634 patients. J Hypertens 2009;27(6):1136–51.

57. Batterink J, Stabler SN, Tejani AM, et al. Spironolactone for hypertension. Cochrane Database Syst Rev 2010;(8):CD008169.

58. Epstein M, Williams GH, Weinberger M, et al. Selective aldosterone blockade with eplerenone reduces albuminuria in patients with type 2 diabetes. Clin J Am Soc Nephrol 2006;1(5):940–51.

59. Bomback AS, Kshirsagar AV, Amamoo MA, et al. Change in proteinuria after adding aldosterone blockers to ACE inhibitors or angiotensin receptor blockers in CKD: a systematic review. Am J Kidney Dis 2008;51(2):199–211.

60. Yancy CW, Jessup M, Bozkurt B, et al. 2016 ACC/AHA/HFSA focused update on new pharmacological therapy for heart failure: an update of the 2013 ACCF/AHA guideline for the management of heart failure. J Am Coll Cardiol 2016;68(13):1476–88.

61. Cooper LB, Lippmann SJ, Greiner MA, et al. Use of mineralocorticoid receptor antagonists in patients with heart failure and comorbid diabetes mellitus or chronic kidney disease. J Am Heart Assoc 2017; 6(12). https://doi.org/10.1161/JAHA.117.006540.

62. Bakris GL, Agarwal R, Chan JC, et al. Effect of finerenone on albuminuria in patients with diabetic nephropathy. JAMA 2015;314(9):884.

63. Thomopoulos C, Parati G, Zanchetti A. Effects of blood-pressure-lowering treatment on outcome incidence in hypertension. J Hypertens 2017;35(5):922–44.

64. Iribarren C, Karter AJ, Go AS, et al. Glycemic control and heart failure among adult patients with diabetes. Circulation 2001;103(22):2668–73. Available at: http://www.ncbi.nlm.nih.gov/pubmed/11390335. Accessed March 11, 2019.

65. Kramer CK, Ye C, Campbell S, et al. Comparison of new glucose-lowering drugs on risk of heart failure in type 2 diabetes. JACC Heart Fail 2018;6(10):823–30.

66. Gerstein HC, Swedberg K, Carlsson J, et al. The hemoglobin A1c level as a progressive risk factor for cardiovascular death, hospitalization for heart failure, or death in patients with chronic heart failure. Arch Intern Med 2008;168(15):1699.

67. Aguilar D, Bozkurt B, Ramasubbu K, et al. Relationship of hemoglobin A1C and mortality in heart failure patients with diabetes. J Am Coll Cardiol 2009;54(5):422–8.

68. Intensive blood-glucose control with sulphonylureas or insulin compared with conventional treatment and risk of complications in patients with type 2 diabetes (UKPDS 33). UK Prospective Diabetes Study (UKPDS) Group. Lancet 1998;352(9131):837–53. Available at: http://www.ncbi.nlm.nih.gov/pubmed/9742976. Accessed January 6, 2019.

69. Boussageon R, Bejan-Angoulvant T, Saadatian-Elahi M, et al. Effect of intensive glucose lowering treatment on all cause mortality, cardiovascular death, and microvascular events in type 2 diabetes: meta-analysis of randomised controlled trials. BMJ 2011;343:d4169.

70. Zinman B, Wanner C, Lachin JM, et al. Empagliflozin, cardiovascular outcomes, and mortality in type 2 diabetes. N Engl J Med 2015;373(22):2117–28.

71. Wiviott SD, Raz I, Bonaca MP, et al. Dapagliflozin and cardiovascular outcomes in type 2 diabetes. N Engl J Med 2019;380(4):347–57.

72. Cavender MA, Norhammar A, Birkeland KI, et al. SGLT-2 inhibitors and cardiovascular risk. J Am Coll Cardiol 2018;71(22):2497–506.

73. Toyama T, Neuen BL, Jun M, et al. Effect of SGLT2 inhibitors on cardiovascular, renal and safety outcomes in patients with type 2 diabetes mellitus and chronic kidney disease: a systematic review and meta-analysis. Diabetes Obes Metab 2019.

74. Majewski C, Bakris GL. Blood pressure reduction: an added benefit of sodium-glucose cotransporter 2 inhibitors in patients with type 2 diabetes. Diabetes Care 2015;38(3):429–30.

75. Cherney DZ, Perkins BA, Soleymanlou N, et al. The effect of empagliflozin on arterial stiffness and heart rate variability in subjects with uncomplicated type 1 diabetes mellitus. Cardiovasc Diabetol 2014;13(1):28.

76. Fitchett D, Zinman B, Wanner C, et al. Heart failure outcomes with empagliflozin in patients with type 2 diabetes at high cardiovascular risk: results of the EMPA-REG OUTCOME trial. Eur Heart J 2016;37(19):1526–34.

77. Verma S, McMurray JJV. SGLT2 inhibitors and mechanisms of cardiovascular benefit: a state-of-the-art review. Diabetologia 2018;61(10):2108–17.

78. Arnett DK, Blumenthal RS, Albert MA, et al. 2019 ACC/AHA guideline on the primary prevention of cardiovascular disease. J Am Coll Cardiol 2019;26029. https://doi.org/10.1016/j.jacc.2019.03.010.

Management of Acute Hypertensive Heart Failure

Jim X. Liu, MD, Saurav Uppal, MD, Viren Patel, MD*

KEYWORDS

- Acute hypertensive heart failure • Acute heart failure • Hypertension • Ventricular-vascular coupling

KEY POINTS

- Heart failure presents a particularly difficult public health challenge.
- Of the heart failure presentations, acute hypertensive heart failure represents a distinct clinical phenotype and is characterized by sudden-onset systemic hypertension and pulmonary edema.
- The pathophysiology of acute hypertensive heart failure is primarily driven by an abnormal ventricular-vascular relationship, and the medical management is aimed at improving this relationship.

INTRODUCTION

Heart failure presents a difficult and substantial public health challenge resulting in more than 1 million hospitalizations annually with a 1-month readmission rate of 25%.[1] The total cost of heart failure treatment in the United States exceeds $30 billion annually,[1] and 80% of emergency room visits for heart failure result in hospital admission.[2] Patients with heart failure have a particularly poor prognosis as demonstrated by in-hospital mortalities, which range from 2% to 20%.[2] In addition, after hospitalization, 30-day, 1-year, and 5-year mortality was 10.4%, 22%, and 42.3%, respectively.[1]

Fifty-three percent to 73% of all patients presenting to the emergency room with heart failure have a history of hypertension. Hypertension is more common in those with heart failure with preserved ejection fraction (76%) compared with those with heart failure with reduced ejection fraction (66%).[3] A study using observational and retrospective data from the STAT registry (Studying the Treatment of Acute hypertensive) on patients receiving intravenous therapy for severe hypertension (blood pressure >180/110 mm Hg) showed that 25.2% of patients in this registry had acute heart failure.[4] In this study, heart failure patients were more likely to be African American and more likely to have comorbidities, such as diabetes, chronic obstructive pulmonary disease, prior history of admissions for hypertension, and history of heart failure. Heart failure patients were more likely to be admitted to the intensive care unit and require positive pressure ventilation. Patients with acute heart failure resulting from hypertensive emergency required more clinical resources than patients with severe hypertension without associated heart failure.[4]

PATHOPHYSIOLOGY OF ACUTE HYPERTENSIVE HEART FAILURE

Acute hypertensive heart failure is a rapidly progressive disorder characterized by hypertension and dyspnea. It is more common in older patients, patients with a history of hypertension, and those with a preserved ejection fraction.[5] The physiologic mechanisms behind acute hypertensive heart failure include an increase in afterload and a decrease in venous capacitance. Acute hypertensive heart failure results in pulmonary edema owing to redistribution of fluid from peripheral vasculature to pulmonary circulation.[6] ADHERE registry data demonstrate that those admitted for heart failure are more often significantly hypertensive and have preserved systolic function.[7] Chronic poorly

Disclosure Statement: Nothing to disclose.
Division of Cardiovascular Medicine, Department of Internal Medicine, The Ohio State University Wexner Medical Center, 473 West 12th Avenue, Suite 200, Columbus, OH 43210, USA
* Corresponding author.
E-mail address: Virenkumar.Patel@osumc.edu

heartfailure.theclinics.com

controlled hypertension can lead to cardiac remodeling with left ventricular (LV) hypertrophy, LV stiffness, and diastolic dysfunction, which are important factors in precipitation of acute hypertensive heart failure.[6]

The primary driving pathophysiological abnormality in acute hypertensive heart failure is an abnormal ventricular-vascular relationship. The ventricular and arterial systems can be thought of as elastic chambers where ventricular and arterial elastance work opposite each other to affect and respond to changes in volume. Dysfunction in ventricular-vascular coupling occurs when there is an imbalance in the system and is often attributed to vascular stiffening.[6] Arterial stiffness increases with age, hypertension, atherosclerosis, diabetes, renal failure, obesity, and heart failure.[8] Of these conditions, chronic hypertension is the most closely associated with increased arterial stiffness.[6] Chronic hypertension leads to decreased vascular compliance because of wall stress and smooth muscle hypertrophy. A decrease in vascular compliance leads to increased resistance to LV forward flow. To maintain the coupling relationship and to disperse transmural stress, the LV hypertrophies, which lead to changes in LV relaxation.[6] These changes in concert with molecular changes in collagen cross-linking and protein expression result in decreased compliance in the ventricle. Vascular elastance and LV elastance are closely coupled to optimize mechanical efficiency and maintain a normal ejection fraction.[9] Maintenance of low ventricular and arterial elastance permits a dynamic range of volume transfer during ejection with minimal change in pressure.[9] A system with elevations in arterial elastance and LV end systolic elastance has decreased cardiac reserve.[6] In noncompliant states, small increases in preload and afterload change arterial elastance, resulting in exaggerated changes to systolic blood pressure. In a stiff LV, cardiac reserve and ability to compensate for increases in arterial elastance are blunted.[6] Increased LV stiffness makes the system particularly sensitive to loading conditions with an exaggerated pressure response to small increases in preload and inability to adapt normal volume with an increase in afterload. The increase in left ventricular end diastolic pressure (LVEDP) and increase in afterload cause changes in the pressure-volume relationship and factors in the development of acute hypertensive heart failure. The inability to augment LV pressure to match vascular resistance leads to a decrease in stroke volume and precipitation of heart failure.[6]

The arterial circulation serves to transport blood and to buffer pulsatile systolic flow while maintaining nonpulsatile diastolic flow.[6] As the arterial system ages and is subject to insult, there is loss of vascular elasticity.[10] Elasticity is lost from both the aorta and the peripheral circulation. As the aorta loses elastance, it loses the ability to dampen systolic ventricular load, redistributing it during diastole. The decreased elastance results in more rapid and forceful pulsatile load to the peripheral vessels.[6] The peripheral arterials, which account for most of the resistance to blood flow, absorb and recoil with the pulsatile flow during systole. As the arterioles recoil, a pulsatile wave is reflected back toward central circulation. Normally this pulsatile flow backwards reaches the ventricle during early diastole immediately after aortic valve closure. Increased vascular stiffness causes this reflected wave to reach the ventricle during late systole, resulting in impedance to outflow and shortened LV ejection time.[6] In a noncompliant ventricle, this increased force results in increased central aortic pressure, which leads to a rapid increase and LVEDP and backward flow into pulmonary circulation. Increased afterload in the setting of impaired ventricular compliance hinders contractile function and leads to an imbalance and ventricular-vascular coupling.[6]

CLINICAL CHARACTERISTICS

Acute heart failure is defined as rapid or gradual changes in signs and symptoms of heart failure that may necessitate hospitalization and change of existing therapy.[11] Patients with acute hypertensive heart failure usually develop sudden onset of symptoms. Symptoms of dyspnea can often be severe, and patients can be tachypneic and tachycardic. In addition, rales are common on auscultation of the lungs. The systolic blood pressure is usually significantly elevated (>180/100). Chest radiograph will be consistent with pulmonary edema, and patients are commonly hypoxemic.[12] Precipitating causes leading to vasoconstriction can be the result of exertion, arterial baroreceptor insensitivity, sympathomimetic substance abuse, medication noncompliance, activation of the renin-angiotensin-aldosterone system, endothelial dysfunction, and stress or anxiety.[6]

MANAGEMENT PRINCIPLES

In general, the treatment of acute heart failure is aimed at improving hemodynamics and relieving congestion regardless of the precipitating cause. Traditionally, this is achieved using various combinations of afterload reduction, diuresis, and inotropic support (Fig. 1). Different phenotypes and patient profiles based on an assessment of perfusion and volume status have been used to

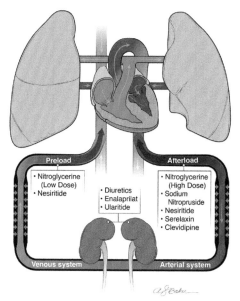

Fig. 1. Depiction of the circulatory circuit and location of action of therapeutic agents used and studied in the management of acute hypertensive heart failure. (Reproduced with the permission of The Ohio State University.)

describe patients presenting with acute heart failure, and therapy is tailored accordingly for each profile.[13] Acute hypertensive heart failure has emerged as a unique phenotype in which the hallmark characteristic is a rapid increase in systemic afterload and preload that lead to pulmonary edema. Because peripheral vasoconstriction is the primary contributing mechanism, interventions targeting this syndrome focus on reducing afterload and preload with vasodilators, whereas diuretics may be used for hypervolemia (**Table 1**).

DIURETICS

Diuretics remain one of the mainstays in the treatment of acute decompensated heart failure. The American College of Cardiology/American Heart Association (ACC/AHA) guidelines for the management of heart failure recommend (class I) that all heart failure patients hospitalized with fluid overload should be treated with intravenous diuretics.[14] Intravenous loop diuretics should be given early because early administration has been associated with better outcomes.[15] For most patients with acute heart failure, initial treatment with intravenous diuretics would be appropriate to reduce congestion. An estimated 90% of all acute heart failure patients fit the "warm and wet" profile, and in this phenotype, the predominant mechanism of decompensation is congestion owing to fluid retention and increased total body volume caused by a

variety of precipitants.[13] Decompensation usually occurs more gradually over days or weeks.

In contrast, patients with acute hypertensive heart failure represent a specific phenotype in which decompensation occurs abruptly and is the result of an acute increase in afterload from severe systemic hypertension. The acute pulmonary edema that occurs is due to vascular volume redistribution from the splanchnic veins to the pulmonary circulation rather than from a strict increase in total body volume.[16,17] Treatment, therefore, relies more on afterload reduction with vasodilators instead of diuresis. Respiratory improvement has been shown to be more associated with the extent of blood pressure reduction rather than the amount of diuresis.[18] Certainly, concomitant volume overload may exist because most patients with acute hypertensive heart failure have underlying chronic hypertension with an activated renin-angiotensin-aldosterone system that predisposes them to fluid retention. As a result, diuretics can be used as needed for volume control, and this decision should be dictated by a careful clinical assessment of the patient's volume status.

Intravenous loop diuretics are typically the drug of choice if diuresis is needed. Furosemide inhibits sodium reabsorption in the ascending limb of the loop of Henle to augment natriuresis and thereby achieve diuresis. The onset of action is usually rapid, and its half-life is relatively short. In addition to diuresis, furosemide also has early venodilatory properties that are independent from its diuretic properties.[19] Studies have demonstrated that intravenous furosemide can increase venous capacitance and decrease preload and pulmonary capillary wedge pressures even before significant diuresis is achieved.[20,21] This venodilation is the result of both direct and indirect effects of furosemide on the peripheral vasculature.[22] This added benefit of furosemide may be considered useful in settings where increased preload is particularly prominent, such as acute hypertensive heart failure. However, as demonstrated in a randomized placebo controlled trial evaluating furosemide in patients presenting with pulmonary edema and severe hypertension, there was no significant difference in reported dyspnea or adverse outcomes when furosemide was added compared with placebo.[23] Even in the general acute heart failure population, the role of diuretics in improving mortality has never been well established, and on the contrary, high doses of diuretics have been associated with worse clinical outcomes.[24] Clinical outcomes may be partly due to the potential harmful effects of diuretics, which include stimulation of the renin-angiotensin system, worsening of glomerular

Table 1
Typical dosing, pharmacokinetics, and limitations of pharmacologic therapy available for the management of acute hypertensive heart failure

Class (Mechanism)	Medication	Usual Dose	Onset of Action	Peak Effect	Duration	Limitations
Diuretics (inhibition of sodium reabsorption)	Furosemide (IV)	20–600 mg/d	5 min	30 min	2 h	• Nephrotoxicity • Ototoxicity • Electrolyte derangements • Sulfa allergy
	Torsemide (IV)	10–200 mg/d	10 min	Within 60 min	6–8 h	
	Bumetanide (IV)	0.5–10 mg/d	2–3 min	15–30 min	2–3 h	
Nitrovasodilators (nitric oxide upregulation and smooth muscle relaxation)	Nitroglycerine (IV)	5–400 μm/min	Immediate	Immediate	3–5 min	• Headache • Increased intracranial pressure • Tachyphylaxis
	Sodium nitroprusside (IV)	5–400 μg/min	<2 min	Immediate	1–10 min	• Cyanide toxicity • Increased intracranial pressure • Invasive hemodynamic monitoring
	Isosorbide mononitrate (PO)	30–120 mg/d	30–45 min	30–60 min	12–24 h	• CNS depression • Increased intracranial pressure • Avoidance in patients with PDE-5 inhibitors
	Isosorbide dinitrate (PO)	20–120 mg/d	1 h	Unknown	Up to 8 h	• Frequent dosing • Increased intracranial pressure • Avoidance in patients with PDE-5 inhibitors
Natriuretic peptides (upregulation of cyclic GMP)	Nesiritide (IV)	0.01–0.03 μm/kg/min	15 min	1 h	>60 min	• Hypersensitivity reaction • May be associated with Azotemia
ACEi (block synthesis of angiotensin II)	Enalaprilat (IV)	0.625–20 mg/d	<15 min	1–4 h	6 h	• Use with caution in renal dysfunction • Angioedema • Cough
Calcium channel blocker (inhibition of L-type calcium channels)	Clevidipine (IV)	1–21 mg/h	2–4 min	30 min	5–15 min	• Hypertriglyceridemia • Pancreatitis

Abbreviations: ACEi, angiotensin-converting enzyme inhibitors; IV, intravenous; PDE-5, phosphodiesterase-5; PO, orally.

filtration rates, and electrolyte disturbances.[25] Therefore, diuretics should be used with caution in acute hypertensive heart failure and are most appropriate for patients with true volume overload.

NITROVASODILATORS

Nitrovasodilators are commonly used in acute heart failure. Up to 51% of patients admitted with acute heart failure receive some form of nitrates.[26] This group of medications, which includes nitroglycerin, sodium nitroprusside, isosorbide mononitrate, and isosorbide dinitrate, acts by providing nitric oxide to activate the guanylate cyclase and cyclic GMP cascade and ultimately results in smooth muscle relaxation and vasodilatation. Because of their effectiveness in reducing afterload and preload, nitrates are considered first-line agents to be used in acute hypertensive heart failure where afterload and preload reduction are the cornerstones of treatment.[27]

Nitroglycerin has become the vasodilator of choice in patients with pulmonary congestion and acute hypertensive heart failure.[28] It is an inexpensive agent with multiple routes of administration, including intravenous, sublingual, and oral spray. Intravenous nitroglycerin is typically the more commonly used route given the ease in titrating dosages, although oral forms may be given in the prehospital setting in patients with acute respiratory distress. The initial intravenous dose is usually 5 μg/min and can be increased up to 400 μg/min as needed.[29] The onset of action is within seconds, and the duration of action is 3 to 5 minutes. At low doses, nitroglycerin primarily causes venous dilatation, but at higher doses greater than 150 to 250 μg/min, both arteriolar and venous dilatation are achieved, including epicardial coronary artery dilatation. Ultimately, the net effect of these hemodynamic changes is a decrease in LV wall tension and filling pressures, an increase in subendocardial blood flow, and a decrease in myocardial oxygen consumption.[30] The value of nitroglycerin, however, may be limited by nitrate tolerance in patients with heart failure and by tachyphylaxis, which can occur within 24 hours of use.[31,32] Furthermore, nitroglycerin may cause headaches, which may make its use less desirable in patients who already have headaches from severe hypertension.

Similar to nitroglycerin, sodium nitroprusside is an intravenous nitrate that rapidly provides vasodilatation. It is generally considered a more potent vasodilator than nitroglycerin because of its ability to cause balanced venous and arterial dilatation as well as dilatation of the pulmonary vasculature.[33]

For these reasons, it is an effective therapy in settings of severe hypertension. With a rapid onset of action of less than 30 seconds and half-life of approximately 2 minutes, sodium nitroprusside allows for rapid vasodilatation and ease in weaning.[34] The typical starting dose is 0.15 μg/kg/min and can be uptitrated to achieve adequate lowering of systolic blood pressure. Because of its potent vasoactive properties, patients receiving sodium nitroprusside generally require invasive blood pressure monitoring in an intensive care setting. Pulmonary artery catheters are also often used for additional close hemodynamic monitoring. Despite its potency, the occurrence of hypotension is uncommon and usually resolves rapidly. Unfortunately, the major limitation in its use is the potential development of cyanide toxicity. Thiocyanate is a toxic metabolite of sodium nitroprusside, and if levels of thiocyanate accumulate, symptoms of toxicity may occur, including altered mental status, nausea, abdominal discomfort, dysphoria, and even death.[35] Factors that increase the risk for cyanide toxicity include underlying renal or hepatic insufficiency, prolonged use of more than 48 hours, and doses higher than 2 μg/kg/min. Therefore, the use of sodium nitroprusside is typically limited to no more than 48 hours. When prolonged infusions are required, cyanide levels may be monitored. If cyanide toxicity is suspected, the infusion should be discontinued or reduced, and sodium thiosulfate may be given.

Despite the hemodynamic benefits provided by nitrates, data and clinical trials evaluating their use and outcomes in acute heart failure are limited. Several studies have evaluated outcomes of nitrates in patients presenting with acute hypertensive heart failure and pulmonary edema, but few have been randomized controlled trials. An extensive Cochrane Review of studies comparing nitrates with alternative agents in acute heart failure revealed no difference in symptom relief or other outcomes, including rates of mechanical ventilation, myocardial infarction, and changes in pulmonary capillary wedge pressure (PCWP).[36] Of the studies reviewed, only 4 were randomized controlled trials, and 2 of the 4 included only acute heart failure patients after myocardial infarction. The other 2 randomized controlled trials failed to show any significant benefit favoring nitroglycerin in terms of symptoms or outcomes.[37,38] One criticism of these 2 trials, however, has been that the doses of nitroglycerin used were much lower than what is typically used in clinical practice, with a median dose of 13 μg/min in 1 trial and a range of 2.5 to 10 μg/min in the other.[28] Studies using higher doses of nitrates have shown more supportive evidence with regards to improvement in symptoms and short-term outcomes. One nonrandomized open-label trial of 29 patients with severe hypertension and heart failure demonstrated that high-dose nitroglycerin was associated with less frequent endotracheal intubation, noninvasive positive airway ventilation, and intensive care admission.[39] Furthermore, a retrospective study showed that early administration of high-dose intravenous nitroglycerin in intermittent boluses was associated with fewer intensive care admissions and shorter hospital stay as compared with continuous nitroglycerin infusion,[40] and a separate randomized trial showed similar results when comparing high-dose isosorbide dinitrate with lower doses.[41] Overall, although nitrates have not been shown to improve long-term outcomes, current limited existing evidence does suggest that they are safe to administer and can offer short-term symptom relief. Current ACC/AHA guidelines provide a weaker (class IIb) recommendation regarding intravenous nitroglycerin and nitroprusside, stating that they may be considered for dyspnea relief in patients with acutely decompensated heart failure.[14]

NATRIURETIC PEPTIDES

Natriuretic peptides are a group of hormones that include atrial natriuretic peptide (ANP), b-type natriuretic peptide (BNP), and urodilatin. ANP and BNP are produced in the atria and ventricles, respectively, and are secreted in response to elevated filling pressures and wall stress. When bound to the A-type natriuretic peptide receptor, ANP and BNP will activate cyclic GMP, like nitrates, and cause downstream effects of vasodilatation and natriuresis.

Nesiritide was the first recombinant form of BNP to be approved for treatment of acute heart failure. Originally approved by the Food and Drug Administration in 2001, nesiritide is identical to endogenous BNP and produces balanced arterial and venous vasodilatation to reduce filling pressures and improve dyspnea.[42] It is administered intravenously as a continuous infusion with typical starting dose of 0.01 μg/kg/min. The therapeutic dose range is narrow (0.01–0.03 μg/kg/min), and unlike nitroglycerin or nitroprusside, frequent dose titrations are not necessary. Although it does lead to natriuresis, the actual diuretic effect of nesiritide is only modest, and its purpose is not to enhance or replace diuretics. Hypotension can occur with prolonged use, particularly in those who are already volume deplete.[37] Therefore, its use is best reserved for patients with congestion and volume overload, which may limit its value in acute hypertensive heart failure, where hypervolemia may not always be present.

Similar to nitrates, evidence in support of nesiritide has been limited. Most data regarding nesiritide in acute heart failure have stemmed from 2 large randomized trials. VMAC was the first randomized trial and compared nesiritide to both nitroglycerin and placebo in patients with acute heart failure.[37] Nesiritide was found to improve dyspnea compared with placebo, but no difference compared with nitroglycerin, at 3 hours after initiation. At 24 hours after initiation, nesiritide lowered PCWP more than nitroglycerin, but there was no difference in dyspnea relief. The ASCEND-HF study was a randomized trial of 7141 patients with acute heart failure comparing nesiritide with placebo.[43] Although there was a modest improvement in self-reported dyspnea with nesiritide, this improvement was not statistically significant. There was also no difference in the primary endpoints of 30-day mortality and rehospitalization. Furthermore, nesiritide was associated with a higher rate of hypotension. Thus, despite its favorable hemodynamic effects and potential to improve subjective dyspnea, the lack of data supporting nesiritide, along with its high costs, limits its usefulness. In current guidelines, nesiritide falls under the same category as nitroglycerin and nitroprusside and receives a class IIB recommendation to be used for dyspnea relief in acute heart failure.[14]

ANGIOTENSIN-CONVERTING ENZYME INHIBITORS

Angiotensin-converting enzyme (ACE) inhibitors are well-proven medications in the management of chronic hypertension and chronic systolic heart failure, but there has also been an interest in their use for acute hypertensive heart failure. As a class, ACE inhibitors decrease arterial resistance and increase venous capacitance by blocking the synthesis of angiotensin II. This inhibition of the renin-angiotensin system makes ACE inhibitors a logical treatment choice for acute hypertensive heart failure with pulmonary edema, which is generally characterized by high renin levels. Enalaprilat is an ACE inhibitor available in intravenous form and can be given with initial recommended doses of 0.625 mg to 1.25 mg administered over 5 minutes. Blood pressure lowering is typically achieved in 15 to 30 minutes, and repeat doses can be given after 1 hour if needed for a maximum daily dose of 20 mg.[44] Caution must be used when given to patients on chronic diuretics or with renal impairment, because enalaprilat is excreted renally and may cause significant hypotension in patients who are already volume deplete.

The safety and efficacy of enalaprilat used for acute hypertensive heart failure have been demonstrated in a few studies. In a retrospective study evaluating its use in acute hypertensive heart failure in the emergency department, intravenous enalaprilat bolus was administered to 103 patients with mean systolic blood pressure of 195 mm Hg.[45] Systolic blood pressure decreased by 30 mm Hg at 3 hours after receiving enalaprilat. Only 2 patients developed hypotension, and there was no significant change in renal function at 72 hours. As a result the authors to conclude that enalaprilat can safely and effectively reduce systemic blood pressure in acute hypertensive heart failure. Enalaprilat was compared with placebo in a randomized controlled trial in patients with acute cardiogenic pulmonary edema.[46] In this study, there was a significant reduction in PCWP seen in patients receiving a single dose of enalaprilat compared with placebo. Although studies suggest that enalaprilat can safely reduce afterload and preload, evidence regarding clinical and long-term outcomes is lacking.

NOVEL THERAPIES

Ularitide is a synthetic version of urodilatin, an endogenous natriuretic peptide produced in the kidneys. Urodilatin is secreted in response to increased pressure and, like ANP and BNP, binds to natriuretic peptide receptor A to cause vasodilatation and natriuresis. In contrast to ANP and BNP, urodilatin is more resistant to enzymatic degradation and is able to exert its effects more in the distal renal collecting ducts.[27,47] Phase 1 and 2 clinical trials have demonstrated the ability of ularitide to reduce PCWP, reduce systemic vascular resistance, and improve dyspnea without worsening renal function.[48–50] A phase 3 randomized placebo-controlled trial of 2157 patients found that a 48-hour infusion of ularitide provided a greater reduction in systolic blood pressure and in BNP levels.[51] However, there was no difference in the primary outcome of death from cardiovascular causes at 15 months. In addition, hypotension occurred more frequently in patients receiving ularitide.

Serelaxin is recombinant human relaxin-2, which is a vasoactive peptide normally secreted by the placenta to regulate the hemodynamic changes of pregnancy. Relaxin-2 increases the production of nitric oxide and reduces vasoconstriction caused by endothelin-1.[52,53] These effects lead to increased arterial compliance, cardiac output, and renal blood flow.[54] Phase 2

and early phase 3 trials have suggested improvement in dyspnea and clinical outcomes in acute heart failure patients receiving serelaxin.[55,56] In RELAX-AHF, an international double-blind, placebo-controlled trial, 1161 patients with acute heart failure were randomized to 48-hour infusions of serelaxin or placebo. The serelaxin treatment arm was found to have a significant improvement in dyspnea, and there were fewer cardiovascular deaths at 180 days, although this was not a primary endpoint.[56] However, the most recent phase 3 RELAX-AHF2 trial, a larger trial with 180-day cardiovascular mortality as the primary endpoint, showed no difference in mortality between serelaxin and placebo.[57]

Clevidipine is a late-generation, short-acting dihydropyridine calcium channel blocker that is currently approved for the acute management of severe hypertension. Although other dihydropyridine calcium channel blockers, such as intravenous nicardipine, have been effective in treating hypertensive crises, they have generally been avoided in acute heart failure because of their potential negative inotropic effects and stimulation of the renin-angiotensin system.[58,59] Compared with other dihydropyridine calcium channel blockers, clevidipine holds the unique properties of having a rapid onset of action with short duration, being more arterial selective, and having no negative effects on cardiac function.[27,60] These properties have made clevidipine an attractive therapeutic target for acute hypertensive heart failure. In a subset analysis of patients with severe hypertension treated with clevidipine, nearly all patients who were also in acute heart failure had a successful decrease in systolic blood pressure to the intended target range, and there were no adverse events found, suggesting that clevidipine is both safe and efficacious in reducing blood pressure in acute heart failure.[61] A subsequent phase 3 randomized open-label trial studied clevidipine versus standard of care in patients with acute heart failure presenting to the emergency department with dyspnea and systolic blood pressure ≥ 160 mm Hg.[62] The clevidipine-treated group had more success in achieving target blood pressure and at faster rates. Clevidipine also improved dyspnea more than standard of care, but there were no differences in adverse events or 30-day mortality.

The soluble guanylate cyclase signaling pathway represents another potential therapeutic target for vasodilators. When activated by nitric oxide, soluble guanylate cyclase leads to an increase in cyclic GMP. Cinaciguat is an agent that activates soluble guanylate cyclase independent of nitric oxide. Consequently, cinaciguat can produce vasodilatation even in patients who have developed tolerance to nitrates.[63] Although early cinaciguat studies showed promising hemodynamic benefits with PCWP reduction, there were clinically significant episodes of hypotension.[64,65] Subsequent randomized placebo-controlled trials were either terminated prematurely because of hypotension or not completed because of recruitment difficulties.[66] There have been no additional acute heart failure studies involving cinaciguat, but another soluble guanylate cylase modulator, vericiguat, has shown early favorable results in chronic heart failure.[67]

SUMMARY

Acute hypertensive heart failure represents a distinct clinical phenotype in the heart failure spectrum and is characterized by sudden-onset systemic hypertension and pulmonary edema. Increased afterload is the predominant pathophysiologic mechanism. Consequently, vasodilators are the treatment of choice, with diuretics used adjunctively for hypervolemia. Nitrovasodilators and nesiritide are commonly used, and although they can effectively improve hemodynamics and symptoms, each agent has its own limitations. Furthermore, evidence supporting their benefit for long-term outcomes is lacking, which has led to weak recommendations for their use in acute heart failure from current major society guidelines. Newer vasodilators using novel mechanisms are being investigated.

REFERENCES

1. Yancy CW, Jessup M, Bozkurt B, et al. 2013 ACCF/AHA guideline for the management of heart failure: a report of the American College of Cardiology Foundation/American Heart Association Task Force on Practice Guidelines. J Am Coll Cardiol 2013; 62(16):e147–239.
2. Peacock WF, Cannon CM, Singer AJ, et al. Considerations for initial therapy in the treatment of acute heart failure. Crit Care 2015;19:399.
3. Fonarow GC, Stough WG, Abraham WT, et al. Characteristics, treatments, and outcomes of patients with preserved systolic function hospitalized for heart failure: a report from the OPTIMIZE-HF Registry. J Am Coll Cardiol 2007;50(8):768–77.
4. Peacock F, Amin A, Granger CB, et al. Hypertensive heart failure: patient characteristics, treatment, and outcomes. Am J Emerg Med 2011;29(8): 855–62.
5. Cotter G, Metra M, Milo-Cotter O, et al. Fluid overload in acute heart failure–re-distribution and other mechanisms beyond fluid accumulation. Eur J Heart Fail 2008;10(2):165–9.
6. Viau DM, Sala-Mercado JA, Spranger MD, et al. The pathophysiology of hypertensive acute heart failure. Heart 2015;101(23):1861–7.
7. Adams KF Jr, Fonarow GC, Emerman CL, et al. Characteristics and outcomes of patients hospitalized for heart failure in the United States: rationale, design, and preliminary observations from the first 100,000 cases in the Acute Decompensated Heart Failure National Registry (ADHERE). Am Heart J 2005;149(2):209–16.
8. Ooi H, Chung W, Biolo A. Arterial stiffness and vascular load in heart failure. Congest Heart Fail 2008;14(1):31–6.
9. Borlaug BA, Kass DA. Ventricular-vascular interaction in heart failure. Heart Fail Clin 2008;4(1):23–36.
10. O'Rourke MF. Arterial aging: pathophysiological principles. Vasc Med 2007;12(4):329–41.
11. Gheorghiade M, Filippatos G, De Luca L, et al. Congestion in acute heart failure syndromes: an essential target of evaluation and treatment. Am J Med 2006;119(12 Suppl 1). S3–s10.
12. Braunwald's heart disease: a textbook of cardiovascular medicine, 2-Volume Set - 9780323463423 | US Elsevier Health Bookshop. Elsevier. 2018. Available at: https://www.us.elsevierhealth.com/braunwalds-heart-disease-a-textbook-of-cardiovascular-medicine-2-volume-set-9780323463423.html. Accessed February 1, 2018.
13. Gheorghiade M, Pang PS. Acute heart failure syndromes. J Am Coll Cardiol 2009;53(7):557–73.
14. Yancy CW, Jessup M, Bozkurt B, et al. 2013 ACCF/AHA guideline for the management of heart failure: executive summary: a report of the American College of Cardiology Foundation/American Heart Association Task Force on practice guidelines. Circulation 2013;128(16):1810–52.
15. Peacock WF, Fonarow GC, Emerman CL, et al. Impact of early initiation of intravenous therapy for acute decompensated heart failure on outcomes in ADHERE. Cardiology 2007;107(1):44–51.
16. Gelman S, Mushlin PS. Catecholamine-induced changes in the splanchnic circulation affecting systemic hemodynamics. Anesthesiology 2004;100(2): 434–9.
17. Gandhi SK, Powers JC, Nomeir AM, et al. The pathogenesis of acute pulmonary edema associated with hypertension. N Engl J Med 2001;344(1):17–22.
18. Schreiber W, Woisetschläger C, Binder M, et al. The nitura study–effect of nitroglycerin or urapidil on hemodynamic, metabolic and respiratory parameters in hypertensive patients with pulmonary edema. Intensive Care Med 1998;24(6):557–63.
19. Jhund PS, McMurray JJ, Davie AP. The acute vascular effects of frusemide in heart failure. Br J Clin Pharmacol 2000;50(1):9–13.

20. Dikshit K, Vyden JK, Forrester JS, et al. Renal and extrarenal hemodynamic effects of furosemide in congestive heart failure after acute myocardial infarction. N Engl J Med 1973; 288(21):1087–90.

21. Franciosa JA, Silverstein SR. Hemodynamic effects of nitroprusside and furosemide in left ventricular failure. Clin Pharmacol Ther 1982;32(1):62–9.

22. Pickkers P, Dormans TP, Russel FG, et al. Direct vascular effects of furosemide in humans. Circulation 1997;96(6):1847–52.

23. Holzer-Richling N, Holzer M, Herkner H, et al. Randomized placebo controlled trial of furosemide on subjective perception of dyspnoea in patients with pulmonary oedema because of hypertensive crisis. Eur J Clin Invest 2011;41(6):627–34.

24. Butler J, Forman DE, Abraham WT, et al. Relationship between heart failure treatment and development of worsening renal function among hospitalized patients. Am Heart J 2004;147(2):331–8.

25. Felker GM, O'Connor CM, Braunwald E, Heart Failure Clinical Research Network Investigators. Loop diuretics in acute decompensated heart failure: necessary? Evil? A necessary evil? Circ Heart Fail 2009;2(1):56–62.

26. Follath F, Yilmaz MB, Delgado JF, et al. Clinical presentation, management and outcomes in the acute heart failure global survey of standard treatment (ALARM-HF). Intensive Care Med 2011;37(4):619–26.

27. Singh A, Laribi S, Teerlink JR, et al. Agents with vasodilator properties in acute heart failure. Eur Heart J 2017;38(5):317–25.

28. Collins S, Martindale J. Optimizing hypertensive acute heart failure management with afterload reduction. Curr Hypertens Rep 2018;20(1):9.

29. Divakaran S, Loscalzo J. The role of nitroglycerin and other nitrogen oxides in cardiovascular therapeutics. J Am Coll Cardiol 2017;70(19):2393–410.

30. Brown BG, Bolson E, Petersen RB, et al. The mechanisms of nitroglycerin action: stenosis vasodilatation as a major component of the drug response. Circulation 1981;64(6):1089–97.

31. Elkayam U, Kulick D, McIntosh N, et al. Incidence of early tolerance to hemodynamic effects of continuous infusion of nitroglycerin in patients with coronary artery disease and heart failure. Circulation 1987;76(3):577–84.

32. Dupuis J, Lalonde G, Lemieux R, et al. Tolerance to intravenous nitroglycerin in patients with congestive heart failure: role of increased intravascular volume, neurohumoral activation and lack of prevention with N-acetylcysteine. J Am Coll Cardiol 1990;16(4):923–31.

33. Mullens W, Abrahams Z, Francis GS, et al. Sodium nitroprusside for advanced low-output heart failure. J Am Coll Cardiol 2008;52(3):200–7.

34. Stevenson LW. Management of acute decompensated heart failure. In: Mann DL, Felker GM, editors. Heart failure: a companion to Braunwald's heart disease. 3rd edition. Philadelphia: Elsevier; 2016. p. 514–34.

35. Grossman E, Lip GYH. Hypertensive crisis. In: Dimarco J, editor. Cardiology. 3rd edition. Philadelphia: Elsevier Ltd; 2010. p. 607–18.

36. Wakai A, McCabe A, Kidney R, et al. Nitrates for acute heart failure syndromes. Cochrane Database Syst Rev 2013;(8):CD005151.

37. Publication Committee for the VMAC Investigators (Vasodilatation in the Management of Acute CHF). Intravenous nesiritide vs nitroglycerin for treatment of decompensated congestive heart failure: a randomized controlled trial. JAMA 2002;287(12):1531–40.

38. Beltrame JF, Zeitz CJ, Unger SA, et al. Nitrate therapy is an alternative to furosemide/morphine therapy in the management of acute cardiogenic pulmonary edema. J Card Fail 1998;4(4):271–9.

39. Levy P, Compton S, Welch R, et al. Treatment of severe decompensated heart failure with high-dose intravenous nitroglycerin: a feasibility and outcome analysis. Ann Emerg Med 2007;50(2):144–52.

40. Wilson SS, Kwiatkowski GM, Millis SR, et al. Use of nitroglycerin by bolus prevents intensive care unit admission in patients with acute hypertensive heart failure. Am J Emerg Med 2017;35(1):126–31.

41. Cotter G, Metzkor E, Kaluski E, et al. Randomised trial of high-dose isosorbide dinitrate plus low-dose furosemide versus high-dose furosemide plus low-dose isosorbide dinitrate in severe pulmonary oedema. Lancet 1998;351(9100):389–93.

42. Colucci WS, Elkayam U, Horton DP, et al. Intravenous nesiritide, a natriuretic peptide, in the treatment of decompensated congestive heart failure. Nesiritide Study Group. N Engl J Med 2000;343(4):246–53.

43. O'Connor CM, Starling RC, Hernandez AF, et al. Effect of nesiritide in patients with acute decompensated heart failure. N Engl J Med 2011;365(1):32–43.

44. Grossman E, Ironi AN, Messerli FH. Comparative tolerability profile of hypertensive crisis treatments. Drug Saf 1998;19(2):99–122.

45. Ayaz SI, Sharkey CM, Kwiatkowski GM, et al. Intravenous enalaprilat for treatment of acute hypertensive heart failure in the emergency department. Int J Emerg Med 2016;9(1):28.

46. Annane D, Bellissant E, Pussard E, et al. Placebo-controlled, randomized, double-blind study of intravenous enalaprilat efficacy and safety in acute cardiogenic pulmonary edema. Circulation 1996;94(6):1316–24.

47. Anker SD, Ponikowski P, Mitrovic V, et al. Ularitide for the treatment of acute decompensated heart failure: from preclinical to clinical studies. Eur Heart J 2015;36(12):715–23.

48. Mitrovic V, Lüss H, Nitsche K, et al. Effects of the renal natriuretic peptide urodilatin (ularitide) in patients with decompensated chronic heart failure: a double-blind, placebo-controlled, ascending-dose trial. Am Heart J 2005;150(6):1239.

49. Mitrovic V, Seferovic PM, Simeunovic D, et al. Haemodynamic and clinical effects of ularitide in decompensated heart failure. Eur Heart J 2006; 27(23):2823–32.

50. Kentsch M, Ludwig D, Drummer C, et al. Haemodynamic and renal effects of urodilatin bolus injections in patients with congestive heart failure. Eur J Clin Invest 1992;22(10):662–9.

51. Packer M, O'Connor C, McMurray JJV, et al. Effect of ularitide on cardiovascular mortality in acute heart failure. N Engl J Med 2017;376(20):1956–64.

52. Nistri S, Bani D. Relaxin receptors and nitric oxide synthases: search for the missing link. Reprod Biol Endocrinol 2003;1:5.

53. Dschietzig T, Bartsch C, Richter C, et al. Relaxin, a pregnancy hormone, is a functional endothelin-1 antagonist: attenuation of endothelin-1-mediated vasoconstriction by stimulation of endothelin type-B receptor expression via ERK-1/2 and nuclear factor-kappaB. Circ Res 2003;92(1):32–40.

54. Teichman SL, Unemori E, Teerlink JR, et al. Relaxin: review of biology and potential role in treating heart failure. Curr Heart Fail Rep 2010;7(2):75–82.

55. Teerlink JR, Metra M, Felker GM, et al. Relaxin for the treatment of patients with acute heart failure (Pre-RELAX-AHF): a multicentre, randomised, placebo-controlled, parallel-group, dose-finding phase IIb study. Lancet 2009;373(9673):1429–39.

56. Teerlink JR, Cotter G, Davison BA, et al. Serelaxin, recombinant human relaxin-2, for treatment of acute heart failure (RELAX-AHF): a randomised, placebo-controlled trial. Lancet 2013;381(9860):29–39.

57. ClinicalTrials.gov. Efficacy, safety and tolerability of serelaxin when added to standard therapy in AHF (RELAX-AHF-2). 2013. Available at: https://clinicaltrials.gov/ct2/show/NCT01870778. Accessed February 3, 2019.

58. Aroney CN, Semigran MJ, Dec GW, et al. Inotropic effect of nicardipine in patients with heart failure: assessment by left ventricular end-systolic pressure-volume analysis. J Am Coll Cardiol 1989; 14(5):1331–8.

59. Packer M, Lee WH, Medina N, et al. Prognostic importance of the immediate hemodynamic response to nifedipine in patients with severe left ventricular dysfunction. J Am Coll Cardiol 1987; 10(6):1303–11.

60. Kieler-Jensen N, Jolin-Mellgård A, Nordlander M, et al. Coronary and systemic hemodynamic effects of clevidipine, an ultra-short-acting calcium antagonist, for treatment of hypertension after coronary artery surgery. Acta Anaesthesiol Scand 2000; 44(2):186–93.

61. Peacock F, Varon J, Ebrahimi R, et al. Clevidipine for severe hypertension in acute heart failure: a VELOCITY trial analysis. Congest Heart Fail 2010; 16(2):55–9.

62. Peacock WF, Chandra A, Char D, et al. Clevidipine in acute heart failure: results of the a study of blood pressure control in acute heart failure-a pilot study (PRONTO). Am Heart J 2014;167(4):529–36.

63. Stasch JP, Schmidt P, Alonso-Alija C, et al. NO- and haem-independent activation of soluble guanylyl cyclase: molecular basis and cardiovascular implications of a new pharmacological principle. Br J Pharmacol 2002;136(5):773–83.

64. Lapp H, Mitrovic V, Franz N, et al. Cinaciguat (BAY 58-2667) improves cardiopulmonary hemodynamics in patients with acute decompensated heart failure. Circulation 2009;119(21):2781–8.

65. Erdmann E, Semigran MJ, Nieminen MS, et al. Cinaciguat, a soluble guanylate cyclase activator, unloads the heart but also causes hypotension in acute decompensated heart failure. Eur Heart J 2013;34(1):57–67.

66. Gheorghiade M, Greene SJ, Filippatos G, et al. Cinaciguat, a soluble guanylate cyclase activator: results from the randomized, controlled, phase IIb COMPOSE programme in acute heart failure syndromes. Eur J Heart Fail 2012;14(9):1056–66.

67. Pieske B, Maggioni AP, Lam CSP, et al. Vericiguat in patients with worsening chronic heart failure and preserved ejection fraction: results of the SOluble guanylate Cyclase stimulatoR in heArT failurE patientS with PRESERVED EF (SOCRATES-PRESERVED) study. Eur Heart J 2017;38(15):1119–27.

UNITED STATES POSTAL SERVICE ®

Statement of Ownership, Management, and Circulation
(All Periodicals Publications Except Requester Publications)

1. Publication Title	2. Publication Number	3. Filing Date
HEART FAILURE CLINICS	025 – 055	6/18/2019

4. Issue Frequency	5. Number of Issues Published Annually	6. Annual Subscription Price
JAN, APR, JUL, OCT	4	$261.00

7. Complete Mailing Address of Known Office of Publication (Not printer) (Street, city, county, state, and ZIP+4®)

ELSEVIER INC.
230 Park Avenue, Suite 800
New York, NY 10169

Contact Person
STEPHEN R. BUSHING
Telephone (Include area code)
215-239-3688

8. Complete Mailing Address of Headquarters or General Business Office of Publisher (Not printer)

ELSEVIER INC.
230 Park Avenue, Suite 800
New York, NY 10169

9. Full Names and Complete Mailing Addresses of Publisher, Editor, and Managing Editor (Do not leave blank)

Publisher (Name and complete mailing address)

TAYLOR BALL, ELSEVIER INC.
1600 JOHN F KENNEDY BLVD. SUITE 1800
PHILADELPHIA, PA 19103-2899

Editor (Name and complete mailing address)

STACY EASTMAN, ELSEVIER INC.
1600 JOHN F KENNEDY BLVD. SUITE 1800
PHILADELPHIA, PA 19103-2899

Managing Editor (Name and complete mailing address)

PATRICK MANLEY, ELSEVIER INC.
1600 JOHN F KENNEDY BLVD. SUITE 1800
PHILADELPHIA, PA 19103-2899

10. Owner (Do not leave blank. If the publication is owned by a corporation, give the name and address of the corporation immediately followed by the names and addresses of all stockholders owning or holding 1 percent or more of the total amount of stock. If not owned by a corporation, give the names and addresses of the individual owners. If owned by a partnership or other unincorporated firm, give its name and address as well as those of each individual owner. If the publication is published by a nonprofit organization, give its name and address.)

Full Name	Complete Mailing Address
WHOLLY OWNED SUBSIDIARY OF REED/ELSEVIER, US HOLDINGS	1600 JOHN F KENNEDY BLVD. SUITE 1800 PHILADELPHIA, PA 19103-2899

11. Known Bondholders, Mortgagees, and Other Security Holders Owning or Holding 1 Percent or More of Total Amount of Bonds, Mortgages, or Other Securities. If none, check box ▶ ☐ None

Full Name	Complete Mailing Address
N/A	

12. Tax Status (For completion by nonprofit organizations authorized to mail at nonprofit rates) (Check one)
The purpose, function, and nonprofit status of this organization and the exempt status for federal income tax purposes:
☒ Has Not Changed During Preceding 12 Months
☐ Has Changed During Preceding 12 Months (Publisher must submit explanation of change with this statement)

PS Form **3526**, July 2014 [Page 1 of 4 (see instructions page 4)]   PSN: 7530-01-000-9931   PRIVACY NOTICE: See our privacy policy on www.usps.com.

---

13. Publication Title	14. Issue Date for Circulation Data Below
HEART FAILURE CLINICS	JULY 2019

15. Extent and Nature of Circulation			Average No. Copies Each Issue During Preceding 12 Months	No. Copies of Single Issue Published Nearest to Filing Date
a. Total Number of Copies (Net press run)			56	38
b. Paid Circulation (By Mail and Outside the Mail)	(1)	Mailed Outside-County Paid Subscriptions Stated on PS Form 3541 (Include paid distribution above nominal rate, advertiser's proof copies, and exchange copies)	15	17
	(2)	Mailed In-County Paid Subscriptions Stated on PS Form 3541 (Include paid distribution above nominal rate, advertiser's proof copies, and exchange copies)	0	0
	(3)	Paid Distribution Outside the Mails Including Sales Through Dealers and Carriers, Street Vendors, Counter Sales, and Other Paid Distribution Outside USPS®	9	11
	(4)	Paid Distribution by Other Classes of Mail Through the USPS (e.g., First-Class Mail®)	0	0
c. Total Paid Distribution (Sum of 15b (1), (2), (3), and (4))		▶	24	28
d. Free or Nominal Rate Distribution (By Mail and Outside the Mail)	(1)	Free or Nominal Rate Outside-County Copies Included on PS Form 3541	32	10
	(2)	Free or Nominal Rate In-County Copies Included on PS Form 3541	0	0
	(3)	Free or Nominal Rate Copies Mailed at Other Classes Through the USPS (e.g., First-Class Mail)	0	0
	(4)	Free or Nominal Rate Distribution Outside the Mail (Carriers or other means)	0	0
e. Total Free or Nominal Rate Distribution (Sum of 15d (1), (2), (3) and (4))		▶	32	10
f. Total Distribution (Sum of 15c and 15e)		▶	56	38
g. Copies not Distributed (See Instructions to Publishers #4 (page #3))		▶	0	0
h. Total (Sum of 15f and g)		▶	56	38
i. Percent Paid (15c divided by 15f times 100)		▶	42.86%	73.68%

* If you are claiming electronic copies, go to line 16 on page 3. If you are not claiming electronic copies, skip to line 17 on page 3.

16. Electronic Copy Circulation	Average No. Copies Each Issue During Preceding 12 Months	No. Copies of Single Issue Published Nearest to Filing Date
a. Paid Electronic Copies ▶		
b. Total Paid Print Copies (Line 15c) + Paid Electronic Copies (Line 16a) ▶		
c. Total Print Distribution (Line 15f) + Paid Electronic Copies (Line 16a) ▶		
d. Percent Paid (Both Print & Electronic Copies) (16b divided by 16c × 100) ▶		

☒ I certify that 50% of all my distributed copies (electronic and print) are paid above a nominal price.

17. Publication of Statement of Ownership

☒ If the publication is a general publication, publication of this statement is required. Will be printed in the OCTOBER 2019 issue of this publication.   ☐ Publication not required.

18. Signature and Title of Editor, Publisher, Business Manager, or Owner

STEPHEN R. BUSHING - INVENTORY DISTRIBUTION CONTROL MANAGER   Date 6/18/2019

I certify that all information furnished on this form is true and complete. I understand that anyone who furnishes false or misleading information on this form or who omits material or information requested on the form may be subject to criminal sanctions (including fines and imprisonment) and/or civil sanctions (including civil penalties).

PS Form **3526**, July 2014 (Page 2 of 4)   PRIVACY NOTICE: See our privacy policy on www.usps.com.

Moving?

Make sure your subscription moves with you!

To notify us of your new address, find your **Clinics Account Number** (located on your mailing label above your name), and contact customer service at:

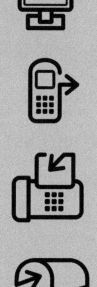

Email: journalscustomerservice-usa@elsevier.com

800-654-2452 (subscribers in the U.S. & Canada)
314-447-8871 (subscribers outside of the U.S. & Canada)

Fax number: 314-447-8029

Elsevier Health Sciences Division
Subscription Customer Service
3251 Riverport Lane
Maryland Heights, MO 63043

*To ensure uninterrupted delivery of your subscription, please notify us at least 4 weeks in advance of move.

Printed and bound by CPI Group (UK) Ltd, Croydon, CR0 4YY

03/10/2024

01040308-0018